NANOMATERIALS-BASED SENSING PLATFORMS

Towards the Efficient Detection of Biomolecules and Gases

NANOMATERIALS-BASED SENSING PLATFORMS

Towards the Efficient Detection of Biomolecules and Gases

Edited by
Aneeya K. Samantara, PhD
Sudarsan Raj, PhD
Satyajit Ratha, PhD

AAP APPLE ACADEMIC PRESS

First edition published 2022

Apple Academic Press Inc.
1265 Goldenrod Circle, NE,
Palm Bay, FL 32905 USA

4164 Lakeshore Road, Burlington,
ON, L7L 1A4 Canada

CRC Press
6000 Broken Sound Parkway NW,
Suite 300, Boca Raton, FL 33487-2742 USA

2 Park Square, Milton Park,
Abingdon, Oxon, OX14 4RN UK

Library and Archives Canada Cataloguing in Publication

Title: Nanomaterials-based sensing platforms : towards the efficient detection of biomolecules and gases / edited by Aneeya K. Samantara, PhD, Sudarsan Raj, PhD, Satyajit Ratha, PhD.
Names: Samantara, Aneeya Kumar, editor. | Raj, Sudarsan, editor. | Ratha, Satyajit, editor.
Description: First edition. | Includes bibliographical references and index.
Identifiers: Canadiana (print) 20210280220 | Canadiana (ebook) 20210280328 | ISBN 9781774630372 (hardcover) | ISBN 9781774638590 (softcover) | ISBN 9781003199304 (ebook)
Subjects: LCSH: Biosensors. | LCSH: Nanostructured materials.
Classification: LCC R857.B54 N36 2022 | DDC 610.28—dc23

Library of Congress Cataloging-in-Publication Data

Names: Samantara, Aneeya Kumar, editor. | Raj, Sudarsan, editor. | Ratha, Satyajit, editor.
Title: Nanomaterials-based sensing platforms : towards the efficient detection of biomolecules and gases / edited by Aneeya K. Samantara, Sudarsan Raj, Satyajit Ratha.
Description: 1st edition. | Palm Bay, FL : AAP, Apple Academic Press, 2022. | Includes bibliographical references and index. | Summary: "Sensors are effective tools to carry out cost-effective, fast, and reliable sensing for a wide range of applications. This volume, Nanomaterials-Based Sensing Platforms: Towards the Efficient Detection of Biomolecules and Gases, presents a brief history behind the sensing technology and also emphasizes a broad range of biosensing techniques based on optical and electrochemical response methods. Starting from the traditional enzyme-based biosensing method to functionalized nanostructure-based sensors, this book also provides a detailed overview of some of the advanced sensing methodologies based on photonic crystal cavity-based sensing devices. The authors have compiled the book keeping in mind the extraordinary success history of nanomaterials, their current strategical exploitation, and an unprecedented pool of possibilities they hold for the future. Many of the technologies have been developed recently for the sensing of various bio-analytes and molecules, some of which have been included in this book through dedicated chapters in a highly organized manner. The book looks at the various sensors, such as for biosensing, electrochemical sensing, gas sensing, photo-electrochemical sensing, and colorimetric sensing, all of which have shown potential. This volume will be valuable for professors, scientists, graduate students, industry professionals, researchers, and libraries. Many universities, institutes, and colleges are offering courses on nanotechnology, nanoscience, materials sciences, and this volume will be a helpful ancillary text"-- Provided by publisher.
Identifiers: LCCN 2021036492 (print) | LCCN 2021036493 (ebook) | ISBN 9781774630372 (hardback) | ISBN 9781774638590 (paperback) | ISBN 9781003199304 (ebook)
Subjects: MESH: Biosensing Techniques | Nanostructures | Electrochemical Techniques | Gases--analysis
Classification: LCC R857.E52 (print) | LCC R857.E52 (ebook) | NLM QT 36.4 | DDC 610.28--dc23
LC record available at https://lccn.loc.gov/2021036492
LC ebook record available at https://lccn.loc.gov/2021036493

ISBN: 978-1-77463-037-2 (hbk)
ISBN: 978-1-77463-859-0 (pbk)
ISBN: 978-1-00319-930-4 (ebk)

Dedicated to our parents

About the Editors

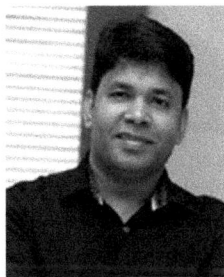

Aneeya Kumar Samantara, PhD

Postdoctorate, School of Chemical Sciences,
National Institute of Science Education and
Research, Bhubaneswar, Odisha–752050, India,
E-mail: cmrjitu@gmail.com

Aneeya Kumar Samantara, PhD, is a National Postdoctorate Fellow at the National Institute of Science Education and Research, Odisha, India. Dr. Samantara's research interests include the synthesis of metal chalcogenides and graphene composites for energy storage/conversion applications and designing of electrochemical sensors for detection of different bioanalytes. To his credit, he has authored over 25 peer-reviewed papers published in international journals, as well as books and book chapters. He earned his PhD in Chemistry at the CSIR-Institute of Minerals and Materials Technology, Odisha, India. Before joining the PhD program, he completed a Master of Science in Advanced Organic Chemistry from Ravenshaw University, India, and Master of Philosophy (MPhil) from Utkal University, India.

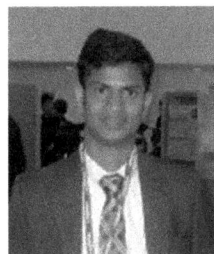

Sudarsan Raj, PhD

Research Associate,
Advanced Materials Technology,
CSIR-Institute of Minerals and Materials
Technology, Bhubaneswar, Odisha–751013, India,
E-mail: rajcbnu@gmail.com

Sudarsan Raj, PhD, is currently working as a Research Associate at the CSIR-Institute of Minerals and Materials Technology, Odisha, India. He was previously working as a postdoctoral research scientist at Nagoya University, Japan. He did his PhD in Materials Engineering from Chonbuk National University, South Korea. Before that, he completed his MSc in Analytical Chemistry from Berhampur University, Odisha, India.

His research output includes over 15 authored and co-authored peer-reviewed international journal articles and book chapters. His research interest includes nanoparticle synthesis for LEDs, solar cells, gas sensors, Automobile exhaust catalysts, and value-added beach sand minerals.

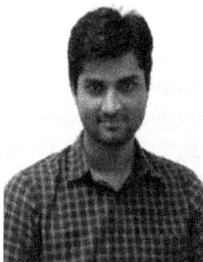

Satyajit Ratha, PhD
School of Basic Sciences,
Indian Institute of Technology,
Bhubaneswar, Odisha–752050, India,
E-mail: satyajitratha89@gmail.com

Satyajit Ratha, PhD, has pursued his PhD at the Indian Institute of Technology Bhubaneswar, India. Prior to joining IIT Bhubaneswar, he received his Bachelor of Science, First Class Honors, from Utkal University in 2008 and a Master of Science from Ravenshaw University in 2010. Dr. Ratha research interests include two-dimensional semiconductors, nanostructure synthesis, applications, energy storage devices, and supercapacitors. He has authored and co-authored about 21 peer-reviewed international journal articles and 10 books.

Contents

Contributors

Chinmayee Acharya
Department of Bio-Technology, North Orissa University, Baripada, Odisha–757003, India

Ayonbala Baral
Post-Doctorate Fellow, Department of Metallurgical and Energy Engineering,
Kunming University of Science and Technology, Kunming–650093, China

Tapan Kumar Behera
Department of Chemistry, North Orissa University, Baripada, Odisha–757003, India,
E-mail: tapankumarbeherachemistry@gmail.com

Sabyasachi Dash
Post-Doctorate Fellow, Department of Pathology and Laboratory Medicine,
Weill Cornell Medicine, New York–10065, USA, E-mail: sda4003@med.cornell.edu

Sandeep Kaushik
Post-Doctorate Fellow, I3Bs-Research Institute on Biomaterials, Biodegradables, and Biomimetics,
University of Minho, Barco, Guimarães, Portugal

Ajeet Kumar
Post-Doctorate Fellow, TIFAC-Center of Relevance and Excellence in Fiber Optics and Optical
Communication, Department of Applied Physics, Delhi Technological University, Delhi–110042, India

Sudha Kumari
Assistant Professor, Department of Physics, National Institute of Technology, Raipur,
Chhattisgarh–492010, India, E-mail: kumari.sudha93@gmail.com

Priyabrat Mohapatra
Department of Chemistry, C.V. Raman College of Engineering, Bhubaneswar, Odisha–752054, India

Snehalata Pradhan
Department of Botany, Government College Koraput, Landiguda, Odisha–764021, India

Sudarsan Raj
Institute of Materials and Systems for Sustainability, Nagoya University, Nagoya, Japan,
E-mail: rajcbnu@gmail.com

Satyajit Ratha
School of Basic Sciences, Indian Institute of Technology Bhubaneswar, Argul, Khordha–752050,
Odisha, India, E-mail: satyajitratha89@gmail.com

Surjit Sahoo
School of Basic Sciences, Indian Institute of Technology Bhubaneswar, Argul, Khordha–752050,
Odisha, India, E-mail: surjit488@gmail.com

Sapan Mohan Saini
Associate Professor, Department of Physics, National Institute of Technology, Raipur,
Chhattisgarh–492010, India

Than Singh Saini
Post-Doctorate Fellow, Optical Functional Materials Laboratory, Toyota Technological Institute, Nagoya–468-8511, Japan, E-mail: tsinghdph@gmail.com

Aneeya K. Samantara
School of Chemical Sciences, National Institute of Science Education and Research, Bhubaneswar, Odisha–752050, India, E-mail: aneeya1986@gmail.com

Pramod Kumar Satapathy
Department of Chemistry, North Orissa University, Baripada, Odisha–757003, India

Lakkoji Satish
Research Associate, Department of Chemistry, Ravenshaw University, Cuttack, Odisha–753003, India, E-mail: lakkojisatish@gmail.com

Narendra Singh
Centre for Advanced Studies, Dr. A.P.J. Abdul Kalam Technical University, Lucknow, Uttar Pradesh, India; Department of Chemical Engineering, Indian Institute of Technology Kanpur, Kanpur–208016, Uttar Pradesh, India, Tel.: +91-9936337743, E-mail: narendra.hbti.be@gmail.com

Ravindra Kumar Sinha
Post-Doctorate Fellow, TIFAC-Center of Relevance and Excellence in Fiber Optics and Optical Communication, Department of Applied Physics, Delhi Technological University, Delhi–110042, India; CSIR-Central Scientific Instrument Organization, Chandigarh–160030, India

Meenakshi Srivastava
Centre for Advanced Studies, Dr. A.P.J. Abdul Kalam Technical University, Lucknow, Uttar Pradesh, India

Abbreviations

0D	zero-dimensional
1D	one-dimensional
2D	two-dimensional
3D	three-dimensional
A/D	analog to digital
AA	ascorbic acid
AC	acetaminophen
ACh	acetylcholine
ADHD	attention deficit hyperactivity disorder
AFM	atomic force microscopy
Ag	silver
Al	aluminum
AQ	anthraquinone
Au	gold
BOD	biological oxygen demand
C_2H_5OH	ethanol
CD	cyclodextrin
CDRs	complementarity-determining regions
CH_4	methane
Chits	chitosan
Cl_2	chlorine
CNF	carbon nanofiber
CNTs	carbon nanotubes
CO	carbon monoxide
CO_2	carbon dioxide
CPC	circular photonic crystal
CPs	conducting polymers
CR-GO	chemically reduced graphene oxide
CR-GO/GC	reduced graphene oxide modified glassy carbon
CTCs	circulating tumor cells
Cu_2O	cuprous oxide
Cu_2ZnSnS_4	CZTS
CuO	copper oxide

CV	cyclic voltammetry
DA	dopamine
DC	direct current
DLS	dynamic light scattering
DNA	deoxyribonucleic acid
DPV	differential pulse voltammetry
DTT	dithiothreitol
ECG	electrocardiography
EEG	electroencephalography
EGFR	epidermal growth factor receptor
ELISA	enzyme-linked immunosorbent assay
EM	electromagnetic
F_c	constant fragment
FDA	Food and Drug Administration
FDTD	finite difference time domain method
FESEM	field emission scanning electron microscope
FET	field-effect-transistors
fMWCNTs	functionalized multi-wall carbon nanotubes
FOM	figure of merit
FRET	fluorescence resonance energy transfer
FWHM	full width at half maximum
$g\text{-}C_3N_4$	graphitic carbon nitride
GC	glassy carbon
GCE	glassy carbon electrode
GLAD	glancing angle deposition
Glu	glucose
GNP	graphene nanoplatelet
GNs	graphene nanosheets
GO	graphene oxide
GOD-HFs	glucose oxidase and hydroxyl fullerenes
GO_x	glucose oxidase
H_2	hydrogen
H_2S	hydrogen sulfide
hCG	human chorionic gonadotrophin
HCHO	formaldehyde
His	histidine
HIV	human immunodeficiency viruses
HPV	human papillomavirus

HRP	horseradish peroxidase
HS	hollow spheres
IDA	imidodiacetic acid
IEC	international electrochemical committee
IgG	immunoglobulin gamma
Igs	immunoglobins
In_2O_3	indium oxide
ISE	ion-selective electrode
ITO	indium tin oxide
Lac	laccase
LAMP	loop-mediated isothermal amplification
LD	levodopa
LED	light-emitting diode
LIG	laser-induced graphene
LNAs	locked-nucleic acids
LOD	limit of detection
LPG	liquefied petroleum gas
LSPR	localized surface plasmon resonances
MEMS	micro-electro-mechanical system
MIP	molecular imprinted polymers
miRNA	microRNA
MMP	matrix metallopeptidases
Mo	molybdenum
MON	metal oxide nanostructures
MOS	metal oxide semiconductor
MoS_2	molybdenum disulfide
MWCNTs	multi-walled carbon nanotube
NaCl	sodium chloride
NF	nafion
NGs	nano-generators
NH_3	ammonia
NHS	N-hydroxysuccinimide
NiCNFs	nickel nanoparticle loaded carbon nanofibers
nm	nanometer
NMOF	nano-metal-organic frameworks
NO	nitric oxide
NO_2	nitrogen dioxide
NPs	nanoparticles

NRs	nanorods
NTA	nitrilotriacetic acid
NW	nanowires
PCC	photonic crystal cavity
PDA	polydopamine
PDDA	poly diallyl dimethyl ammonium chloride)
PDMS	poly dimethyl siloxane
PI	polyimide
PI-BN	polyimide-boron nitride
PL	photoluminescence
PNA	peptide nucleic acid
PPd NS	porous pd nanostructures
ppm	parts per million
Ppy	polypyrrole
PSA	prostate-specific antigen
PSS	poly(sodium 4-styrene sulfonate)
Pt	platinum
Pt-DENs	dendrimer-encapsulated Pt nanoparticles
PVP	polyvinylpyrrolidone
QCM	quartz crystal microbalance
QDs	quantum dots
rGO	reduced graphite oxide
RI	refractive index
RIS	refractive index sensitivity
RIU	refractive index unit
RNA	ribonucleic acid
RRE	rev responsive element
SEM	scanning electron microscope
SIPs	surface imprinted polymers
SMOs	semiconductor metal oxides
SnO_2	tin oxide
SNR	signal to noise ratio
SOI	silicon-on-insulator
SPP	surface plasmon polarities
SPR	surface plasmon resonance
SPs	surface plasmons
SQUID	superconducting quantum interference devices
SWCNT	single-walled carbon nanotubes

TB	tuberculosis
TE	transverse electric
TEM	transmission electron microscope
THF	tetrahydrofuran
Thi	thionine
TIR	total internal reflection
TM	transverse magnetic
TR	tyramine
UA	uric acid
UV	ultraviolet
V_H	variable heavy
WO_3	tungsten oxide
XRD	X-ray diffraction
ZnO	zinc oxide

Preface

The growing interest in the early and reliable detection of several bio-molecules is due to the fact that the increasing set of bio-analytes are rather hard to detect and are of extremely small dimension, which requires the implementation of precise detection techniques. Traditional methods use enzyme-based methods to carry out the detection process. The most commonly used biosensors make extensive use of labels (such as enzymes and fluorescent or radioactive molecules attached to the targeted analyte). Thus, the final sensing output is completely dependent on the number of labels present in the analyte. These label-based detection techniques are thus labor- and cost-intensive as well as time-consuming. In addition, labeling of biomolecules can block active binding sites and alter the binding properties. As a result, this may adversely affect the affinity-based interaction between the recognition elements and the target molecules.

However, label-free biosensing techniques-based on optical and/or electrochemical recognition techniques are free from any such biomarkers or labels. Rather, they make use of several intrinsic properties such as molecular weight, size, charge, electrical impedance, dielectric permittivity, or refractive index (RI), to detect their presence in a sample. Since there will be no biomarkers or labels here, the detection process will be much faster in comparison to traditional enzyme-based biosensing. Also, this would allow for the real-time and reliable detection of a wide range of analytes depending upon their specific set of inherent physicochemical properties.

Optical biosensors, especially SPR-based techniques, are of significant importance. And if combined with the latest fiber-optical systems, this could readily provide an effective tool to carry out a cost-effective, fast, and reliable sensing platform for a wide range of applications. This book deals with the brief history behind the sensing technology and also emphasizes a broad range of biosensing techniques-based on optical and electrochemical response methods. Starting from the traditional enzyme-based biosensing method to functionalized nanostructure-based sensors; this book also provides a detailed overview of some of the advanced sensing methodologies-based on photonic crystal cavity (PCC)-based sensing devices.

—Aneeya Kumar Samantara, PhD
Sudarsan Ra, PhD
Satyajit Ratha, PhD

Introduction

Detection of biomolecules and the underlying mechanism of the interactions among them are critical for several fields of interest such as cell biology, the pharmaceutical industry, and medical diagnosis, etc. The different kinds of interactions shown by the biomolecules, analytes, and protein molecules provide basic yet important information regarding the functions of a typical cell. This can be exploited by scientists to find out whether specific interactions can be guided to perform the proliferation of cancerous cells. This could also help in the diagnosis of the concerned cancerous cell growth. However, the development of such techniques would require high-precision and fast response sensing devices. Most of the analytes consist of drug compounds, DNA oligomers, peptides, viral particles, enzymes, etc., that have ultra-small dimensions and are also present in a very low concentration in a given specimen. Also, larger bioanalytes such as bacteria, cells are generally stained with fluorescent dyes to mark them. But, the process itself results in the death of the specimen. Therefore, for larger and smaller analytes, fabrication of a precise and non-invasive sensing technique is imperative considering the growing demand for reliable, fast, and responsive medical diagnosis.

This book introduces key fundamental aspects of several biosensing techniques with a brief overview of the processes involved and their future perspectives. It contains eight chapters comprising various materials and methods that are critical for the development of next-generation sensing devices.

The first chapter provides detailed information regarding the current trends and the future development of biosensing techniques, along with few excerpts on the application part. This will provide us a clear picture about the current state of the biosensing techniques and whether significant improvement and/or upgradations are being made to make the same more effective in the long run. The second chapter emphasizes on the application of nanostructured materials for biosensing applications. Materials like graphene (GN) and carbon nanotube (CNT) are well-known for their excellent physicochemical properties and can revolutionize the sensing technique. Also, there has been a specific mention about quantum dots (QDs) which has drawn significant interest due to its unique optical properties. In the third chapter, we will be dealing with some of the advanced sensing techniques-based on photonic crystal cavity (PCC)-based sensors and their wide range of applications. This chapter provides insights regarding some of the self-assembly techniques and fabrication methods that could help researchers to understand the potential of such cavity-based sensors for biomolecule detection. The fourth chapter consists of information regarding the sensing activities of metal oxide-based nanostructures towards the detection of gas molecules. The fifth chapter provides information regarding optical biosensors for diagnostic applications. Here, a detailed overview of the detection methods based on advanced techniques such as surface plasmon resonance (SPR) has been provided along with an emphasis on the rise of gold nanoparticles (AuNPs) as biosensors. The sixth chapter discusses the synthesis of materials and fabrication of various types of metal-free sensing platforms and elaborately presented the electrochemical sensing performance. On the other hand, the seventh chapter covers the gas sensing performances of various noble metal-based nanostructures. The eighth chapter concludes the book and discusses different aspects of noble metal-based sensing platforms for the electrochemical detection of various bio-analytes.

The above chapters provide a lucid understanding of the background and working principles of bio-sensing techniques-based on both traditional label-based and latest label-free methods. Furthermore, advanced concepts such as photonic crystal cavity-based sensing and nanostructure-based materials have been discussed in detail for a better understanding of the futuristic development in the field of biosensing.

CHAPTER 1

Biosensors: Current Trends and Future Perspectives

SABYASACHI DASH[1] and SANDEEP KAUSHIK[2]

[1]*Department of Pathology and Laboratory Medicine, Weill Cornell Medicine, New York–10065, USA, E-mail: sda4003@med.cornell.edu*

[2]*I3Bs-Research Institute on Biomaterials, Biodegradables, and Biomimetics, University of Minho, Barco, Guimarães, Portugal*

ABSTRACT

A biosensor is an analytical device employed to sense analytes and associated changes in a given biochemical environment. The output is interpreted in the form of electronic signals read by an appropriate recognition system and an electrochemical transducer. The past few decades have witnessed the evolution of biosensors as well recognized sensitive and selective devices to record subtle changes in analytes of a various chemical or biological system. Due to such potential, biosensors have been implemented across disciplines of pure and applied sciences in some form or the other. Since their birth in the early 1960s, Extensive research and development has happened globally to enhance our existing knowledge on these devices. However, only a handful of biosensors have been commercialized and actively used, for example, the glucose monitors and pregnancy test kits. This chapter will provide details on the inception, evolution, current applications and the probabilistic future of this technology in the context of human health and disease.

1.1 BIOSENSORS AND THEIR UNDERLYING PRINCIPLE

1.1.1 *HISTORICAL PERSPECTIVE ON THE BIRTH OF BIOSENSORS*

In simple words, Biosensors can be defined as analytical devices that convert a biological or biochemical response to an electronic output. Biosensors have witnessed remarkable progress since their inception. Within the past 40 years, the direct or indirect applications of biosensors supported by research in both pure and applied sciences have established the impact of these devices. The history of biosensors dates to as early as the year 1906 when M. Cremer demonstrated that the concentration of an acid in a liquid is proportional to the electric potential between parts of the fluid located on opposite sides of a glass membrane (Cremer, 1906). Later, Søren Peder Lauritz Sørensen introduced the concept of pH, percentage of hydrogen ion concentration, in 1909, and an electrode for pH measurements was published in the year 1922 by W. S. Hughes. Between 1909 and 1922, Griffin and Nelson demonstrated enzyme immobilization on a surface of aluminum hydroxide and charcoal (1916). In 1956 Professor LeLand C. Clark, also known as the "father of biosensors," published his work on the development of the first true biosensor, an oxygen probe that could sense the changing oxygen concentrations in a given biochemical environment (2006). This electrode was named as "Clark Electrode" after Professor Clark (Heineman et al., 2006). Employing this invention, the first demonstration was performed using a dialysis membrane containing the enzyme glucose oxidase (GO_x) wrapped over the oxygen detection probe. In this demonstration, observers witnessed the ability of the probe to detect the changes in oxygen concentration in proportion to the activity of the enzyme GO_x (Heineman et al., 2006; Bhalla et al., 2016). Thus, the first biosensor was an "enzyme electrode" marking the activity observed during the scientific demonstration (Heineman et al., 2006; Bhalla et al., 2016). Later in 1967, Updike and Hicks used a similar principle employing the immobilization of enzyme GO_x in a gel (polyacrylamide gel) onto the surface of an oxygen electrode to facilitate rapid quantitative measurement of oxygen concentration (Bhalla et al., 2016). Soon, this innovation sparked a great interest and curiosity in the global scientific community. Only 2 years later, Guilbault and Montalvo developed glass electrode-based sensors to measure urea concentration (Guibault and Montalvo, 1969). Subsequently, from 1970 several authors began accepting and reproducing the idea of biosensors, based on the coupling of enzyme and electrochemical sensors. A new set of sensors were proposed in 1971-based on a novel principle called ion-selective electrode (ISE) to detect the activity of beta-glucosidase enzyme for the formation of benzaldehyde and cyanide (Rechnitz and Llenado, 1971). This marked a transformative approach in the field where researchers attempted to employ various targets as receptors including, tissues, microorganisms, cellular organelles, cell surface receptors, enzymes, antibodies, nucleic acids, etc. (Bhalla et al., 2016). On the other hand, probable transducers included, electrochemical, optical, thermometric, magnetic, and others (Bhalla et al., 2016).

1.1.2 BIOSENSORS FOR DISEASE

The progress made within a decade of the first "biosensor" led the scientific and medical community to collaborate towards a common idea-Can these "biosensors" or sensing devices be used in detection and diagnosis of various human diseases? Little did the scientific community foresee the power of these simple yet innovative devices during that time. Nevertheless, the idea majorly focused towards developing simplified, cost-effective and user-friendly devices. Due to this, biosensor technology has continued to evolve into an ever-expanding and multidisciplinary domain of innovation-driven science since its birth.

1.1.3 SENSORS VS. BIOSENSORS: WORKING PRINCIPLE

The working principle of a biosensor could be imagined similar to that of a classical sensing device (Figure 1.1(A)). Hence, the question is-What exactly is unique about biosensors and how different they are from the conventional sensing devices? Thus, it is important to gain a deeper insight to their structural components which makes them of functionally unique. The functional anatomy of a conventional sensing device includes components that will involve a sensing unit, a converter unit to convert the sensed signal into a digital format, and a display unit to interpret this converted signal to a user-friendly readable format (Figure 1.1(A)). So, to begin with the first component is a *sensor*: a device that can sense physical changes including, temperature, mass, humidity, light, and pressure. This change measured and captured by the sensor is analog in nature. To ensure proper interpretation, it is important to change the analog signal into a specific electronic potential difference termed as "voltage." This analog signal is sensitive to fluctuations and constant changes that can be captured using a *transducer*, the second component of the sensing device. The transducer enables analog to digital (A/D) signal conversion that is efficient enough to capture and convert even the smallest of fluctuations in the analog readings. The transducers can be semiconductors, diodes or transistors (for temperature changes), capacitors (to measure pressure changes) or photodiodes or photoresistors (to detect light-based changes) (Yoon, 2016). Thereafter, the recorded signal is processed with a network of electronic components constituting an amplifier to capture signal changes, an electronic processor and a readable display unit to record the changes detected by the user (Figure 1.1(A)).

Although, the overall structure of a biosensor primarily overlaps with the principle of a general sensing device as described above however it differs significantly with a few unique features (Figure 1.1(B)). For example, the sensor used in a "biosensor" module is a sensitive biochemical element called *bioreceptor*, also otherwise known as a biomimetic material (Figure 1.1(B)). Bioreceptors prove superior in determining the differences in biochemical analytes (tissue changes, microbes, nucleic acid changes, etc.), which the conventional sensors (for temperature, pressure, etc.), fail to detect (Bhalla et al., 2016; Yoon, 2016). For example, to detect *E. coli* in a given sample, a voltage signal will be generated only when the bioreceptor (for instance, anti-*E. coli* antibody) will recognize and bind to the bacteria. As of today, the commonly used bioreceptors include nucleic acids (DNA, RNA) and antibodies that target proteins of interest. Second, the transducer of a biosensor primarily features electrochemical (measures voltage differences), optical, thermal (change of temperature) and piezo-electric (to measure antigens, nucleic acids, biomolecules, enzymes) (Yoon, 2016). Like the conventional sensing device, the third unit is the electronic module comprising of the electronic unit to record the changes detected by the user (Figure 1.1(B)).

1.2   CHARACTERISTICS OF A BIOSENSOR

A biosensor constitutes of unique components integral for its function. Therefore, the device should include components that harness optimized properties for the efficient detection of the analyte and its associated changes with minimal error.

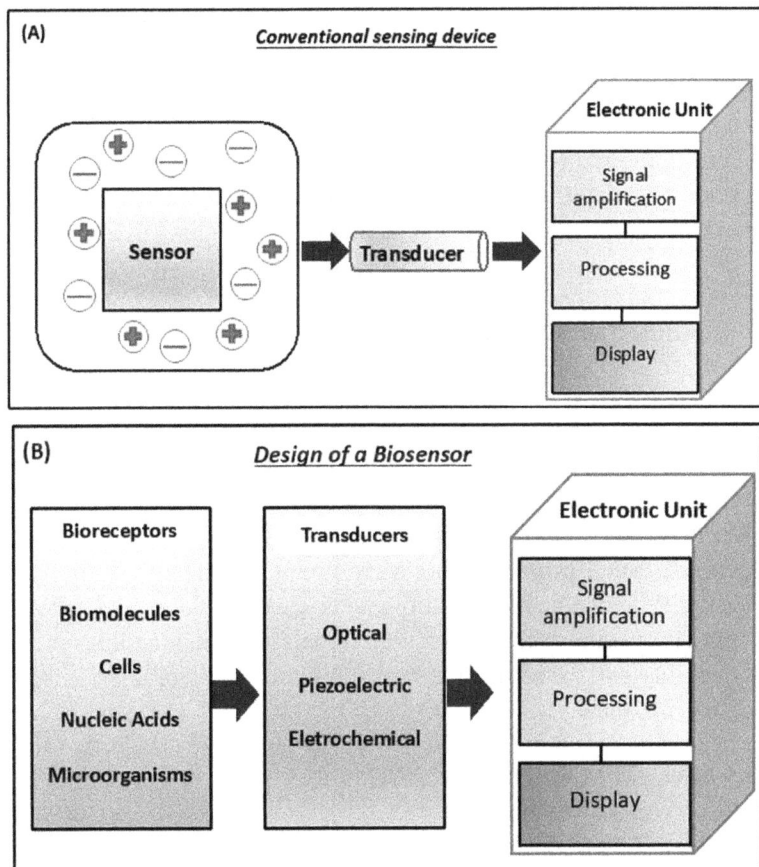

FIGURE 1.1 Schematic representations of functional components of biomolecule sensing devices. (A) Classical sensing device-sensor senses the charge-based changes in environment which are recorded by the transducer in connection. Thereafter, the transducer signals the charge recorded to the electronic unit for subsequent processing of data. (B) Design of a biosensor-sensors can include biomolecules to microorganisms which recognize the changes-based on the environment or specific analyte. The signal is thereafter processed by the specific type of transducer-based on the sensing method and transferred to the electronic unit for data processing and analysis.

Source: Adapted with permission from: Bhalla, Jolly, Formisano, and Estrela (2016).

1.2.1 SPECIFICITY AND SELECTIVITY

Selectivity and specificity enable a bioreceptor to detect a specific analyte in a given sample containing various biomolecules and other constituents

(Yoon, 2016; Holzinger and Goff, 2014). One can imagine the interaction of an antigen with the antibody which is of very specific and selective in nature. Considering this example, antibodies can be considered as bioreceptors that are clamped (attached) on the transducer's surface. A buffering solution (containing salts) with the antigen when exposed to the transducer allows the antibodies to interact only with its target antigens (Yoon, 2016). Hence, these features are an important consideration for designing of a biosensor.

1.2.2   PRECISION AND ACCURACY

Precision ensures to provide similar results each time an analyte is measured while accuracy ensures the digital readings obtained with a mean value nearest to the true value when an analyte is measured in multiple replicates (Bhalla et al., 2016). This property is further characterized by the reproducibility to generate identical responses for experiments conducted in replicates. Such properties are very much dependent on the quality of transducer and electronic components used in the given biosensor. Therefore, the accuracy in the obtained signals or digital readings provides high reliability and robustness towards the functioning of a biosensor.

1.2.3   LINEAR RANGE OF SENSING

The linearity or linear range of a biosensor can be defined as the range of analyte concentration changes to which the biosensor responds linearly. It is the feature that is indicative of the accuracy of the detected changes in the analyte (Gupta et al., 2017). This unique property of the biosensor helps to recognize the smallest of any change associated with the analyte during a given response of the biosensor (Gupta et al., 2017).

1.2.4   BIOSENSING STABILITY

Stability defines the degree of susceptibility to ambient changes occurring within the vicinity of the biosensing system (Bhalla et al., 2016; Yoon, 2016; Gupta et al., 2017). These changes can potentially induce drifts or biases in the output signal during measurement of analyte-associated changes. This results in error in the end results obtained. Stability of a biosensor also helps to record changes with the analyte in long experimental conditions. Factors including the functioning of transducers and electronics, affinity of the bioreceptor (interaction between analyte and bioreceptor) may influence the stability of a biosensor. Therefore, appropriate tuning of electronics is required to ensure a stable response of the sensor.

1.2.5 SENSITIVITY

The sensitivity of a biosensor defines its ability to detect the least amount of analyte and associated changes (Gupta et al., 2017). This is important since the concentrations of various analytes occur in the range of nanograms to femtograms in a given biological system.

1.3 TYPES OF BIOSENSORS

The classification of biosensors broadly depends on the transducers used in its design (Yoon, 2016; Kubicek-Sutherland et al., 2017). This is because of the transducers that enable the isolation and immobilization of the analyte to its electrical component. Therefore, biosensors can be categorized-based on the biological or the transduction elements used in their designing (Kubicek-Sutherland et al., 2017). Biological elements include enzymes, antibodies, tissue samples, microorganisms, etc., while transducers include components that are based on the recognition of mass, electrochemical, and optical properties (Figure 1.2).

1.3.1 OPTICAL BIOSENSORS

Optical biosensors utilize optical fibers to allow detection of analytes-based on absorption, fluorescence or scattering of light (Yoon, 2016; Kubicek-Sutherland et al., 2017). This type of biosensor enables the measurement of both catalytic and affinity reactions. Biochemical or molecular reactions induce a change in the fluorescence or absorbance concurrent with a change in refractive index (RI) of the surface-immobilized with varied density of bioreceptors and analytes. Optical biosensors can be utilized for *in vivo* applications, including the precision of recording the changes inside a living biological cell.

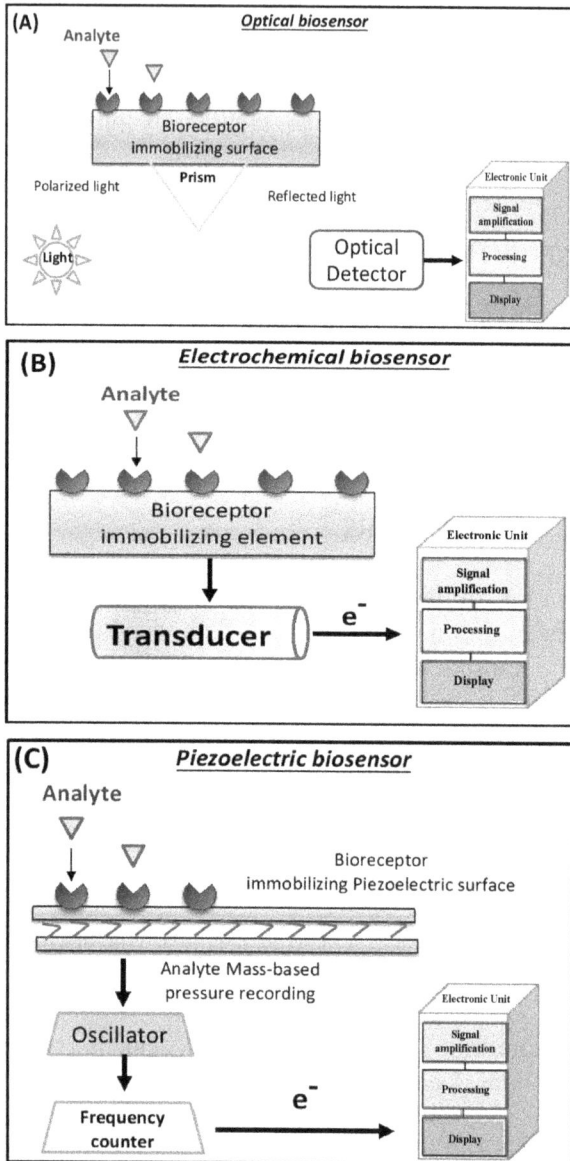

FIGURE 1.2   Classification of commercially available biosensors-based on the transducing element. (A) Optical biosensor-allows the detection of analytes-based on the properties of light. (B) Electrochemical biosensor-transduction of electrical signals produced as a result of bioreceptor-analyte interaction allows efficient detection of analyte-associated changes. (C) Piezoelectric biosensor-functions-based on the principle of mass-based production of mechanical force produced due to the interaction of analyte-bioreceptor interaction.

1.3.2 ELECTROCHEMICAL BIOSENSORS

These families of biosensors constitute sensing molecules that are immobilized by covalently bonding to the surface of an appropriate probe (Kubicek-Sutherland et al., 2017). This probe surface holds the sensing molecules or bioreceptors in a static manner to avoid bioreceptor loss and to exclude interference in signals. These immobilized bioreceptors react specifically with analytes in the given sample producing an electrical signal. This electrical signal is directly proportional to the concentration of the analyte. Based on this principle, electrochemical biosensors can employ a variety of transducing materials such as potentiometric, amperometric, and impedimetric transducers that enable efficient conversion of the chemical information into a measurable signal recorded by the electronic detection system (Yoon, 2016).

1.3.3 PIEZOELECTRIC BIOSENSORS

These classes of biosensors are also known as mass-based biosensors. The function of these biosensors is based on the principle of mechanical force generated due to the mass of the analytes bound to the bioreceptors immobilized on the piezoelectric surface (Kubicek-Sutherland et al., 2017). Upon interaction, it generates a range of vibrations thus recorded by the oscillator and frequency counter module. The piezoelectric surface in this kind acts as the mass to frequency transducer which translates the interactions between the analyte and the bioreceptors in the form of electrical signal recorded by the detection unit (Yoon, 2016). Due to their working principle, these sensors are also referred to as "acoustic wave" or "microbalance" sensors. The maximum amplitude of vibration generated allows the surface detection through the formation of bulk acoustic waves in the range of 10 and 50 megahertz.

1.4 CURRENT APPLICATIONS OF BIOSENSOR TECHNOLOGY

Over time, several biosensors including enzyme-based, immunosensors, tissue-based, DNA biosensors, piezoelectric, and thermal biosensors have been developed by many research groups (Mehrotra, 2016; Kozitsina et al., 2018; Bahadir and Sezgintürk, 2015). These biosensors have offered avenues for detection and analysis of a wide range of analytical agents ranging from small cellular biomolecules to microorganisms to modern-day detection of cancer. These miniaturized innovative devices offer the possibilities towards the implementation of advanced technology to improve the instrumentation features, thereby making these devices user-friendly. Over time, biosensors have evolved from a classical electrochemical analytical device to highly proficient detection devices with improved sensitivity and selectivity. Additionally, an extensive amount of information can be gathered from electronic libraries regarding the applications of commercial biosensors being used today. To assist the readers in-brief, some of the elegant and routinely used commercial biosensors have been highlighted in Figure 1.3.

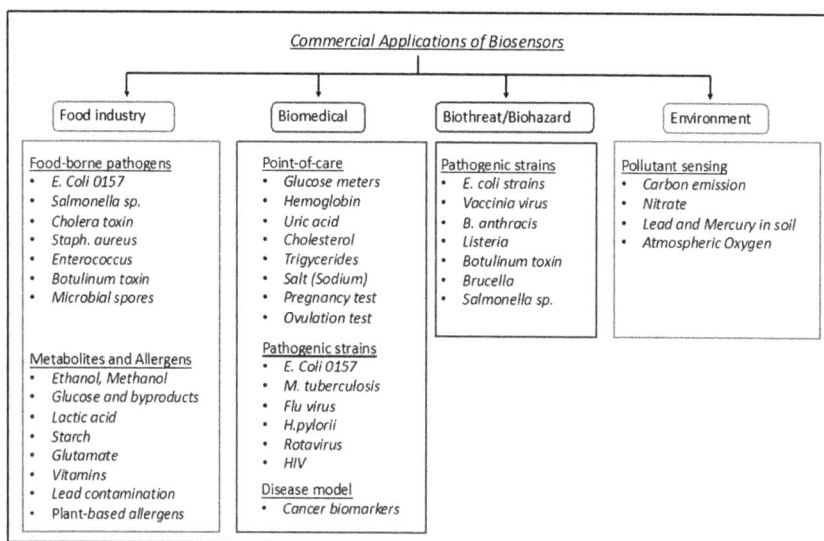

FIGURE 1.3 Commercial applications of biosensors-schematic representation of various commercial biosensors widely used in day-to-day life across various industries. Some of the commonly used biosensors are described along with few examples hereafter in this chapter.

1.4.1 *ENZYME-BASED BIOSENSORS*

Leyland Clark invented the first functional model of glucose sensing device that relied primarily on the enzymatic activity of GO_x enzyme

(Heineman et al., 2006; Bhalla et al., 2016). As technology evolved, the utility of this device also found its niche in primary health care, such as the blood glucose detection tests. The principle of the device remained the same where it was capable of detecting the changes associated with blood glucose levels driven by the enzymatic conversion of glucose to gluconolactone and hydrogen peroxide in the presence of oxygen. The presence of electrode enables the detection for fluctuations in the levels of dissolved oxygen in the blood sample which is correlative of the levels of blood glucose levels. This principle serves as a powerful tool that triggered the use of enzymes in biosensor devices. Current research indicates diabetes as one of the serious health concerns for the rapidly growing economy, which has been predicted to affect more than 300 million people by 2045 (Davis and Altintas, 2017). An interesting observation is that in 2009 approximately half of the world biosensor market was focused towards developing point of care devices whose 32% included only blood glucose monitoring devices. Enzymes serve as excellent sensors due to their high selectivity and specificity towards their substrate. In addition, their catalytic activity ensures the longevity of the biochemical reaction thus triggered. Despite these advantages, these biomolecules also have certain limitations. For instance, as of today, we lack knowledge on enzymes for every substrate available. Many enzymes are precious and difficult to extract using biochemical procedures. Further, many enzymes lose their activity and stability upon extraction from their respective sources. Moreover, detection of enzyme turnover could be confounded by non-specific interference of other metabolic substrates leading to false readings. These limitations were some of the usual characteristics of first-generation biosensors. Subsequent integration of appropriate technology and measures led to the birth of second generation of glucose biosensors. These biosensors were developed involving small redox-active molecule, *for instance*, a ferrocene derivative that functioned as a carrier of electrons between the enzyme and an electrode. The molecule reacts with the enzyme with high affinity and sensitivity, thereby blocking the interference of baseline levels of oxygen in the system. This mechanism produces lower potential difference that provides appropriate and reliable glucose readings (Figure 1.4).

Soon after, technology enthusiasts provided the prototype for third-generation biosensors. The uniqueness of third-generation biosensors includes the direct connection of the enzyme to the electrode using redox polymers that provide conductivity. Recently, metal nanoparticles (NPs), carbon nanotubes (CNTs) and graphene (GN) have also been utilized as base materials in the designing of glucose biosensing devices to enhance the efficiency of the enzyme-electrode function. Thereafter, glucose dehydrogenase-based sensors have also been established as an alternative to GO_x. Using this principle as a proof-of-concept, other sensors have been developed engaging enzymes including cholesterol oxidase, lactate oxidase, peroxidase enzymes. Similarly, biosensors have also been developed to detect the conversion of urea to ammonia via pH-dependent activity of the enzyme urease. The enzyme-dependent change in local pH serves as the signal to be captured by the sensing device. The signal is thus captured by employing potentiometric or optical methods such as by combining urease with an appropriate optical dye. In another example, cholesterol esters can be determined using electrodes that contain cholesterol metabolizing enzymes (esterase and oxidase).

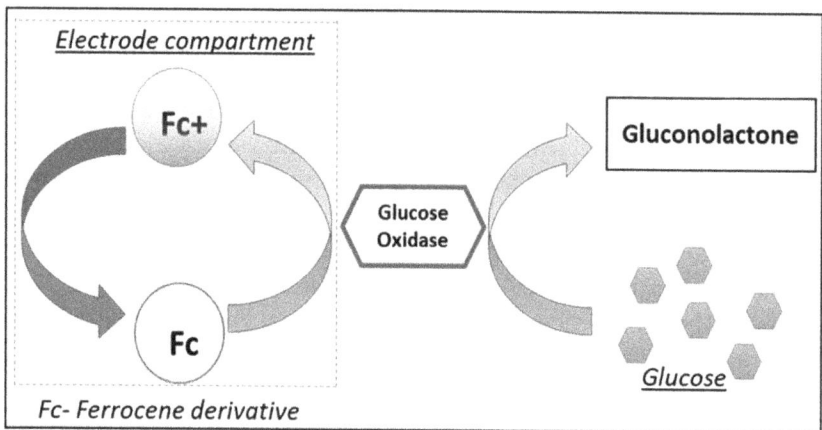

FIGURE 1.4   Schematic of a second-generation glucose biosensor. The ferrocene derivative immobilized on the sensing electrode acts as the electron shuttle in the presence of catalytically active glucose oxidase enzyme resulting in signal for detection of glucose in the sample.

1.4.2   ANTIBODY-BASED BIOSENSORS

Biochemically, antibodies are proteins produced naturally by living systems which regulate the immune system in a living organism. Antibodies are also termed as immunoglobins (Igs), soluble glycoproteins present abundantly in the serum. Their main role is to provide defense to the host against foreign pathogens, allergies, and associated immune reactions. To understand the working principle for an antibody-based biosensor, it is important to gain knowledge on the structure of an antibody. In addition, it is important to note that there are five classes of antibodies-based on their structural differences, i.e., IgM, IgD, IgG, IgE, and IgA. The general structure of an Ab is represented in Figure 1.5(A). For the benefit of readers to understand this structure, one can imagine the structure of an antibody-like the English alphabet "Y." This structure can be broadly divided into two parts. First is F_{ab} region responsible for antigen-binding and second is the constant fragment represented as (F_c). An antibody constitutes two heavy chains and two are light chains making a total of four polypeptide chains. These polypeptide chains are connected by disulfide bonds. Furthermore, this heavy chain is composed of subunits that includes one variable region (variable heavy or V_H) and three constant regions (C_{H1}, C_{H2} and C_{H3}). On the other hand, the light chain has only one variable region (V_L) and one constant region (C_L). The variable fragment (F_v) region harboring the complementarity-determining regions (CDRs) is contained within the F_{ab} region of the antibody. These CDRs contain antigen-binding sites of a given antibody and provide specificity against an antigen. In contrast, the Fc region is responsible for mediating effector functions, for instance, Ab-immune response that involves a wide array of cellular responses (Yoon, 2016; Neethirajan et al., 2018).

Antibodies harness specificity and affinity for diverse analytes, which makes them a natural choice as efficient molecular receptors and probes in biosensor technology. Antibodies can be produced or raised by inoculating or injecting appropriate laboratory animals (for instance, mice, rats, rabbits, guinea pigs) with a given antigen. This leads to production of antibodies against this antigen in the given animal model. Thereafter the antibodies generated naturally within the organism (animal model) can then be harvested from these animals employing biochemical extraction procedures. After developing the required antibodies, these can be immobilized onto a bioreceptor interface conjugated to a functional transducer to design a biosensor, represented in Figure 1.5(B).

Given the idea of an antibody-based biosensor, one can imagine that these molecules can be utilized as sensors either in analyte or in immobilized form. However, the structure that we learnt provides us the idea that the antigen or analyte should essentially interact with the Fab regions. Now, this interaction can only be facilitated if the F_{ab} region is well exposed to

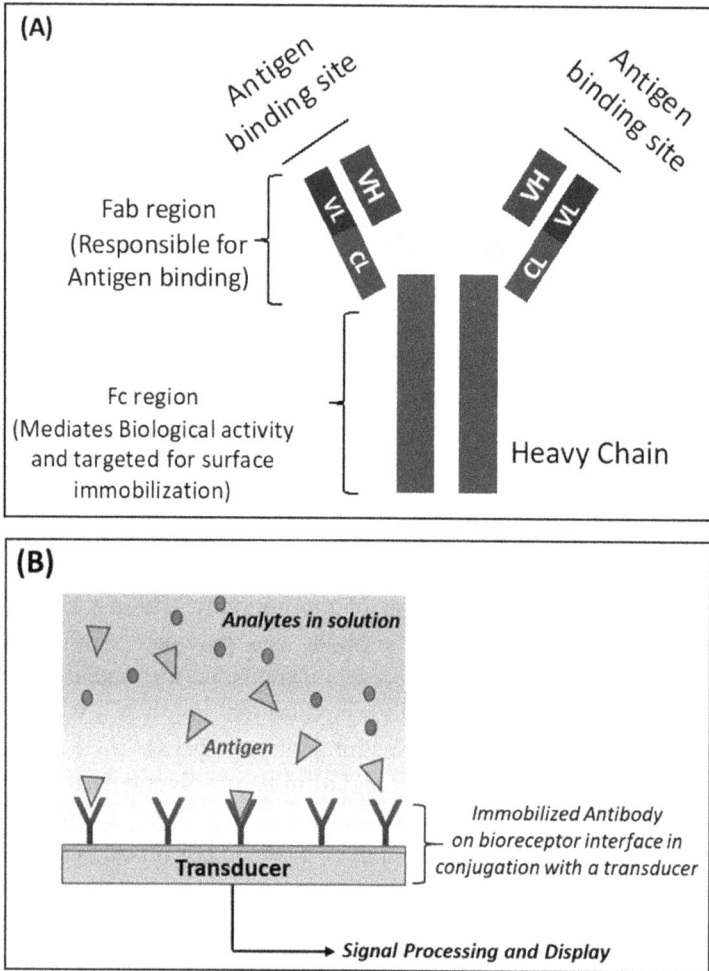

FIGURE 1.5   (A) Simple representation for the structure of an antibody. (B) General working principle of an antibody-based biosensor-Immobilized antibodies recognize specific antigens present in the analyte mixture. Immobilized antibodies could be bound to a fluorescent or colorimetric substrate to provide appropriate signal upon a successful antigen-antibody reaction.

the surface, allowing sufficient access to the antigenic surface for interactions. Therefore, it leads to the idea for surface adsorption of antibodies for their efficient immobilization. Physical forces including, non-covalent forces, electrostatic, hydrophobic interactions or van der Waals forces can also be utilized to immobilize antibodies on a given surface such as the poly-(2-cyano-ethylpyrrole)-coated gold electrode which has been shown to increase the efficiency of immunologic activity by allowing 3-dimensional open orientations of the antibody structure. Many research groups have also attempted to immobilize antibodies-based on entrapment methods using platinum wire substrate. Some of the commonly used conducting polymers (CPs) for immunosensor fabrication include poly-acetylene, polythiophene, polyaniline, polyindole, and polypyrrole due to their higher level of biocompatibility in aqueous solutions. Recently, polyquinone was also shown as an additional conducting polymer that provides coupling and transduction abilities for better sensitivity during analyte sensing. Subsequently, silica sol-gel-based antibody entrapment has also been used for enhanced antigen attachment. However, this method relies on the immunosensor sensitivity-based on antigen entrap-ment. Changes in the active site structure or 3-dimensional confirmation can lead to poor immunological activity or recognition efficiency. It is important to keep in mind that these commonly used coupling methods are confounded by technical limitations such as limited control over the antibody orientations and mass-based transfer through membranes or gels. As a result, these challenges affect the correct immobilization efficiency, which occurs via the Fc region, thus leading to poor antigen-binding site accessibility (Yoon, 2016).

Another method for antibody immobilization includes covalent bonding on various solid surfaces to facilitate long-term storage. The covalent bindings include surface modification so as to expose various reactive groups such as hydroxy, thiol, carboxy, or amino groups on the solid surfaces. To achieve this, various surface modification techniques have been implemented that include chemical modification, photo-chemical grafting, plasma gas discharge and ionizing radiation grafting. The side chains of Ab containing lysine residues are an attractive target for covalent immobilization. This method also leads to chances of error where the modifications might interact with nearby amine residues and alter the antibody activity. One way to reduce chances of error associated with antibody activity is by coupling the terminal carboxyl groups on gold surfaces with the amine groups of Abs. In addition, the presence of excess amounts of lysine residues might lead to increased noise due to the previous non-specific effects of covalent targeting. One of the substitute methods can be targeting the thiol groups that provide uniformity immobilization patterns. This method of immobilization typically involves thiol-disulfide exchange chemistry when the complex is exposed on an immobilizing surface. Using this strategy, antibody fragment have been observed to orient in their physiological pattern providing a significant increase in antigen binding ability when compared to amine group modifications. Using this idea, an impedimetric immunosensor was developed with high sensitivity and selectivity for the detection of peptides derived from avian influenza virus by immobilizing the F_{ab} fragment of the antibody fragment on a gold electrode surface. Despite the robustness and advantages of covalent immobilization, the lack of a definite orientation remains one of the existing challenges. Hence, several non-physical immobilization strategies can be implemented such as the precoating of sensor surface with biotin-avidin complex or intermediate binding proteins including Protein A or G provide improved specificity for antibody function. These proteins allow high affinity and binding specificity against the F_c region of antibodies, making the antibody molecules immobilize on the coated surface. Antibody-based sensing methods are often confounded by technical limitations. To overcome this, recombinant Abs that exhibit high physical and chemical stability are being developed. These molecules also allow an easy access to the antigen, making them a much reliable alternative to natural antibodies. However, one of the confounding challenges with this system is the interference of redox-active species produced because of the antigen-antibody reaction. To overcome this challenge, sandwich immunoassays are used where the antibody is coated on a surface and the antigen in the given sample or solution can react. Thereafter, this complex is detected by the addition of a labeled conjugated-secondary antibody to provide a colorimetric or fluorescent signal indicative of the interaction between the antibody and the antigen. Subsequently, label-free detection methods have been developed that allow detection of antibody-antigen interactions. These methods include electrochemical techniques such as AC impedance, optical techniques such as surface plasmon resonance (SPR) and mass-sensitive techniques such as quartz crystal microbalance (QCM).

It is also important to note that some antibody-antigen bindings can be very strong and irreversible in nature under physiological conditions. This would result in a lack of substrate turnover leading to saturated signals. Such cases demand altering the conditions, for instance, by changing the pH of the environment can lead to dissociation of the complex, however will also account for permanent loss of their activities. Based on these ideas, employing immunoassay-based lateral analyte flow strategy, the first commercially available home pregnancy test was launched. This device detects the presence of human chorionic gonadotrophin (hCG) in the urine samples (Figure 1.6).

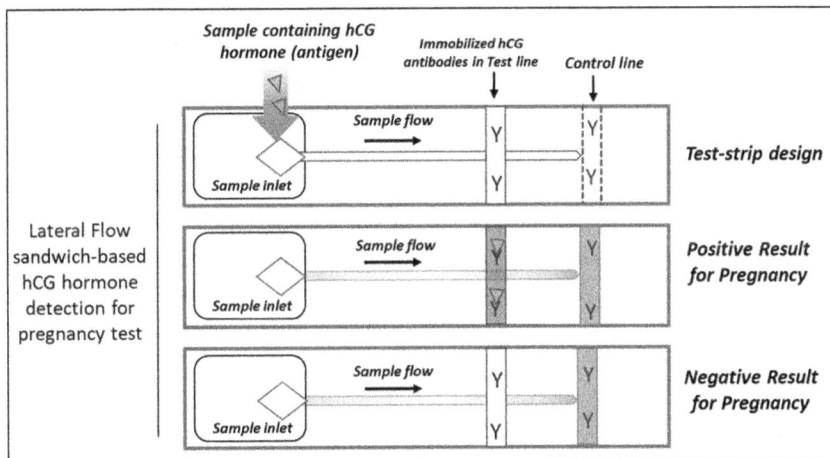

FIGURE 1.6 Working principle of pregnancy detection biosensor. Pregnancy detection kits are based on lateral flow of analytes or sample. The sample is added in the inlet area and flows-based on lateral capillary movement to the regions containing antibodies conjugated with a chromophore or fluorophore against human hCG hormone. Reaction of the hCG (antigen) with these specific conjugated antibodies in the test line results in a suitable signal allowing the user to know their status-based on the number of blue lines observed.

The test detects the presence of this hormone by showing a blue line indicative of whether the patient or subject is pregnant or not pregnant. Later, improved models have emerged that employ optical sensor-based strategies to measure the intensity of the colorimetric signal (for instance, the blue line) to provide an estimate of the time since conception proportional to the amount of hormone being produced.

1.4.3 PEPTIDE-BASED BIOSENSORS

In simple words, peptides are the polymers of amino acids that serve as the backbone of protein structure. Several proteins are selective and can bind to respective targets with higher order of specificity. Therefore, their amino acid sequences responsible for this feature can be designed and mimicked in the concept of biosensor designing. Usually, shorter length peptides introduce less complexity reducing the chance of errors. Furthermore, these shorter peptides can be easy to handle and will display simpler 3-dimensional (tertiary) confirmation important with regards to substrate binding. Moreover, the structural simplicity allows easy synthesis followed by manipulation using fluorescent labeling without altering their biochemical activity. For example, peptide-based sensors can be effective tools for studying the activity of certain enzymes, for example, proteases. Proteases possess the ability to hydrolyze peptide bonds, and these enzymes have been shown to be implicated in various diseased outcomes. In this strategy, a peptide sequence is engineered to contain a fluorescent unit and a fluorescence quencher at its protease-sensitive opposite terminals as outlined in Figure 1.7. Enzymatic degradation of these probes by the protease results in enhanced fluorescent emission. This emission can be correlated with the enzymatic activity.

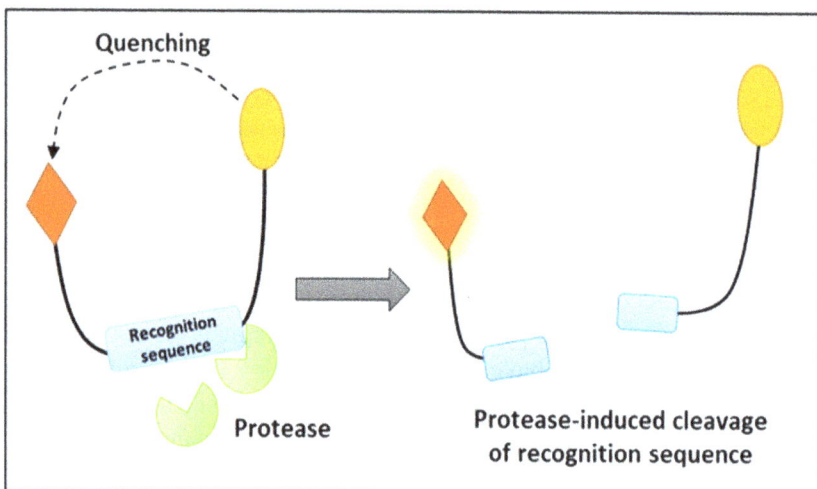

FIGURE 1.7 Principle of protease-based biosensing technology. Strategy employs a fluorophore (in orange under the control of a quencher in yellow present in close proximity). Upon cleavage of the recognition peptide by a protease, the fluorophore is free whose signal can be detected in the form of fluorescent emission.

Source: Reproduced with permission from: Pazos, Vázquez, Mascareñas, and Vázquez (2009). © Royal Society of Chemistry.

One such example includes matrix metallopeptidases (MMP-2 and MMP-9) that have been implicated in several inflammatory responses including tumor metastasis. In addition, some peptides can also be used to determine proteinase activity. For instance, peptides are coated on quantum dots (QDs) that are conjugated to dye molecules are widely used in fluorescence resonance energy transfer (FRET) reactions. This unique and highly sensitive technique allows to study intermolecular distance between two biomolecules present in a given system. This technique also allows to assess the activity of a variety of other enzymes such as kinases. In an interesting example, peptide degradation by proteases was implemented for *in vivo* imaging of tumors. This strategy makes use of a protease specific peptide sequence. The imaging strategy could also prove beneficial for studying enzymes where the fluorochrome is attached to the carrier backbone through specific linker sequences. This selection of linker sequences is based on the peptide-specific enzymes. Employing similar principle, fluorophores have also been implemented in the design of kinase-specific sensors. Structurally, these sensors constitute a kinase recognition sequence and a fluorescence reporter system finely situated near the amino acid residue that is phosphorylated. When phosphorylated, the sensor experiences a conformational change that allows a change in the fluorescent emission. Imperiali's group was the first to develop such a sensor in the year 1998, based on the binding of Mg^{2+} ion to Sox amino acid immobilized to the sensing surface (Pazos et al., 2009). The sensor involves a kinase recognition sequence, including the amino acid sequence (See/Tyr/Thr), susceptible to undergo phosphorylation and a peptide sequence (D-Pro-Gly) that can induce beta-turns responsible for conformational flexibility (Figure 1.8). This carefully designed structural assembly pre-organizes the binding site for the interaction with Mg^{2+}. Thus, based on the binding affinities of the metal ions in the presence or absence of peptide chain phosphorylation determines the emission of fluorescent signal (Figure 1.8).

1.4.4 MOLECULAR IMPRINTED POLYMERS (MIP)-BASED BIOSENSORS

Until now, we have discussed various types of biosensors made on the principles of biological molecules such as enzymes, peptides, nucleic acids, and antibodies. Unlike many others, these molecules also exhibit challenges such as cost of production, challenges related to purification and extraction, quality, and long-term stability. Therefore, a new and emerging approach has been to use synthetic materials that could mimic the behavior and biochemical features of bioactive molecules, for instance, enzymes, and antibodies. This idea has led to the birth of molecularly imprinted polymers (MIPs), which possess the ability to overcome the challenge associated with biological molecules. In MIP designing, the analyte (usually a biological molecule) is mixed with polymerizable monomers that will initiate polymerization and crosslinking to entrap the analytes, which will act as templates (Figure 1.9). Removal of the analyte produces the formation of pores within the polymer structure. These pores contain the internal surface groups which will react with the analyte.

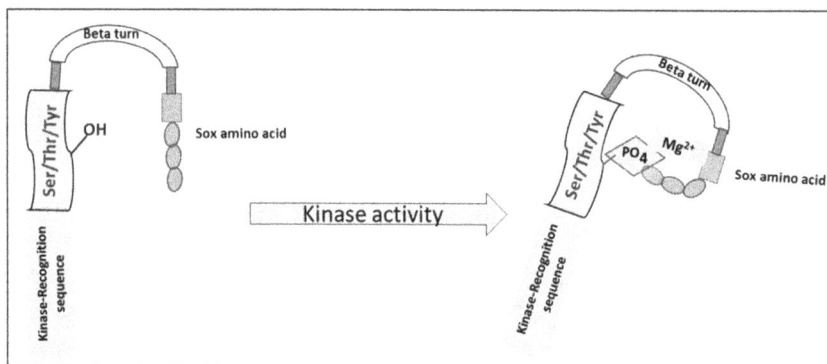

FIGURE 1.8   Modular design of kinase-based biosensing technology. Phosphorylation of the Ser/Thr/Tyr peptide attracts Mg^{2+} binding allowing the beta-turn mediated structural flexibility of the polypeptide resulting in enhanced and fluorescence of the Sox amino acid.
Source: Reproduced with permission from: Pazos, Vázquez, Mascareñas, and Vázquez (2009). © Royal Society of Chemistry.

Several advantages can be assigned with MIP's over biological materials, including higher stability at room temperature, a longer half-life ranging in years, easy availability, low cost of production and their usability in aqueous solutions without compromising their activity or efficiency. One such example is the deposition of inorganic polymers containing glucose onto a QCM surface utilizing a gel-based process. When glucose was washed out, the change (increase) in mass was sensed by the system when exposed to glucose. Other strategies of immobilization include electrochemical deposition of polymers onto electrode surfaces in the presence of a template. For instance, to detect atropine (an anticholinergic drug), a QCM chip can be coated electrochemically with poly(o-phenylenediamine). Similar principles have been efficiently used in the detection of viruses in tobacco plant. One important observation is that once these MIPs are crosslinked, they become insoluble. Therefore, recent strategies include the use of nanoparticle-based MIPs, which have higher solubility than the previous designs. For instance, nano-sized MIPs are used in high throughput ELISA (enzyme-linked immunosorbent assay) assays for an array of analytes with detection limits as low as 1 picomolar. MIP-based nano-biomimetic sensors have also been developed for the detection of pathogens, toxins, and drugs.

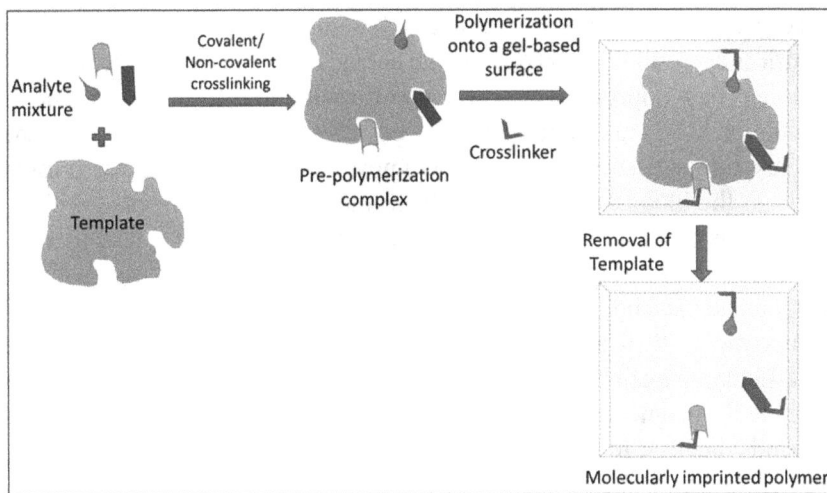

FIGURE 1.9 Designing of molecularly imprinted biosensors. Complex formed by the interaction of analytes and a given template (target) is subjected to polymerization in the presence of suitable crosslinkers to form a solid structure. Removal of template results in accessible binding sites within the polymer that allow selective recognition for the imprinted analytes.
Source: Reproduced with permission from: Davis and Altintas (2017). © John Wiley and Sons.

1.4.5 NUCLEIC ACID-BASED BIOSENSORS

All living cells contain DNA (deoxyribonucleic acid) that serves as the genetic messenger responsible for life. In simple words, it can be considered as a uniquely encrypted information storage blueprint. DNA undergoes a series of highly coordinated biological processes to produce RNA is also known as ribonucleic acid (RNA). RNA acts as a messenger molecule and participates in further events leading to the synthesis of proteins that are critical for life. Chemically, it is important to note that both DNA and RNA are biomolecules composed of nucleic acid bases (adenine, cytosine, guanine, and thymine (in DNA) which is replaced by uracil (in RNA), and sugar-phosphate backbone. It is known that cancer is associated with DNA-mutations that accumulate over a period of time and trigger a network of cellular and molecular processes, eventually leading to carcinogenesis. Given this reason, analyzes of these mutations allow the clinicians to detect and diagnose the disease at various stages. These genetic mutations can also be detected in the freely circulating tumor cells (CTCs) in the bloodstream of cancer patients. These CTCs are of high significance in studying the origin and spread of cancers that offer avenues to design new approaches towards non-invasive diagnosis and prognosis of a tumor. CTCs are tumor cells that get released into the blood from the primary tumor tissue. Although it is known that these CTCs are present freely in the bloodstream of the patient, the challenge associated with its detection is due to their low abundance and heterogeneity. Thus, modern tools targeting the nucleic acid composition (DNA and RNA chemistry of tumor cells) have been of tremendous help. Using PCR-based methods that include digital PCR and next-generation sequencing platforms have made the efficient detection and analysis of these DNA and RNA level changes, possible for diagnosis of the disease. The rare and complex nature of CTCs demands the need for new tools to be developed for a smooth and detailed analysis at single-cell level.

Emerging knowledge on nucleotide interactions has led to the development of smart strategies for nucleotide sensing. In nucleic acid-based sensors, oligonucleotide strands are immobilized on a suitable transducer which serves as the electrode and facilitates interaction with the complementary oligonucleotides or analytes (especially biomolecules) in a sample. The recognition of the immobilized oligonucleotide and nucleotides in the sample occurs based on complementary nucleotide interactions. A few examples include-detection of RNA molecules in tumor samples selectively based on oxidation of guanine nucleotide. One such innovation can be credited to the peptide nucleic acid (PNA) technology. Smart and advanced nucleic acid recognition process involving Peptide Nucleic Acid (PNA) aptamers can augment the efficiency of DNA-based biosensors. PNA is a synthetic nucleic acid analog whose sugar-phosphate backbone is replaced with pseudo-peptide composed of repeating N-(2-aminoethyl)-glycine derivatives linked via peptide bonds. This backbone is uncharged in native conditions and provides stability when PNA forms a complex with charged nucleic acid molecules like DNA or RNA. PNAs can be used as probes to capture complementary sequences in a given DNA or RNA molecule of interest. The hybridization principle of PNA molecules with complementary nucleotides follows the classical Watson-Crick base-pairing rules that involve hydrogen bonds between complementary nucleotides. Aptamers are short oligonucleotides, usually 40–60 nucleotides in length. They are chemically synthesized and can be easily modified and integrated with a variety of nanomaterials, including CNTs, gold or iron-oxide NPs. Immobilized oligonucleotide probes are utilized in food safety procedures to detect complementary nucleotides present in several pathogenic bacteria including *Brucella abortus*, *Escherichia coli*, and *Staphylococcus aureus* (Neethirajan et al., 2018; Bunney et al., 2017). Some of the current clinical applications of nucleic acid-based sensing technologies are highlighted in Figure 1.10 and Table 1.1.

The other advantage of PNA includes thermal and pH stability meaning it is stable in temperature and pH conditions that often lead to degradation of DNA or RNA. PNAs are chemically synthesized using classical solid-phase peptide synthesis protocols and purified and characterized via chromatographic and spectroscopic methods. Considering these biophysical properties of PNAs, they are identified as excellent candidates for use in nucleic acid-biosensing applications. PNA oligomers have found application in the detection of tumor cells and to deliver sequence-specific anti-nucleic acid molecules which could act as drugs. However, PNA's are merely water-soluble as a result lead to inefficient cellular uptake by mammalian cells. To address these issues, various modifications have been tested, including changing the backbone from glycine derivatives to other chiral amino acids. Fluorescently labeled PNA bonded to the nano-metal-organic frameworks (MOF) are used in the detection of small RNA molecules that serve as biomarkers for cancer detection. Graphitic carbon nitride ($g-C_3N_4$) nanosheets can also be used to design assays to exploit the quenching of fluorescently labeled PNA probes. Cationic polythiophene derivatives can also be used as an active layer for a QCM surface modification to detect nucleic acid levels in human serum-plasma samples that could provide early diagnosis for a given disease.

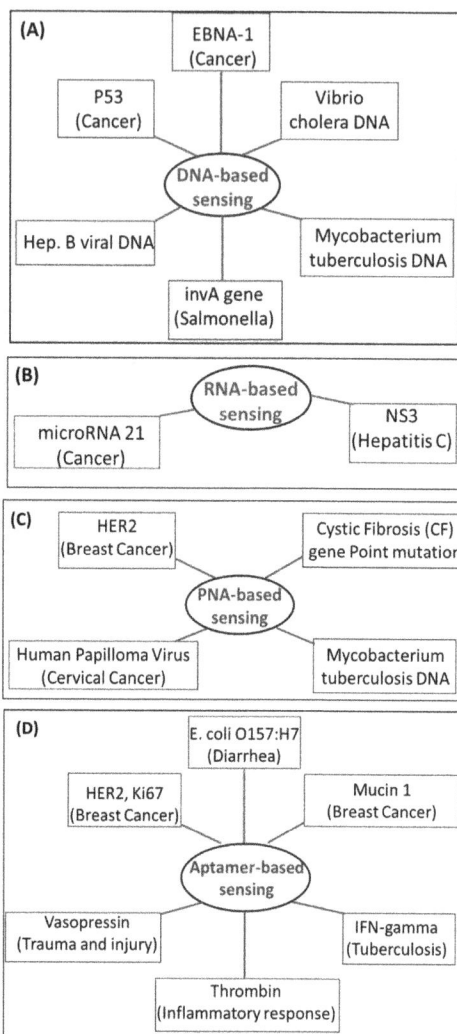

FIGURE 1.10 Current clinical applications of nucleic-acid-based sensing technology. Nucleic acid-based sensing technology has proven advantageous with time. These biosensors have gained popularity in the field of biomedical sciences in the context of disease detection and diagnosis. In this figure illustrated, (A) indicates the utility of DNA-based biosensors; (B) RNA-based sensing; (C) Peptide nucleic acid-based sensing; and (D) aptamer-based sensing of specific complementary nucleotides in various clinical and biological samples towards the diagnosis of complex human diseases as well as detection of pathogenic strains of bacteria and viruses. Due to high sensitivity and selectivity, nucleic acid-based biosensing technology is rapidly gaining commercial success by drawing attention as a powerful and inexpensive clinical diagnostic.

TABLE 1.1 List of Commercial Nucleic Acid-Based Biosensors Available as of Date and Used in Various Biomedical and Clinical Applications

Commercial Product	Target Nucleic Acid	Application
Genechip by Affymetrix	DNA-based	Single nucleotide polymorphisms in human diseases
GeneLyzer by Toshiba	Electrochemical DNA chip	Detection of pathogenic strains of bacteria and DNA-viruses
BAX by Dupont	DNA-based	Detection of *E. coli* O157:H7, *Listeria*, *Enterobacter*, *Campylobacter*, *Vibrio* and *Salmonella*
ACCUPROBE by Biomirieux ANSR by Neogen	DNA-based	*Campylobacter*, *Salmonella*, and *Listeria* in clinical samples
APTIMA virology by Hologic	RNA-based	Detection of HIV, HCV
APTIMA STI by Hologic	RNA-based	Detection of sexually transmitted diseases caused by chlamydia, gonorrhea, *Mycoplasma genitalium*, trichomoniasis, herpes and Zika virus

For the electrochemical detection of nucleic acids, methods include specific procedures for signal enhancement by combining nanostructured materials and biomolecules along the use of PNA probes. Similarly, field-effect transistors (FETs) that are GN-based have been widely used to detect the presence of nucleic acids. In addition, coating the surface with gold nanoparticles (AuNPs) enhanced the signal due to improved binding efficiency of antigens with low non-specificity. Combining microfluidics and voltammetry-based biosensing leads to efficient capture of CTCs by antibody-modified magnetic NPs as studied using samples collected directly from patient blood. In addition, electrochemical biosensing-based on the screening of KRAS gene mutations in DNA obtained from serum samples of patients has also been used for cancer diagnosis. As per this principle, a PNA-based probe complementary against the mutated KRAS gene target associated with various forms of cancer such as lung, colorectal, and ovary is immobilized on nanostructured gold microelectrodes. Thereafter exposing a mixture of PNA clamps to the human serum sample allows hybridization at the sequences closely related to the sequence of target gene KRAS. In principle, this facilitates interaction of the immobilized PNA probe specifically with KRAS gene's mutated sequence. Therefore, the detection of mutation in the DNA sequences of specific genes has been an important breakthrough in cancer disease diagnosis directly from patient samples using the PNA-based electrochemical DNA sensing technology.

Another rapid diagnostic method for the detection of genetic level changes is using PCR-based target DNA amplification. However, PCR-based methods are often encountered with sample contamination and generates artifacts or noise due to recombination between homologous regions of DNA. Therefore, new approaches for the highly sensitive detection of changes at the DNA level changes are currently under investigation. Hence, biosensors offer attractive alternatives to presently available platforms. Biosensor-based technology allows for the sensitive, rapid, and cheap detection strategies for nucleic acid targets. One such example is the plasmonic biosensors that exploit the unique properties of metal NPs for detection of DNA-associated changes using PNA probes. Plasmonic biosensors have been implicated in the detection of point mutations in non-amplified human genomic DNA. In this strategy, AuNPs are coupled with PNA probes including methyl-group specific antibodies to detect methylated-DNA, indicative of epigenetic modifications. Similarly, pyrrolidinyl-PNA is another modified and rigid PNA derivative containing a D-prolyl-2-aminocyclo-pentanecarboxylic acid (ACPC) backbone. This acpc-PNA conjugate exhibits preference for antiparallel binding and a higher affinity towards DNA over RNA. When compared with traditional PNA, this method allows higher retention of affinity and selectivity. For example, combination of anthraquinone (AQ)-labeled acpc-PNA probes with voltammetric-based biosensing allows efficient detection of human papillomavirus (HPV) type 16 DNA.

The PNA-based biosensing technology has been constantly research-driven evolution that has led to the development of diagnostics for early detection of cancers, including non-small cell lung cancer. PNA clamping is also useful to detect genetic mutations in patients with non-small cell lung cancer. PNA-clamps in combination with loop-mediated isothermal amplification (LAMP) confer higher sensitivity in the detection of point mutations, often seen in rare and complex human diseases. Specifically, PNA clamping can be combined with direct sequencing of nucleic acids that could provide detection of gene mutations along with full nucleotide sequences even in samples with very low frequency of mutations, also referred as rare mutations. Thus, the combination of PNA probes and biosensors using nanostructured materials can be the next milestone towards improvement of detection platforms. Most of the advanced optical and electrochemical approaches here discussed take advantage of the neutral charge of PNA and exploit nanostructured materials to enhance the detected signal. Moreover, biosensing platforms using PNA with sensitivity for detection as low as femtomolar (fM) range are already available and can identify both small circulating nucleotides and genetic mutations.

1.5   NON-INVASIVE BIOSENSING TECHNOLOGY

Although we have now discussed the classical concept of biosensors and their contribution in various domains, it is also important to acknowledge that we have not made much progress in the context of novel therapeutics, antimicrobial, and drug delivery systems. One of the inventions along this line can be credited to the electrochemical biosensors that have enabled the efficient detection of avian influenza virus. Emerging evidence also indicates the utility and advantage of affinity-based biosensors in sports medicine for doping analysis where sports professionals are subjected to a health screening for the presence of performance-enhancing drugs in their bloodstream or body fluids. Not to elude, the current market is highly focused on a wide variety of wearable electrochemical biosensors. These devices have also been considered a fashion statement lately endorsed by various celebrities and sports personalities. An array of wearable biosensors has been developed in the past few years that focus on non-invasive and real-time monitoring of electrolytes and metabolites in body fluids, including sweat, tears, or saliva as active indicators of the wearer's health status. The initial phases of point-of-care or portable biosensing devices witnessed tremendous progress in electrochemical sensing technology. This gave birth to commercial hand-held analyzers, for instance, the ACCU-CHEK by Roche Diagnostics, Inc.; iSTAT by Abbott, Inc.; or Lactate Scout by the Sports Resource Group, Inc.; that allow reliable detection of metabolites and electrolytes (Figure 1.11). However, these devices were confounded by challenges. For instance, the blood samples from individuals can only be obtained by the prick of a sterile needle which was an ongoing challenge for both existing and new users. This also means that for the measurement of a given analyte, the user might need to go through repetitive blood drawings leading to a lack of interest for minimally invasive methods. Therefore, the current trend demands the need for non-invasive sensing devices with higher accuracy and precision.

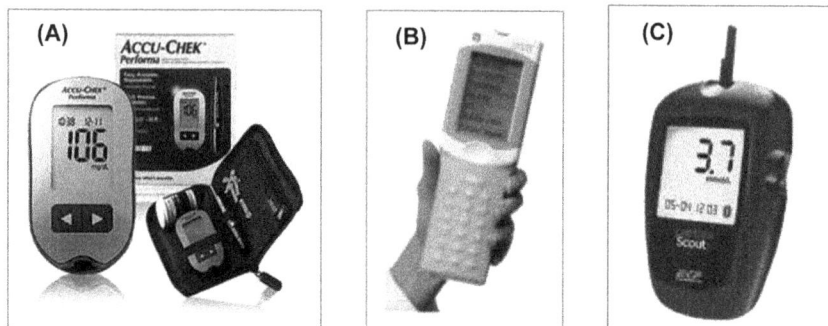

FIGURE 1.11   Minimally invasive point-of-care biosensors. (A) ACCU-CHEK by Roche diagnostics Inc. developed to detect the levels of glucose in blood. (B) iSTAT by Abbott, Inc. helps analyze the levels of soluble nutrients in blood. (C) Lactate Scout by the Sports Resource Group, Inc. helps analyze the levels of lactic acid in the blood stream.
Source: Images of the products have been acquired from the respective product websites.

Like previously illustrated wearable non-invasive devices, electrochemical sensors can be designed competent enough to detect target analytes present in secretory body fluids such as in tears, saliva, and sweat. One such example is the electrochemical sensors that users can wear on their skin called epidermal biosensors. These class of biosensors are electrochemical in nature that offers promise for improved and efficient glucose monitoring in a non-invasive manner, despite their technical limitations. One of the first U.S. Food and Drug Administration (FDA) approved commercial non-invasive wearable biosensor was the GlucoWatch® biographer (developed by Cygnus Inc.) in the early 2000s (Tierney et al., 2001). The watch allows measurement of real-time glucose concentrations in skin interstitial fluid by electrochemical methods based on the principle of reverse iontophoresis. Skin fluid acts as a buffer for many cells and acts as a nutrient supplier through diffusion from the capillary that enables the sensory activity of this wearable device. The GluoWatch® electrochemically detects the levels of glucose present in the interstitial fluid via enzymatic oxidation in the presence of sensing electrode containing enzyme GO_x. Clinical trials performed with this device resulted in precision data that is suitable for home blood glucose monitoring. Despite the gaining populating of this glucose-sensing watch, the device was retracted from the market due to its inherent technological flaws. These included reported skin irritation, long warm-up duration for the device prior to use. Therefore, efforts have been taken and many are underway focusing on reliable, efficient non-invasive glucose monitoring platforms without the interference of existing challenges (Kim et al., 2018; Tierney et al., 2001). Hence, the currently available non-invasive wearable devices hold scope towards continuous monitoring of health parameters, including tracking physical exercise, heart rate, and blood pressure and assessing other physical performance parameters. These devices are robust enough to provide valuable real-time information, educating users to be aware of their health status (Figure 1.12).

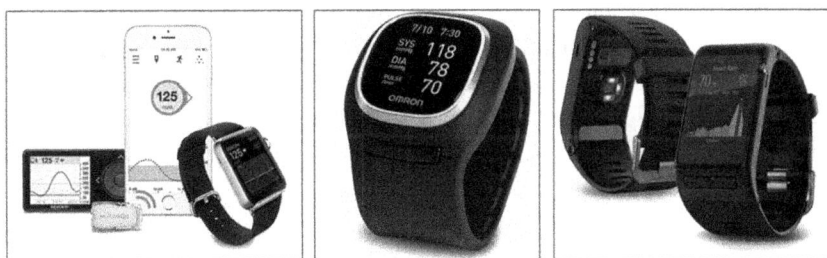

FIGURE 1.12 Emerging non-invasive wearable sensing devices. Pictorial representation of various wearable non-invasive sensing devices constituting applications including heart rate monitoring, blood glucose estimation and sleep cycles.

Source: Image reference-Google images: wearable non-invasive biosensors.

Other recent advances include wearable biosensors that allow continuous monitoring of the health state of individuals from their body sweat in a real-time manner with molecular-level insight. Similar to the skin-based sensing technology, the sweat-based biosensors also utilize iontophoresis interface for efficient analyte sensing. The process involves the delivery of stimulating agonists to the sweat glands in the presence of electrical current. Novel fabrication methods infusion with electro-chemical techniques have led to the birth of new age chemical sensors that have been compatible to perform physical measurements (such as heart rate, EEG (electroencephalography), ECG, etc.), these sensors have shown technological advantage by providing added information on analytical information to the user in a real-time manner. Textile materials and skin-based tattoo platforms have emerged as a novel platform for the integration of wearable electrochemical biosensors. In addition to the user-friendly smart technology, these devices have been successful in contributing towards a growing fashion trend. The knowledge on the impact of mechanical and physical parameters that could affect the read-out and functional efficiency of these modern-day textile- and tattoo-based sensors is of grave importance that remains an area of active investigation. One of the latest inventions can be credited to the wireless ring-based wearable chemical sensor for quick and efficient sensing of explosive and nerve-agent threats that could be present either in vapor or liquid phase. The underlying principle of this ring-based sensing device is based on electrochemical sensing. This device constitutes two major parts: first includes a set of printed electrochemical sensors, and second is the miniaturized electronic system-based on battery power for signal processing and data transmission (Sempionatto et al., 2017; Kim et al., 2018; Windmiller and Wang, 2013). Engaging state-of-the-art technology and efficient amalgamation of disciplines, researchers have made tremendous progress towards the development of wearable chemical sensors that can conveniently monitor analyte-associated changes in these biofluids, as illustrated in Figure 1.13.

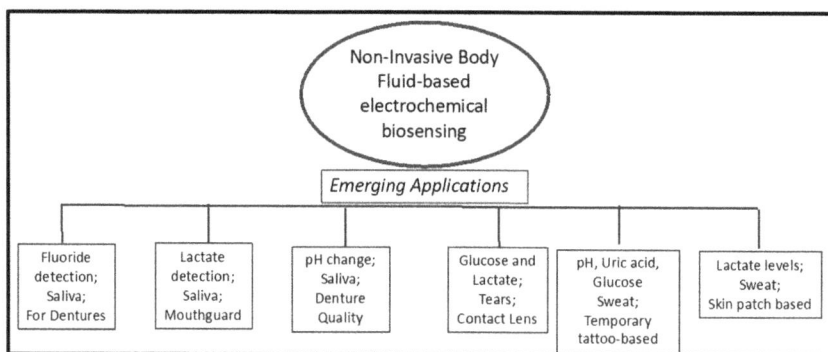

FIGURE 1.13 Current and emerging applications for non-invasive wearable sensors-based on electrochemical biosensing technology.

The constantly growing interest in wearable sensors offers scope for shift in the access for a healthcare facility, for instance, from centralized hospital-based patient care to mobile-based point of care for the user. With extensive efforts from various research groups around the globe, tremendous advances have been made in the field since the inception of this technology. However, the need of higher-order biosensors to cater for emerging health needs remains an area of active investigation.

1.6 CONCLUSION AND FUTURE DIRECTIONS

The advances made in the field has allowed biosensors to gain access in an array of applications ranging from point-of-care health-based applications, environmental monitoring, food safety, and quality control, biomarker discovery, forensic applications, and bioremediation (Bahadir and Sezginturk, 2015). Developments introduced using microfabrication-based technologies in combination with nanotechnology; and amalgamation of knowledge among life science and engineering experts has helped the field of biosensors to progress significantly over time. As of today, immobilized bioreceptor conjugate-based sensing systems are the gold standard in biosensor technology. However, current research is focused on the development of novel affinity reagents such as synthetic receptors to replace immobilized bioreceptor conjugates by peptide and oligonucleotide aptamer. Additionally, synthetic analogs such as PNAs and locked-nucleic acids (LNAs) have been developed as probes to detect and quantify both DNA as well as RNA including, small RNAs such as microRNA (miRNA) sensing in cell and tissue-based systems. It is obvious that our future will encounter advanced level of medical diagnostics that will involve state-of-the-art biosensors. The progress in electrochemical DNA-based biosensors and arrays is one such example that has been revolutionary when compared with technology that existed during the early 2000s. The next generation of biosensors demands the extensive integration of CNTs, SPR, QDs and Piezoelectric sensing devices in molecular diagnostics. It can be predicted that with time-evolving DNA biosensors might eliminate the utilization of PCR-based diagnostics. Therefore, the development of commercially viable biosensors demands the integration of suitable strategies to enhance its stability and efficiency.

It is important to acknowledge the contributions of academic research towards the evolution of biosensors. However, it should be noted that only a countable number of biosensors has achieved commercial success globally. This batch of success also includes the widely used pregnancy test kits and electrochemical blood-glucose detection devices. With critical thinking, we must embark upon the obstacles responsible for the low rate of commercial success for biosensor technology such as, difficulties in translating academic research into commercially viable prototypes in industrial setting; complex regulatory protocols in clinical applications; difficulty in gathering subject knowledge experts in the field of biosensor technology who understand both engineering and life sciences. The federal regulatory bodies should promote biosensors and make them accessible to the public, unlike any electronic gadget, for instance, a smartphone. Given the success of commercial glucose sensors, biosensor research can be very gainful for industrial growth and sustainability. In parallel, it demands a considerable amount of time to develop a commercially viable device-based on a proof-of-concept model designed using academic research. Not to ignore, this simple-sounding idea of biosensor development does involve a multitude of risks that oppose the participation of start-ups and industrial investors. These risks include inevitable mandatory issues such as: identification of an appropriate and stable market for a specific analyte; superior-level advantages over existing methods for analyzes of any given analyte; durability and performance of the biosensor over a period; stability, costs, and ease of manufacturing each component of the biosensor; clear knowledge on the ethics and potential hazards associated with the developed biosensor. Although, the integration of state-of-art technology and knowledge experts over the past few years has helped dissolve many intellectual and technical barriers (Turner, 2013; da Silva Neves et al., 2018; Neethirajan et al., 2018). Currently, well-established companies are opting for high-level investments for ideas and prototypes that overcome the above-discussed challenges to a greater extent and harness great potential in the health care sector. This is bringing the industry closer to academia to provide commercially viable products. Engineering and physical scientists nowadays possess a better understanding of basic biomolecular processes, while biochemists and molecular biologists have greater awareness for the capabilities of different technologies. The collaboration of experts across varied disciplines from the onset of biosensing development projects to build-up of a prototype are indicative of attractive pipelines that can certainly bring advanced and novel products to the market.

Increased longevity is the prime factor driving the advances made so far in the health care industry. The world's population of mid-aged individuals has at-least doubled since the 1980s and is expected to reach 2 billion by 2050. Globally, the net result of massive healthcare spending for various infectious and non-infectious diseases is projected in multi-billion dollars. This rapidly growing health care market urges the need for efficient technology to offer more economical solutions with a point-of-care approach enabled by biosensors that can be accessible over-the-counter to the public. The current worth for diagnostics already estimates at approximately US$40 billion per year. These numbers can be correlated with the massive transformation dictated since the launch of portable glucose biosensors that were impactful for disease management, till date. Similarly, sensors developed towards the diagnosis of non-communicable kidney diseases in aging-population have also shown promise in the recent times. Affinity biosensors have also been found their utility towards detection of diseases associated with cardiovascular disorders and cancer-based on molecular markers. Lastly, developments have also been made to capture the dynamics at the nucleotide levels where nucleic acid-based biosensors such as mutation detectors (with efficiency to detect mutations at single nucleotide level) and gene chips, have played a critical role in the emergence of personalized medicine. These ideas govern us towards a strong commercial future for biosensor technology. As technology has advanced, patient-focused approach predominates demanding new ideas and designs towards point-of-care technologies. For instance, wearable, and distributed sensors have been the latest attraction that is supported by a constant demand from patients and medical professionals. Furthermore, the idea of implantable sensors has witnessed reality and is currently used by diabetic patients. Wearable biosensors present several technical challenges including, lack of an appropriate analyte to capture its changes and correlation with *in-vivo* concentrations and variability within the samples. Similarly, the interference of body sweat leads to a poor correlation in the measurements recorded. Hence it can be stated that the idea of wearable technology is no doubt a reality, but with the given challenges, it requires constant attention towards a better and efficient commercial product. Therefore, the current healthcare market attracts comprehensive non-invasive technologies allowing scope for better investments. Another profound challenge is the emerging demand for intelligent technology to cater the growing elderly population. While the current biosensor platform has been efficient in short-term health care needs, the next generation of biosensors should arguably focus on the management of chronic disease conditions and provide early warning for acute health ailments.

The enormous success we have made so far is indicative of the future possibilities of biosensor technology. The access of patient data driven by artificial intelligence, can be projected to be the future of biosensor technology. The expanding market thus generated will stimulate and foster the development of novel, inexpensive sensors that can overcome the existing economic barriers to meet the ever-growing needs of consumers.

In this galaxy of opportunities predicting the future of biosensor will require harnessing of evolving technology, vision from the biomedical, engineering-design, and user communities to produce functional systems in required numbers and affordability to meet the needs of users.

KEYWORDS

- **biosensors**
- **complementarity-determining regions**
- **human chorionic gonadotrophin**
- **non-invasive wearable technology**
- **point-of-care**
- **transducer**

REFERENCES

Bahadır, E. B., & Sezgintürk, M. K., (2015). Applications of commercial biosensors in clinical, food, environmental, and biothreat/biowarfare analyses. *Analytical Biochemistry, 478*, 107–120.

Bandodkar, A. J., & Wang, J., (2014). Non-invasive wearable electrochemical sensors: A review. *Trends Biotechnol., 32*, 363–371.

Bhalla, N., Jolly, P., Formisano, N., & Estrela, P., (2016). Introduction to biosensors. *Essays Biochem., 60*, 1–8.

Bunney, J., Williamson, S., Atkin, D., Jeanneret, M., Cozzolino, D., Chapman, J., Power, A., & Chandra, S., (2017). The use of electrochemical biosensors in food analysis. *Curr. Res. Nutr. Food Sci., 5*, 183–195.

Cremer, M., (1906). About the cause of the electromotive properties of the tissue, at the same time a contribution to the theory of polyphasic electrolytes. *Z. Biol., 47*, 562–608.

Da Silva, N. M. M. P., González-García, M. B., Hernandez-Santos, D., & Fanjul-Bolado, P., (2018). Future trends in the market for electrochemical biosensing. *Current Opinion in Electrochemistry, 10*, 107–111.

Davis, F., & Altintas, Z., (2017). General introduction to biosensors and recognition receptors. In: *Biosensors and Nanotechnology* (pp. 1–15).

Griffin, E. G., & Nelson, J. M., (1916). The influence of certain substances on the activity of invertase. *J. Am. Chem. Soc., 38*, 722–730.

Guilbault, G. G., & Montalvo, J. G., (1969). *J. Am. Chem. Soc., 91*, 2164–2165.

Gupta, B. D., Shrivastav, A. M., & Usha, A. P., (2017). *Optical Sensors for Biomedical Diagnostics and Environmental Monitoring.* CRC Press. ISBN-13: 978-1-4987-8906-6.

Heineman, W. R., Jensen, W. B., Leland, C., & Clark, Jr., (1918–2005). *Biosens. Bioelectron, 2006, 8,* 1403–1404.

Holzinger, M., Goff, A., & Cosnier, S., (2014). Nanomaterials for biosensing applications: A review. *Frontiers in Chemistry, 2,* 63.

Hughes, W. S., (1922). The potential difference between glass and electrolytes in contact with the glass. *J. Am. Chem. Soc., 44,* 2860–2867.

Kim, J., Campbell, A. S., & Wang, J., (2018). Wearable non-invasive epidermal glucose sensors: A review. *Talanta, 177,* 163–170.

Kozitsina, A. N., Svalova, T. S., Malysheva, N. N., Okhokhonin, A. V., Vidrevich, M. B., & Brainina, K. Z., (2018). Sensors based on bio and biomimetic receptors in medical diagnostic, environment, and food analysis. *Biosensors, 8,* 35.

Kubicek-Sutherland, J., Vu, D., Mendez, H., Jakhar, S., & Mukundan, H., (2017). Detection of lipid and amphiphilic biomarkers for disease diagnostics. *Biosensors, 7,* 25.

Lara, S., & Perez-Potti, A., (2018). Applications of nanomaterials for immunosensing. *Biosensors, 8,* 104.

Lee, T. M., (2008). Over-the-counter biosensors: Past, present, and future. *Sensors (Basel), 8,* 5535–5559.

Mehrotra, P., (2016). Biosensors and their applications: A review. *J. Oral Biol. Craniofac. Res., 6,* 153–159.

Neethirajan, S., Ragavan, V., Weng, X., & Chand, R., (2018). Biosensors for sustainable food engineering: Challenges and perspectives. *Biosensors, 8,* 23.

Nelson, J. M., & Griffin, E. G., (1916). Adsorption of invertase. *J. Am. Chem. Soc., 38,* 1109–1115.

Pazos, E., Vázquez, O., Mascareñas, J. L., & Vázquez, M. E., (2009). Peptide-based fluorescent biosensors. *Chem. Soc. Rev., 38,* 3348–3359.

Pilehvar, S., Wilhelm, A., Wilhelm, A., King, K., & Emaminejad, S., (2018). Emerging wearable technologies for personalized health and performance monitoring. *Micro- and Nanotechnology Sensors, Systems, and Applications X, 10639,* 106391B.

Rechnitz, G. A., & Llenado, R., (1971). Improved enzyme electrode for amygdalin. *Anal. Chem., 43,* 1457–1461.

Sempionatto, J. R., Mishra, R. K., Martín, A., Tang, G., Nakagawa, T., Lu, X., Campbell, A. S., Lyu, K. M., & Wang, J., (2017). Wearable ring-based sensing platform for detecting chemical threats. *ACS Sensors, 2,* 1531–1538.

Tierney, M. J., Tamada, J. A., Potts, R. O., Jovanovic, L., & Garg, S., (2001). Cygnus research team. Clinical evaluation of the GlucoWatch(R) biographer: A continual, non-invasive glucose monitor for patients with diabetes. *Biosens. Bioelectron., 16,* 621–629.

Turner, A. F., (2013). Biosensors: Sense and sensibility. *Chem. Soc. Rev., 42,* 3184–3196.

Windmiller, J. R., & Wang, J., (2013). Wearable electrochemical sensors and biosensors: A review. *Electroanalysis, 25,* 29–46.

Yoon, J. Y., (2016). *Introduction to Biosensors: From Electric Circuits to Immune Sensors.* Springer.

CHAPTER 2

Functionalized Nanomaterials for Biosensing Application

LAKKOJI SATISH[1] and AYONBALA BARAL[2]

[1]*Department of Chemistry, Ravenshaw University, Cuttack, Odisha–753003, India, E-mail: lakkojisatish@gmail.com*

[2]*Department of Metallurgical and Energy Engineering, Kunming University of Science and Technology, Kunming–650093, China*

ABSTRACT

A biosensor is a device developed from biological materials and transducers for the detection of analytes such as metabolites, pollutants, microbial load, etc., in which the biochemical signals are converted into physicochemical signals that can be easily measured. Most of the analytes are biological in nature, such as DNAs of bacteria or viruses, and proteins produced from the immune system (antibodies, antigens). Also, the analytes could be simple molecules like pollutants. Currently, nanotechnology plays a vital role in biosensor development. Nanostructured materials have gained significant attention owing to their distinct physicochemical properties due to the quantum size effects. These materials have shown extraordinary results in the improvement of biosensor's performance through new signal transduction technologies. Moreover, nanomaterials are promising candidates for sensing with high sensitivity and low detection limits. These materials support a large amount of bio-receptor units which can be immobilized in a smaller space. Several nanomaterials such as nanoparticles (NPs), nanotubes, nanorods (NRs), and nanowires (NWs) that are being used in bio-sensing, exhibit faster detection and reproducibility. Specifically, carbon nanotube (CNT), gold nanoparticles (AuNPs), magnetic NPs, and quantum dots (QDs), etc., have been investigated for sensing purposes. In this review, we provide a brief overview of biosensors, including general introduction and recent advances in bio-sensing strategies relating to the cross-disciplines of chemistry and biology. Also, we highlight some smart applications of bio-functional nanomaterials in ultrasensitive bioanalysis.

2.1   INTRODUCTION

A biosensor is a sensing device utilized for the detection of a specific substance or analyte. The work of a biosensor is to convert the biological interactions into a measurable form with the usage of a transducer. Biosensors are used for sensing biological materials such as proteins, antibodies, immunological molecules, enzymes, and so on. There are three key components in a biosensor, which are bio-receptor, transducer, and detector. Analytes are identified by another biologically sensitive material called bio-receptor, which serves as a template for the material to be detected. Several materials are available as bioreceptors, for instance, antigens which can be used to detect antibodies. Transducer is helpful for the conversion of interactions between bio-receptor and bioanalyte into a measurable form (generally an electrical form). In this measurement system, the magnitude of the generated electrical signal is proportional to the analyte concentration. This can be read and studied by a detector system, which receives and amplifies the electrical signal. A graphical representation of the biosensing system is provided in Figure 2.1.

The first biosensor was discovered in the 1950s with the development of electrochemical oxygen biosensors. These oxygen biosensors are used for the determination of glucose. Professor L. C. Clark Jnr. is called the father of the biosensing concept because, for the first time, he invented an oxygen-based sensing device that consists of a cathode (platinum, where oxygen reduction takes place) and a reference electrode (silver/ silver chloride). Clark and Lyons integrated this electrode with glucose oxidase (GO_x) which is kept in a dialysis membrane and used for the determination of glucose concentration in solutions (Clark and Lyons, 1962). The biosensor was prepared with a thin layer of GO_x in contact with an oxygen electrode where GO_x catalyzes the oxidation of glucose to gluconic acid. In this system, oxygen consumption was estimated by electrochemical reduction occurring at the platinum electrode, as observed in the Clark oxygen electrode. Clark's invention was commercialized in 1975 with the successful launch of a glucose analyzer-based on

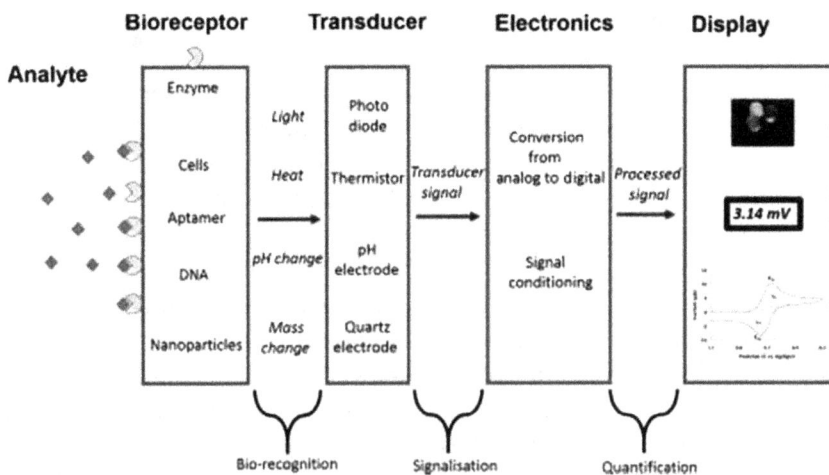

FIGURE 2.1 Schematic representation of a biosensor.
Source: Reproduced with permission from: Bhalla and Singh (2016). © 2016 The Author(s). Published by Portland Press Limited on behalf of the Biochemical Society.

amperometric detection of hydrogen peroxide by the Yellow Springs Instrument Company (Ohio) (Turner et al., 1987). A few most important inventions in bio-sensing were provided here in a yearly manner. Guilbault and Montalvo developed a biosensor for the determination of urea (major urine component) in 1970 (Guilbault and Montalvo, 1970). They studied the hydrolysis of urea into ammonia and carbon dioxide by using the urease enzyme, and the concentration of ammonia is determined with the help of an ammonium ion-selective liquid membrane electrode. Ph. Racinee and W. Mindt successfully developed a lactate electrode in 1973 (Malhotra and Ali, 2017). In the following years, the first microbe-based biosensor was developed by Divies by using Acetobacter xylinum and oxygen electrode (Reshetilov et al., 2010). In 1975, a fiber optic sensor for the estimation of carbon dioxide or oxygen was reported by Lubbers and Opitz (Lubbers and Opitz, 1975). Further extending the work, an optical biosensor was developed for alcohol detection by the immobilization of alcohol oxidase on the end of a fiber-optic oxygen sensor (Meshram et al., 2018). In the early 1970s, the concept of designing immunosensors was developed by the arrangement of antibodies on a piezoelectric/ potentiometric transducer. Liedberg et al. successfully commercialized this technique in 1980 (Rishpon and Buchner, 2005; Agarwal, 2005). They reported the usage of surface plasmon resonance (SPR) phenomenon for real time monitoring of affinity reactions. BI Acore (Pharmacia, Sweden) was launched in 1990 on the basis of this technology (Barredo, 2005). Cass et al. reported amperometric glucose biosensor (ferrocene-mediated) for the first time in 1984 (Cass et al., 1984), which was later commercialized by Medi Sense Inc. with a pen-sized meter that is capable of monitoring blood glucose levels. In the past 50 years, significant focus has been given to the development of biosensors covering a wide range of applications. However, there is only a limited number of biosensors that are commercially available. Hence, bio-sensing technology is still an upcoming field that could be made simpler and widely available for commercialization with further progress. Due to the multifunctional nature, this technology has been widely used in different fields including diagnosis, environmental monitoring of toxicants and physical features like humidity, etc.

It is important to notice that several diseases are difficult to detect, and the diagnosis process is both time consuming and costly. With the advancement of biosensors, the whole process has improved efficiently. The application of biosensors in diagnosis includes detection of cancer, diabetes, and allergic reactions, etc. Several clinical applications of biosensors have been reported such as the detection of HIV-AIDS (Fagerstam et al., 1990; Alterman et al., 2001), glucose in diabetic patients (Pickup et al., 2005; Bolincier et al., 1992), detection of urinary tract bacterial infections (Wang, 2002; Drummond et al., 2003), and the diagnosis of cancer (Gao et al., 2004; Harisinghani et al., 2003; Grimm et al., 2004). The usage of nanomaterials in biosensors has been heightened because of the unique physicochemical properties of nanomaterials, which could significantly impact the diagnosis process. In addition, nanomaterials have been used for enzyme immobilization which subsequently helps in recycling of costly enzymes. Also, the sensitivity and accuracy of bio-sensing results have been improved with the introduction of nanomaterials. Magnetic nanoparticles (NPs) have shown promising results in blood-related disorders. They were used in the isolation of heavy metals having similar properties to iron from the blood serum (Haun et al., 2010). Nanobiosensors prepared with the incorporation of nanomaterials in sensing mechanisms, through different techniques, have produced remarkable outcomes (Chamorro-Garcia and Merkoci, 2016).

One of the important bio-sensing applications is related to the environment. The nanomaterial-based bio-sensing is found to be more versatile in terms of both detection and monitoring. The monitoring of pollutants, heavy metals, toxic intermediates, and weather conditions are highly important in order to understand the consequences of severe environmental changes. Moreover, specific and sophisticated compounds need to be used for the isolation of carcinogens which lead to the disruption of hormonal systems in the living organisms (Kim et al., 2002). For instance, Purohit et al. employed biosensors to examine the abiotic conditions required to optimize biological recovery applications (Purohit, 2003). This method can be recommended for the optimization of environmental quality and decontamination of the hazardous compounds. Several biosensors were developed for recognizing inorganic phosphates (Wollenberger et al., 1992; Kulys et al., 1992), nitrates (Larsen et al., 1997), and parameters like biological oxygen demand (BOD) (Rodriguez-Mozaz et al., 2004, 2005). A single sensing device can be developed by using nanomaterials having different applications, integrated into a single operation. Nanobiosensors have been developed and used for the evaluation of several environmental parameters. These applications are observed to be highly economical and energy saving.

Biosensors can also be utilized to optimize various detection processes. One of the applications is to regulate the feeding of nutrient media and substrate mixtures into bioreactors for miscellaneous applications (Clarke, 1985). In addition, biosensors are reported to have triggered enhanced commercial preparations and improved separations on an industrial scale. For example, separation technique is indispensable in metallurgical operations for the removal of impurities present in complexed form combined with ores. Nanobiosensors can selectively isolate these impurities by attempting several configurations of the enzymes.

2.2 BIOSENSING TYPES

Various methods are available which can be used to enhance the quality of the biosensors. These sensing methods monitor the interaction of bio-receptors with target compounds employing appropriate nanomaterials. The key parts of a bio-sensing device are the biological element and a transducer. When the biological element interacts with the analyte, a detectable physicochemical change is produced. The other important component, i.e., transducer, converts the change produced in the biologically active material (which results from the interaction) into a measurable signal.

Biosensors can be classified into different categories on the basis of sensing elements and transduction modes. Different sensing elements are used in biosensors including enzymes, antibodies, DNA, aptamers, biological tissues and organelles and microorganisms (whole-cell biosensors). Moreover, biosensors are categorized based on different transducers like electrochemical (amperometric, conductometric, and potentiometric), optical (absorbance, fluorescence, and chemiluminescence), piezoelectric (acoustic and ultrasonic) and calorimetric. Here, a brief review on different kinds of biosensors has been provided.

2.2.1 CLASSIFICATION OF BIOLOGICAL RECOGNIZERS

Based on different types of immobilized biomolecules, biosensors are divided into the following classes.

2.2.1.1 ENZYMATIC BIOSENSOR

In an enzymatic biosensor, immobilized specific enzymes convert analytes into products that can be read with an appropriate transducer. These sensors evaluate the selective inhibition of enzyme activity by a specific target (Trojanowicz, 2002; Wang et al., 2014). The mode of action of these biosensors mostly relies on the heterogeneous electron transfer between the electrode and the redox center of biomolecules (proteins) (Lad et al., 2008; Nagiev, 2006; Lakard et al., 2011). Some of the examples of this kind of biosensor are as follows. Enzyme, urease can be used to detect urea, where urea is catalyzed by the enzyme to produce ammonia and carbon dioxide, followed by the detection of ammonia potentiometrically by ammonia-ion-selective electrode. Other modes of operation for this electrode are carbon dioxide electrode or a pH electrode. Glucose is the most extensively studied biosensor. GO_x enzyme catalyzes glucose into gluconic acid and hydrogen peroxide by the oxidation reaction. The reduction in the concentration of oxygen could be monitored amperometrically by using an oxygen electrode. The main advantages of enzyme-based biosensors are; high selectivity, specificity, and sensitivity due to catalytic action. The common disadvantages are; high cost and loss of activity during immobilization on transducers.

2.2.1.2   ANTIBODY-BASED BIOSENSOR

These biosensors are also called immunosensors, and employ antibodies as the biological recognition part. Antibodies are highly specific in recognizing analytes and are most commonly used as bio receptors. The highly sensitive nature of antibodies allows detection of microorganisms like *E. coli*, *Salmonella*, *S. aureus*, pesticides, herbicides, etc. The cost and assay time can be reduced by using suitable immunosensors (Shirale et al., 2010; Mistry et al., 2014). Moreover, antibody-based targeting can be used efficiently for different applications like cell-surface labeling and single bacterial cell quantitation. Anti-cancer nanomedicines have been used for treatment by conjugating tumor-specific antibodies (Ezzati and de La Guardia, 2014; Diaconu et al., 2013). For instance, conjugation of antibodies (bio receptor) and viral antigens produces a readable response in conductivity across the immunosensor surface which subsequently helps in analyte detection (Burcu and Kemal, 2015). The main advantages of immunosensors are selectivity, ultra-sensitivity, and strong binding capacity with substrate.

2.2.1.3   OLIGONUCLEOTIDE (DNA/RNA)-BASED BIOSENSOR

In these biosensors, single-stranded oligonucleotide molecules are incorporated into a transducer. The transducer system can be optical, thermometric, electrochemical, piezoelectric, or magnetic (del Valle and Bonanni, 2014; Lazerges and Bedioui, 2013). Unlike monoclonal antibodies (mAbs), the traditional affinity reagent is employed which binds to any target including small molecules, whole cells, and even microorganisms (Han, Liang, and Zhou, 2010). These are considered very important in biosensor development owing to their special characteristics such as small size, high stability, strong binding affinity and specificity, and easy modification. In recent years, they have attracted much attention in research fields focused on gene analysis, genetic disorders, and forensic applications (Odenthal and Gooding, 2007). DNA-based biosensors have been employed to detect specific DNA sequences in human, bacterial, and viral nucleic acids (Zhao et al., 2014; Peng and Miller, 2011). Also, the genes responsible for inherited human diseases or infectious diseases can be detected by DNA biosensors. Several reports are available in literature which shows the detection of genetic mutations using DNA biosensors-based on electrochemical protocols (Lee and

Yook, 2014; Chen et al., 2013; Wang et al., 1997). They provide exciting opportunities for sequence-specific DNA detection. Moreover, these DNA-based biosensors offer many interesting applications in clinical diagnostics and forensic identification (Zhai et al., 1997). Nanomaterials have shown promising results in DNA biosensors due to their high surface-to-volume ratios and biocompatibility nature. Nanomaterials can enhance the number of DNA molecules during immobilization, retaining overall biological activity (Shi et al., 2013). Several nanomaterials, including NPs (e.g., gold, cadmium sulfide, etc.), nanowires (NWs) (e.g., silicon), nanotubes (e.g., carbon nanotubes (CNTs)), etc., have been used in DNA biosensors. These materials can be useful as support for DNA immobilization and also an amplifier for signal enhancement. Song et al. described DNA hybridization using silver NP aggregates as electrochemical aptasensor for signal amplification (2014). In another study, it was observed that gold and graphene (GN)-based DNA biosensor exhibited high sensitivity (Shi et al., 2014). Khimji et al. reported DNA-functionalized polyacrylamide hydrogel-based optical biosensors (Khimji et al., 2013). Various DNA-based biosensors employing NPs are being developed such as gold and magnetic NPs (Yang et al., 2012), Pt nanoparticle (Kwon and Bard, 2012), Pt NPs/CNTs (Dong et al., 2012), and silver NPs (Song et al., 2014).

2.2.1.4   MICROORGANISMS AND CELLS

In a microbial biosensor, microorganisms or the cells (as a whole) integrate with a transducer (Shin, 2011; Zhang et al., 2013; Mulchandani and Rajesh, 2011). These biosensors offer accurate, fast, and sensitive identification of targeted analytes in different research areas such as medicine, environmental monitoring, defense, food processing, and safety (Gäberlein et al., 2000; Ponomareva et al., 2011; Olaniran et al., 2011). These sources are considered economical as compared to many isolated enzymes. They are highly stable at different temperatures and pH conditions and are less prone to inhibition which leads to extended lifetimes. Cells are mostly used in bioreceptors due to their sensitive nature towards the surrounding atmosphere, which reacts to all kinds of stimulants. They are employed to examine the effect of drugs and to monitor several parameters, specifically toxic levels, organic derivatives, and stress conditions. Cells can also be utilized to control herbicides, which are the main aquatic pollutants. In one study, microalgae are entrapped into quartz microfiber and then the modified chlorophyll fluorescence via herbicides is collected from the optical fiber through a fluorimeter. Interestingly, the results show that the detection limit of specific herbicides reached up to sub-ppb concentration level. In some cases, certain cells can be used to monitor Microbial corrosion. Moreover, microorganisms immobilized on nanomaterials which act as transducers play a crucial role in the microbial biosensor fabrication.

2.2.2   CLASSIFICATION-BASED ON SIGNAL TRANSDUCTION

2.2.2.1   ELECTROCHEMICAL METHODS

Among different sensing techniques, electrochemical methods have exceptional advantages including high sensitivity, low cost, interference characteristics, and compatible fabrication technology (Lad et al., 2008; Bertok et al., 2013; Presnova et al., 2009). In this biosensor, electrochemical species such as electrons are consumed or generated after interaction with bio-receptor, and subsequently, a measurable electronic signal is produced, which could be noted by a detector. The generated electrical signal is directly proportional to the analyte concentration (Ronkainen et al., 2010). Based on the electrochemical property, these biosensors can be classified into the following sub-categories like: potentiometric, amperometric, conductometric, and impedimetric biosensors (Trojanowicz, 2014; Hamidi-Asl et al., 2013; Xu and Wang, 2012).

1. **Potentiometric Biosensor:** Potentiometry is one of the oldest instrumental methods and well-established analytical techniques. In these biosensors, ion-selective electrodes are used for transducing the bio-reactions into an electrical signal. Generally, it is comprised of an immobilized enzyme membrane surrounding the probe of a pH meter, where catalyzed reactions generate/ absorb hydrogen ions. The reactions cause a change in pH which can be readily detected, e.g., use of H^+ ions for detecting penicillin utilizing enzyme penicillinase and detecting tri acyl glycerol utilizing enzyme lipase.

2. **Amperometric Biosensor:** The basic principle behind the working of these biosensors is based on the current generated when a potential is applied between two electrodes. They depend on the movement of electrons produced by enzyme-catalyzed redox reactions. Usually,

an enzymatic reaction produces products that transfer electrons to the surface of electrodes and generates a current which could be directly measured (Kaisheva et al., 1992). Here, the concentration of substrate is directly proportional to the magnitude of current. These biosensors are most useful in medical devices having advantages like high sensitivity, low cost, and wide linear range. Moreover, they are fast, precise, and more accurate than the potentiometric ones, e.g., glucose biosensors for diabetes monitoring.

3. **Conductometric Biosensor:** These monitor the changes in the conductance of a system which occurs due to the presence of the analyte. In enzyme-based conductometric devices, the ionic strength of the solution between two electrodes alters as a consequence of an enzymatic reaction. Thus, these devices are more useful in studying enzymatic reactions, where a change in the concentration of charged species in a solution is observed. In another way, the change in the conductance of an electrode can be directly measured by the immobilization of enzymes, antibody-antigen pairs, etc., on the electrode surface. At present, there is a growing interest in the usage of conductometric immunosensors in association with nanomaterials. This sensing technique has not been implemented much, however, there were several examples with practical application. For instance, detection of drugs in human urine and environmental testing of pollutants. Whole cells can also be employed as biorecognition elements by immobilization of cells to a transducer for toxicity analysis.

4. **Impedimetric Biosensor:** These biosensors measure the electrical impedance of the biological system, which provides information about that system (Bahadir and Sezginturk, 2016). They allow recognition of biomolecular activities in a direct manner without using enzyme. In biomedical examinations, these biosensors are widely used in the label-free identification of ciprofloxacin (antibiotic drug) at very low concentrations (Giroud et al., 2009). In another study, impedimetric aptasensor was used to detect cocaine in the urine, saliva, and plasma of humans (Du et al., 2010). These sensors are used less frequently as compared to potentiometric and amperometric biosensors, however, the applications are impressive due to their small, portable, and all-electrical nature (Guan et al., 2004).

2.2.2.2 OPTICAL BIOSENSOR

Optical bio-sensing technique utilizes light for the detection of target molecules. These sensors either determine the light absorption changes between the reactants and products of a reaction, or measure output light by a luminescent process to sense the binding of the target molecule. These are more powerful and versatile as well as highly sensitive to bimolecular targets, e.g., optic lactate sensor utilizing lactate monooxygenase and oxygen. Several optical methods employed in nanobiosensors which include SPR, fluorescence spectroscopy, interferometry, total internal reflectance, light rotation, and polarization (Damborsky et al., 2016). SPR based biosensors are found to be very successful in health science research, fundamental biological studies, drug discovery, and clinical diagnosis (Guo, 2012; Masson, 2017). They could examine a wide range of analyte surface binding interactions, including absorption of small molecules, proteins, antibody-antigen, DNA, and RNA hybridization.

2.2.2.3 PIEZOELECTRIC METHODS

These biosensors depend on the change in the resonant frequency of a piezoelectric quartz oscillator in response to the changes in the surface adsorbed mass (Pohanka, 2017). The crystal surface is coated with a biorecognition element which is planned to link selectively with the targeted analyte. When the analyte binds to the sensing surface of crystals, resulting change in mass of the crystal creates a measurable alteration in the resonance frequency. Further improvement can be achieved by the application of NPs against analyte resulting in mass increment on the sensor. Figure 2.2 shows the principle of such an idea. These biosensors have been widely utilized for the detection of viruses, bacteria, proteins, and nucleic acids due to their extreme sensitivity.

2.2.2.4 CALORIMETRIC BIOSENSOR

These biosensors utilize the temperature changes in the enzyme-catalyzed reactions (Danielsson, 1990). Several enzymatic reactions are associated with the production of heat, which in general is measured by the means of thermistors and helps in analyzing the rate of reaction and hence the analyte concentration. Thermometric biosensors have been used for the serum cholesterol estimation (Ramanathan and Danielsson, 2001). In this process, heat generated by the enzymatic oxidation of cholesterol by the cholesterol oxidase is measured. Likewise, these biosensors can be used to estimate glucose using GO_x, urea using urease, uric acid (UA) using urease and penicillin G using P lactamase.

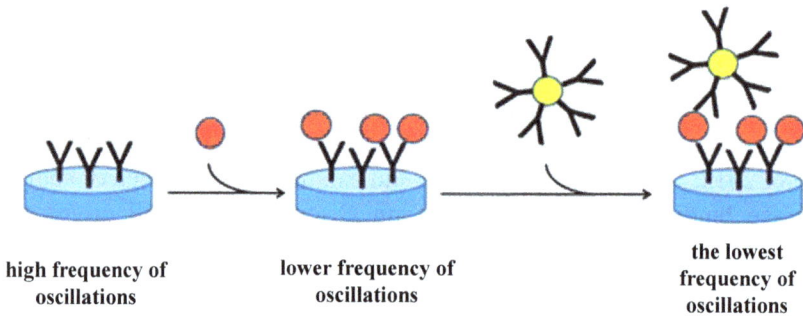

high frequency of   lower frequency of   the lowest
oscillations   oscillations   frequency of
                                                        oscillations

FIGURE 2.2   Piezoelectric immunosensors for the determination of an antigen (red ball) and increase of oscillations by application of a nanoparticle (yellow ball) covered with immunoglobulins (Y shaped). Blue disc represents a piezoelectric crystal.

Source: Reproduced with permission from: Pohanka (2017). (http://creativecommons.org/licenses/by/4.0/).

2.3 NANOBIOSENSORS AND THEIR CLASSIFICATION

Nanomaterials have special chemical and physical properties compared to their bulk counterparts. The exploration of nanomaterial properties that depend on shape and size could further improve the biosensor sensitivity. Several reports are available which explored the electronic properties of metallic nanostructures (Sagadevan and Periasamy, 2014). These include different dimensional nanostructured materials like quantum dots (0D), NWs, and CNTs (1D), and GN sheets (2D), etc. Nanomaterials-based biosensors could provide high sensitivity due to the large surface-to-volume ratios, which allow them to bind with the analytes significantly and modify the bulk electronic properties of the structure. These devices are considered good candidates for in-vivo sensing applications as they could be taken up by cells due to their small size (Chithrani et al., 2006; Wang et al., 2010; Giljohann et al., 2007). Some nanobiosensors, particularly

CNTs have shown extraordinary intrinsic electrical properties and provide improved sensitivity in bio-sensing. Nanobiosensors can be categorized based on the nature of nanomaterials incorporated in biosensing technique, and it is not so easy as in biosensors. A wide range of nanomaterial-based biosensors has been developed, which are defined based on the material used in the method. For example, nanoparticle-based biosensors are named after the use of metallic NPs. Similarly, if NWs are used, they are called nanowire biosensors and if CNTs are used, they termed nanotube biosensors. Some more examples of nanobiosensors and their advantages are given in Table 2.1.

2.3.1 NANOPARTICLE-BASED BIOSENSORS

NPs have specific electronic and electrocatalytic properties that depend on their morphology and size (Jagiello et al., 2016; Adekoya et al., 2018). These biosensors are attractive because their synthesis involves easy and standard chemical techniques rather than advanced fabrication approaches. Therefore, several biological molecules were labeled with metal NPs which retain overall biological activities (Hrapovic et al., 2004). The chemical reactions between biomolecules could be carried out easily by using metallic NPs, which concurrently help immobilization of biomolecules. Considering the noble metals, gold nanoparticles (AuNPs) were utilized mostly in biosensing due to their biocompatibility, improved optical and electronic properties, and relatively simple preparation (Aldewachi et al., 2017; Zeng et al., 2011; Yu et al., 2016). Colloidal AuNPs were employed to improve DNA immobilization on gold electrodes and it was observed that the sensitivity (lower detection limit) increased significantly (Cai et al., 2001). Moreover, biosensors based on enzymes immobilized on AuNPs were used to detect glucose, xanthine, and hydrogen peroxide (Crumbliss et al., 1992; Zhao et al., 1996). In another study, it was reported that horse reddish peroxidase immobilized on gold electrodes loaded with carbon NPs enhanced the sensitivity having a very lower detection limit (Xu et al., 2003). Likewise, enzyme-conjugated nano-sized semiconductor crystals have been used to increase the efficiency of photochemical reactions. Curri et al. reported the oxidation of formaldehyde (HCHO) using nanocrystalline CdS with HCHO dehydrogenase as a catalyst (Curri et al., 2002). Another significant biosensors have been developed with specially designed magnetic NPs which are very useful in biomedical applications and also offer

TABLE 2.1 A List of Nanomaterials Utilized for Improving Biosensing Mechanism

Nanomaterial Type	Benefits	References
Nanoparticles	Aid in immobilization, enable better loading of bioanalyte and possess good catalytic properties	Luo et al. (2006); Katz et al. (2004); Wang (2003)
Nanotubes	Higher enzyme loading, easy to be functionalized, and better electrical communication	Davis et al. (2003); Sotiropoulou et al. (2003); Zhao et al. (2002)
Nanowires	Highly versatile, good electrical and sensing properties, better charge conduction	Cui et al. (2001); Stern et al. (2007); MacKenzie et al. (2009)
Nanorods	Good plasmonic materials which couple sensing phenomenon well and size-tunable energy regulation, can be linked with MEMS, and induce specific field responses	Kabashin et al. (2009); Ramanathan et al. (2006)
Quantum dots	Excellent fluorescence, quantum confinement of charge carriers, and size-tunable band energy	Wang et al. (2002); Zhu et al. (2003); Huang et al. (2005)
Graphene	Good electrical and sensing properties bio- and chemical sensing, High enzyme loading	Pumera (2011); | Pena-Bahamonde et al. (2018)

Source: Reproduced with permission from: Malik et al. (2013). https://creativecommons.org/licenses/by/3.0/

promising results in different analytical applications (Rocha-Santos, 2014). The schematic representation for the detection of analyte concentration in complex solutions through bio-receptor modified magnetic NPs is shown in Figure 2.3. The isolation of magnetically labeled targets has been carried out using magnetic bioassay technique with the help of a magnetometer (Richardson et al., 2001). Superconducting quantum interference devices (SQUID) were reported to screen specific antigens from the mixtures utilizing antibodies conjugated to magnetic NPs. These devices are being employed in order to detect biological targets rapidly (Chemla et al., 2000).

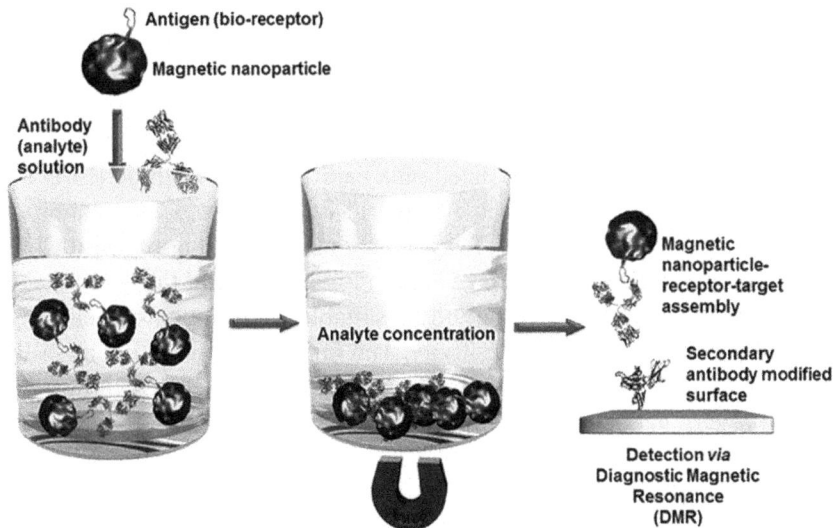

FIGURE 2.3 Scheme of analyte concentration in complex solutions via bioreceptor modified magnetic nanoparticles.

Source: Reprinted from reference: Holzinger, Le Goff, and Cosnier (2014). https://creativecommons.org/licenses/by/3.0/

2.3.1.1 CARBON NANOTUBE (CNT)-BASED BIOSENSOR

CNTs were first evidenced by Sumio Iijima in 1991. Later on, CNTs became the most extensively studied nanostructured materials. CNTs are hollow carbon structures, with one or more walls having a diameter in nanometer-scale range. They are considered more advantageous compared to other nanomaterials due to the extraordinary electrical, magnetic, optical, mechanical, and chemical properties, which make them excel in a broad range of applications including bio-sensing (De Volder et al., 2013; Tilmaciu and Morris, 2015). Moreover, CNTs could be used as platforms for conjugation of compounds at the surface and CNT shells could be opened and filled, retaining overall stability. Also, functionalized CNTs can penetrate into individual cells crossing biological barriers like cell membranes (Tilmaciu and Morris, 2015). These features are of great interest in bio-applications, especially, in intracellular bio-sensing. Various electrochemical CNT-based sensors were used to detect different metabolites, ions, and biomarkers (Wang and Dai, 2015). For example, several CNT-based glucose biosensors were engineered by conjugating GO_x (Lin et al., 2004; Patolsky et al., 2004). In one of the studies, it was observed that single-walled nanotubes exhibit enhanced performance for enzymatic detection of glucose due to high loading of enzyme and electrical conductivity (Azamian et al., 2002). Cholesterol biosensors with high sensitivity have been developed with cholesterol esterase, cholesterol oxidase, and MWNTs immobilized on a carbon paste electrode (Li et al., 2005). Wang et al. described Pt/Au hybrid-functionalized ZnO nanorods (NRs) combined with MWCNT layer, as a matrix for immobilized ChO_x (2012) (general illustration is provided in Figure 2.4). All the components interact with each other and provide a suitable environment for enzyme, and enhance the biosensor sensitivity. The mixing of ZnO NRs, nano-Pt/ Au and MWCNTs, induced signal enhancement that clearly shows the crucial role of nanocomposites in sensing mechanism.

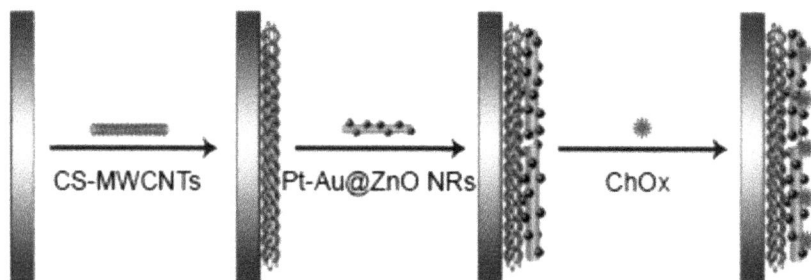

FIGURE 2.4   Preparation of the ChOx/Pt-Au@ZnO nanorod/chitosan MWCNT biosensor. *Source*: Reproduced with permission from: Wang et al. (2012). © Elsevier.

Likewise, the performance of oxidoreductase was found to be higher in both GO_x and flavin adenine dinucleotide precursors (Cai and Chen,

2004). Several review articles highlight the functionalization of CNTs with different biomolecules such as DNA, proteins, oligonucleotide probes, etc., and their significant usage in bio-sensing (Tilmaciu and Morris, 2015; Sireesha et al., 2018; Yang et al., 2015).

2.3.1.2 NANOWIRE BASED SENSORS

Among all other structures, one-dimensional NWs are most promising due to their one-dimensional configuration which improves the electron transportation properties as compared to the bulk materials. Though literature on nanowire-based sensors are very less, few reports have demonstrated the significant results in the detection of biomolecules. Cui and Lieber have described the detection of biological species using silicon NWs doped with boron (Cui and Lieber, 2001). Semiconductor NWs have been used for identifying biological species. In one of the studies, silicon NWs coated with biotin were explored to detect streptavidin molecules from a mixture. Due to their small size and precisely defined dimensions, they are considered ideal candidates for in-vivo diagnostic applications. Wang et al. employed optical fibers coated with antibodies for the detection of toxicants within single cells (Wang, 2002). Xiaotao Cao et al. described Schottky-contacted ZnO NW device for sensitive and selective DNA detection (Cao et al., 2016). Figure 2.5 shows the schematic illustration of the ZnO NW DNA sensor, including the digital and optical images. In another study, Cullum et al. observed highly sensitive and low detection limits in the case of ZnO NWs coated onto the gold electrodes during the detection of hydrazine (2000).

2.3.1.3 QUANTUM DOT (QD) BASED BIOSENSORS

Quantum dots (QDs) are inorganic nanocrystals (also called zero-dimensional materials, approximately 1–10 nm in size) with distinctive photophysical properties such as broad absorption spectra that help in simultaneous excitation of multiple fluorescent colors and narrow size-tunable emission spectra. They are remarkably bright and have high photochemical stability and negligible photobleaching (Kairdolf et al., 2013; Wegner and Hildebrandt, 2015). They have been extensively used in optical biosensors as alternatives to the fluorophores to detect organic compounds, ions, pharmaceutical analytes, and biomolecules (including proteins, nucleic acids, enzymes, carbohydrates, and neurotransmitters) (Ma et al., 2018). Also, they are ideal candidates for the detection of targeted sites in cancer and for multiplexed optical bioanalysis due to their high sensitivity, specificity, cost-effectiveness, and rapid analyte detection. These biosensors are further subdivided, based on the type of molecular beacon conjugated to QDs and transduction signals, into the following categories; QD-based FRET genosensor, and QD-based FRET immunosensor, etc. Zhang and Johnson reported a QD-based nanosensor based on FRET between QD605 and Cy5 for Rev-RRE interaction assay (Zhang and Johnson, 2006) (Figure 2.6). Rev is a key HIV-1 regulatory protein that binds to Rev responsive element (RRE) within env gene of HIV-1 RNA genome, and the binding of Rev to RRE is essential for HIV replication.

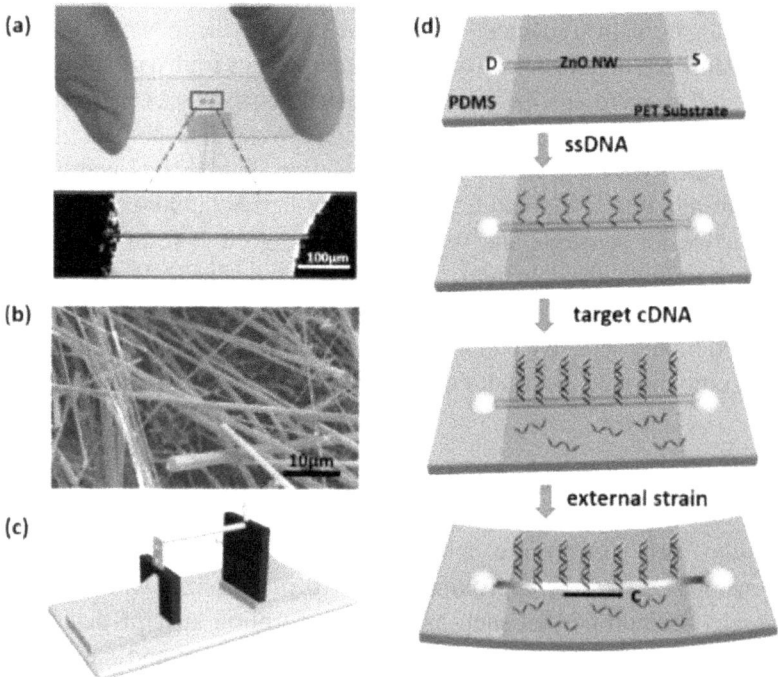

FIGURE 2.5 (a) Digital image and optical microscopy image of the ZnO NW DNA sensor. (b) SEM image of the as-synthesized ZnO NWs. (c) Schematic illustration of the experimental setup. (d) Functionalization and detection process of the ZnO NW DNA sensor under no strain and external strain.

Source: Reproduced with permission from: Cao et al. (2016). © American Chemical Society.

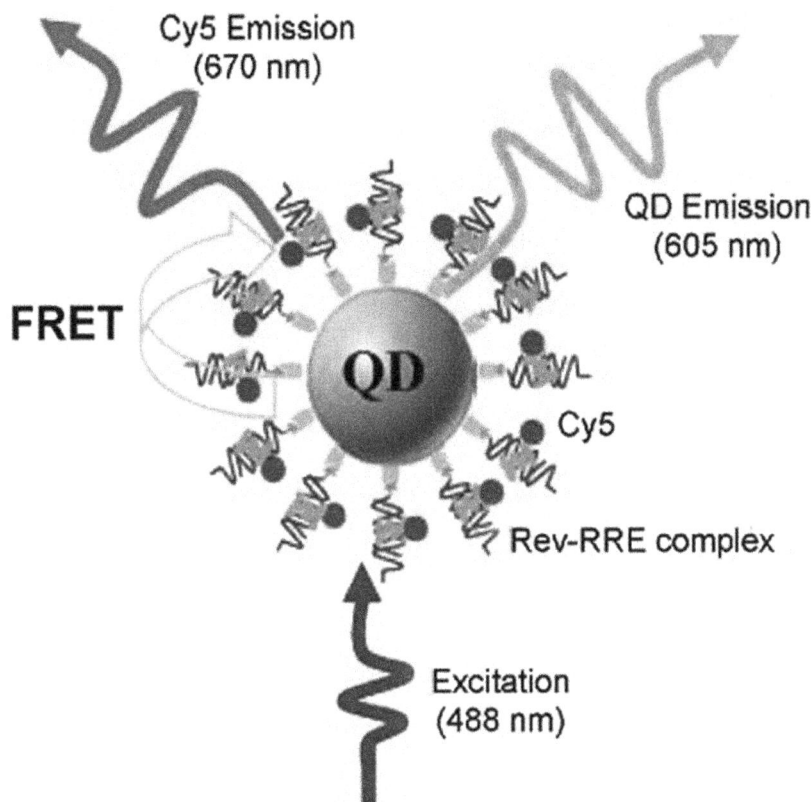

FIGURE 2.6 QD-based FRET genosensor for Rev-RRE interaction assay based on FRET. *Source*: Adapted from reference: Zhang and Johnson (2006). © American Chemical Society.

2.3.1.4 *GRAPHENE (GN) BASED BIOSENSORS*

GN based nanomaterials have shown promising results in sensing applications due to the enhanced signal response (Morales-Narvaez et al., 2017; Chauhan et al., 2017). Also, they are observed to be biocompatible with several biomolecules including enzymes, antibodies, DNA, and cells, etc. (Janegitz et al., 2017). GN has been used in designing biosensors with different transduction modes due to its large surface area, high conductivity, and high immobilization capacity of different biomolecules (Rao et al., 2009). For example, GN's conjugated structure allows electron transfer between the bio-receptor and transducer, subsequently generating high signal sensitivity which is applicable in electrochemical sensors (Kuila et al., 2011). Moreover, these nanomaterials are useful for quenching process in the transducer, which helps to create fluorescent biosensors. It is well known that GN derivatives (GN oxide and reduced GN oxide) possess high fluorescence quenching efficiency (Kasry et al., 2012). It is noteworthy that the antibody biosensors based on GN NPs offer a broad versatility in the detection of pathogens. A general schematic representation of GN modified with antibody for the recognition of pathogens has been provided in Figure 2.7. Since the last decade, different GN-antibody sensors have been developed that possess excellent clinical applications. For example, antibody nano-sensors with GN were employed for the detection of *E. coli* (Huang et al., 2011) and Zika virus (Afsahi et al., 2018). GN oxide has also been utilized for the detection of dengue virus (Navakul et al., 2017) and rotavirus (Jung et al., 2010).

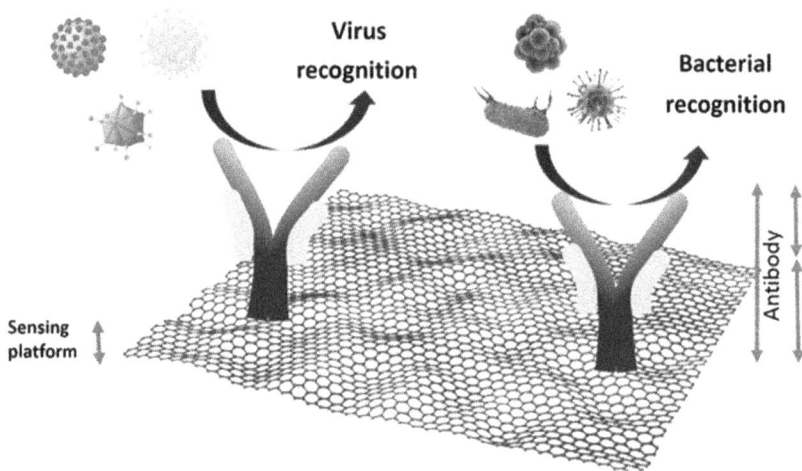

FIGURE 2.7 Scheme of graphene modification with antibodies for the recognition of pathogens.

Source: Reprinted from reference: Peña-Bahamonde, Nguyen, Fanourakis, and Rodrigues (2018). (http://creativecommons.org/licenses/by/4.0/)

2.4 BIOFUNCTIONALIZATION OF NANOMATERIALS

Bio-functionalization is a vital part of modeling the bio-recognition component of a biosensor. It is very important to find out appropriate methods for the functionalization of Nanomaterials which can enhance the sensitivity of the detection signal. The immobilization methods are divided into the following categories on the basis of chemical and physical properties of biomolecule and nanostructure.

2.4.1 NON-COVALENT ASSEMBLY OF NANOMATERIALS WITH BIOMOLECULES

In this method, biomolecules are solubilized in the solvent medium containing the solid support, for a fixed time. After the adsorption of the biomolecules, the unadsorbed part is separated by washing with an appropriate buffer. The process of adsorption involves only weak forces such as van der Waals, electrostatic or hydrophobic interactions, and there is no involvement of any modification in the support. Due to the non-destructive nature, this method has been used frequently for the biofunctionalization of nanomaterials. However, the main disadvantages are; (a) non-specific adsorption of various substances and (b) desorption due to weak binding. A small change in the temperature, pH, and ionic strength might lead to the release of the adsorbed substances from the surface. Here are few examples of bio-sensing devices where adsorption was used for functionalization. Bonnet et al. described an amperometric biosensor based on immobilization of AChE by mere adsorption method (Bonnet et al., 2003). Ekanayake et al. developed an amperometric glucose biosensor, utilizing nano-scale PPy tubes (Ekanayake et al., 2007). Wang et al. produced a disposable H_2O_2 biosensor using HRP adsorbed on AuNPs, which is observed to be highly reproducible, selective, and stable for long time (Wang et al., 2009a). Electrostatic interaction is an alternative method which makes immobilization possible by simply varying the pH of the solution medium. In general, the surface charge of biomolecules depends on the isoelectric point. If the isoelectric point of the biomolecule is less than the pH value of the solution, it carries a surface negative charge, which can bind to a positively charged support. For instance, AuNPs (made by citrate reduction method) were multi-functionalized with antibody and enzyme molecules at pH values higher than the isoelectric point of the citrate ligand. Similarly, carboxylate group decorated QDs can be functionalized with positively charged molecules like cationic polymers as they possess negative charge in neutral or basic buffers (Lei and Ju, 2012). Furthermore, these polymers could be functionalized by a layer-by-layer assembly. In one study, Xu et al. described an amperometric glucose biosensor, where GO_x and dendrimer-encapsulated Pt nanoparticles (Pt-DENs) was adsorbed layer-by-layer on multiwalled CNTs (Xu et al., 2007). The layer-by-layer strategy provides an appropriate environment which retains bioactivity and prevents enzyme leakage. At first, CNTs were functionalized with negatively charged carboxylic groups, and poly(diallyldimethylammonium chloride) (PDDA) and poly(sodium 4-styrenesulfonate) (PSS) monolayers were then adsorbed onto the CNTs surface. After that, alternatively positive charged Pt-DENs and negatively charged GOD molecules were adsorbed onto the PSS/PDDA/CNTs layer. Another important method for protein immobilization is the electrochemical doping. Proteins (positively/negatively charged) could be doped into a conductive polymer film by adjusting the pH. In general, polymers become positively charged during the oxidation. By changing the pH of the solution, negatively charged protein units can be integrated into the conductive polymers in the oxidation procedure. This method was utilized in the development of the biosensors for the detection of cholesterol (Wang and Mu, 1999), choline (Langer et al., 2004), glucose (Shaolin and Huaiguo, 1996), H_2O_2 (Mathebe et al., 2004), etc. Another study by Morrin et al. described an amperometric biosensor for observing H_2O_2 by employing polyaniline NPs synthesized with dodecylbenzylsulfonic acid (2005). Initially, NPs were electrodeposited onto the surface of a glassy carbon (GC) electrode and then HRP was adsorbed electrostatically to the modified nanoparticle surface by electrochemical doping. It was observed that NP based biosensor shows higher signal-to-signal background ratios and shorter response times than earlier polyaniline-based works. A different noncovalent strategy for biomolecule immobilization is entrapment in three-dimensional matrices. Nanomaterials in association with electropolymers can act as intermediates between the enzyme re-dox center and electrode, enabling transfer of electrons. Especially, an electroactive polymer enhances the detection sensitivity as it generates more electrons in electrochemical oxidation that subsequently amplifies the signal. Zhu et al. developed an amperometric glucose biosensor by immobilizing GOD and horseradish peroxidase (HRP) in a PPy film electropolymerized on SWCN coated electrode (2007). In another study, an amperometric biosensor was described for phenol derivatives by electropolymerization procedure in a system comprising CNTs, pyrrole, and HRP (Korkut et al., 2008). Wang and Musameh described an amperometric biosensor based on the co-immobilization of CNTs and GOD within an electropolymerized PPy film (2005).

2.4.2 COVALENT ROUTE FOR BIOFUNCTIONALIZATION OF NANOMATERIALS

Covalent coupling of biomolecules to nanomaterials is a well-known chemical immobilization method. This coupling method has many advantages over noncovalent immobilization (like controllable covalent binding (chemisorption)), which is preferable than unspecific physisorption with reference to stability and reproducibility factors, for surface functionalization. Moreover, the number of functional groups can be managed by fine-tuning the functionalization. Several protocols have been described based on various kinds of chemical reactions for the activation of surfaces. In direct reaction strategy, biomolecule can be directly linked to the functional groups of nanomaterial surfaces with the help of a catalyst. Carbodiimides can be used to link carboxyl groups of nanomaterials with the amino groups of biomolecules (Figure 2.8(A)). Also, N-hydroxysuccinimide (NHS) along with carbodiimide can be employed to improve immobilization efficiency (Figure 2.8(B)). For instance, CNTs are first functionalized with hydrophilic carboxylic acid groups. N-hydroxysuccinimide linkers can be used to covalently bind nanomaterials with biomolecules bearing primary amines. For instance, Rahman et al. utilized this procedure to develop enzyme-based biosensors for glutamate, and lactate detection (Rahman et al., 2009). This strategy has been used in attaching aptamer, DNA, and antibody to the NPs. Moreover, immobilization of proteins could be done covalently on functionalized nanotubes present on an electrode surface. Yu et al. reported an amperometric biosensor for H_2O_2 detection by employing HRP immobilized onto SWCNTs by using EDC (2003). Likewise, amino decorated NPs could be conjugated with biomolecules (peptides, proteins, antibodies, and enzymes) bearing carboxylated groups. For example, Cholesterol oxidase was immobilized onto a two-dimensional monolayer of N-(2-amino-ethyl)-3-aminopropyltrimethoxysilane deposited on ITO-coated glass plates using EDC and NHS (Arya et al., 2007). In another study by Bisht et al. Urease was immobilized on a poly(N-3-aminopropyl pyrrole-copyrrole) film bearing free amino groups through carbodiimide coupling reaction (2005).

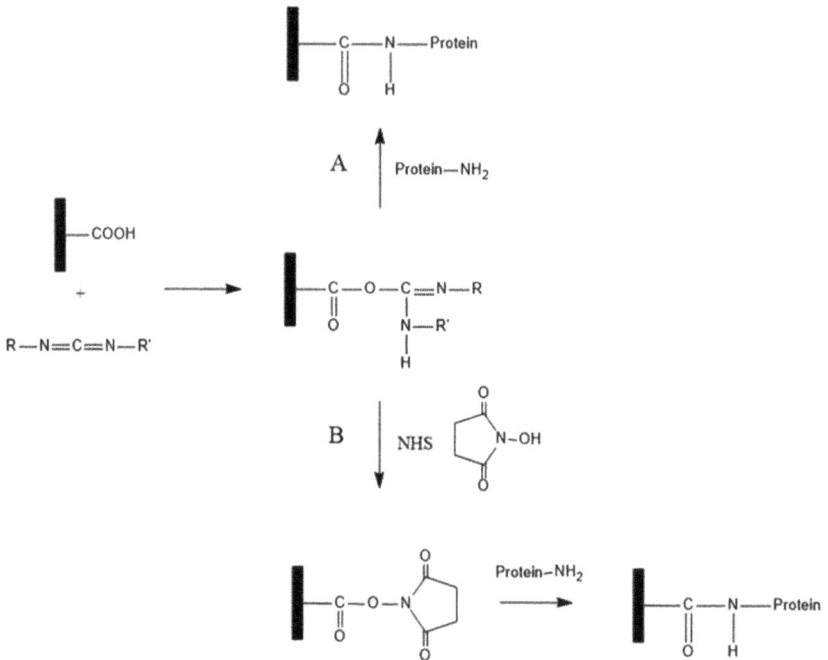

FIGURE 2.8 Protein immobilization on carboxylated surface by carbodiimide coupling (A) without; or (B) with NHS.

Protein immobilization can also be possible with glutaraldehyde, where a Schiff-base reaction occurs initially between an aldehyde group of glutaraldehyde and an amine group of the support. Then, the second aldehyde group reacts with an amine group of the protein (Figure 2.9). In one of the studies, an amperometric biosensor was developed for L-phenylalanine detection using Phenylalanine dehydrogenase which was covalently immobilized on amino-activated cellulose membrane by glutaraldehyde (Villalonga et al., 2008). In another kind of covalent binding reaction, biomolecules containing thiol groups could bind to the nanoparticle surface. This strategy is more advantageous in terms of simplicity and strong attachment. For example, proteins with thiol groups were directly immobilized on gold surface with strong affinity. Also, the protein surface can be modified with thiol groups which would bind to gold surfaces. Traut's reagent could be used to replace the amine groups of GOD (McRipley and Linsenmeier, 1996). Then, the modified enzyme was

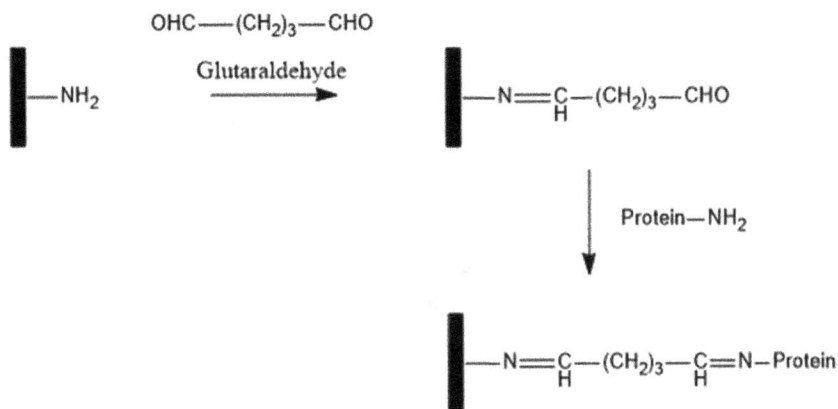

FIGURE 2.9 Protein immobilization on support by glutaraldehyde coupling.

covalently attached to a gold electrode. Another strategy for introducing Cys into the protein sequence is site-directed mutagenesis (Gwenin et al., 2007). Moreover, disulfide bonds can be broken with reagents like dithiothreitol (DTT), which allows coupling reaction. Low-molecular-weight bifunctional linkers are used in covalent-tethered conjugation between biomolecules and NPs. Groups like amine, active ester, and maleimide are commonly used in covalent coupling of biomolecules by carbodiimide mediated esterification and amidation reactions (Veiseh et al., 2010). In a work by Weissleder group, a covalent, bio-orthogonal reaction between a 1, 2, 4, 5-tetrazine and a trans-cyclooctene for small molecule labeling was described (Haun et al., 2010). The cycloaddition reaction is fast, chemoselective, works without a catalyst. This strategy could be adapted to improve binding efficiency and detection sensitivity. Also, this procedure via 1,3-dipolar cycloaddition can be applied in the covalent functionalization of radionuclide-filled SWNTs as radioprobes (Hong et al., 2010). Cu-catalyzed azide-alkyne cycloaddition reaction was employed to conjugate biomolecules with NPs. This was performed by decorating the NP surface with either alkyne or azide and then coupling to biomolecules. The main advantages of these reactions are; fast, efficient, and require mild reaction conditions. In addition, this strategy is highly specific and stable. Krovi et al. described one-step click reaction used for the functionalization of drug-loaded polymer NPs with folate, biotin, and AuNPs for drug delivery (2010).

2.4.3   SPECIFIC AFFINITY INTERACTION OF BIOMOLECULES WITH NANOMATERIALS

It is a highly stable bioconjugation method and considered strongest among the non-covalent strategies. This method is considered as the most effective in bioconjugation of nanomaterials due to strong and specific recognition interactions (such as antigen-antibody, nucleic acid-DNA, lectin-glycan, streptavidin-biotin, aptamer-small biomolecule and hormone-receptor interactions, etc.). Also, the presence of several binding sites in the biomolecules (e.g., antibodies show two Fab (antigen-binding fragment) sites) enables multidirectional growth of nanomaterial structures (Lei and Ju, 2012). Here are few examples of the bioconjugation reactions using this method. The strong affinity between biotin and streptavidin can be used to immobilize biomolecules. Biotinylation is possible with a covalent linking of biotin to the protein by the use of biotin-ester reagents (Nilsson et al., 1997). In addition, proteins could be genetically biotinylated utilizing a biotin acceptor peptide sequence (Zhang and Cass, 2000). Biotinylated proteins were employed in developing chemiluminescent biosensors for the detection of choline and acetylcholine (ACh) (Yao et al., 2002). Similarly, Esseghaier et al. developed an impedimetric biosensor for H_2O_2 detection (Esseghaier et al., 2008). The strong affinity between a metal cation and a chelator could be used to develop biosensors. Some common chelators are nitrilotriacetic acid (NTA), imidodiacetic acid (IDA) and tag poly(histidine). Proteins with histidine (His) residues can be easily linked to support with a metal chelate. Halliwell et al. described a biosensor on the basis of this method for the detection of lactate (Halliwell et al., 2002). Initially, polyaniline-polyacrylate films loaded with Ni^{2+} ions were formed on an electrode which served as the coordination sites for histidine residues available on His-tagged lactate dehydrogenase. Also, NTA can be utilized as a chelator for this purpose. Herein, four of six co-ordinations of Ni^{2+} ions are occupied by the four ligands of NTA chelate, whereas, the other two positions are occupied by the water/buffer molecules. This could be selectively replaced by the His-tag present in the proteins (Andreescu et al., 2001). The same procedure has also been used for the immobilization of His-tagged AChE on functionalized graphite which was employed in SPE fabrication (Andreescu et al., 2003). The graphite was initially modified to introduce the NTA group, which subsequently interacts with the nickel ions. Thereafter, immobilization can be done with the histidine group. Affinity interactions are also possible between the support and sugar moiety present in the enzymes (e.g., AChE, and Con A). Con A is a lectin with various sites possessing stronger affinity for carbohydrates (Andreescu and Marty, 2006). The immobilized lectins are able to bind to the glycosidic enzymes. In contrast to the other procedures, which are based on avidin/biotin and metal ions/chelator, this strategy depends on a tag present naturally in the enzyme, therefore, no modification of enzyme is required. Amperometric biosensors have been developed for acetylthiocholine and insecticide detection on the basis of strong binding affinity between Con A and mannose residues of AChE (Bucur et al., 2004a, b, 2005a).

2.5 CONCLUSION

In summary, this chapter provides a comprehensive view of biosensors and the role of nanomaterials in biosensing technology. Nanomaterials can be successfully used for the development of smart biosensors. Incorporation of nanotechnology in biosensing leads to the development of faster, smarter, cost-effective, and user-friendly biosensors. In addition, the exploration of nanomaterials in biosensing becomes more versatile, robust, and dynamic. Nanomaterial could accomplish better performance by improving the purity and fine-tuning size/shape/conjugation distributions. However, more research is needed to prepare new kinds of nanostructures for use in biosensing. Other than the materials, immobilization method and the detection mode also influence the performance of a biosensor. Although several methods of immobilization are readily available, it is still intriguing to explore innovative immobilization techniques which could be helpful in developing novel and next-generation biosensors. Biosensors based on nanotechnology could be incorporated into biochips which can enhance the functionality. This technique enables biosensors to become small, portable, and highly versatile diagnostic instruments that are easy to use. Further, laser nanosensors are useful in analyzing biomolecules and biomarkers even in individual living cells. Although various nanobiosensors have been developed in the past few decades, the development of low cost and highly sensitive biosensors is still the current interest of research. It is noteworthy to mention that various nanobiosensor models are functional in the lab, but are not functional in practical applications. Therefore, more interdisciplinary research involving different fields like life science, engineering, and pharmacy has to be conducted to create advanced biosensing techniques.

KEYWORDS

- biological oxygen demand
- carbon nanotubes
- poly(diallyl dimethylammonium chloride)
- poly(sodium 4-styrenesulfonate)
- quantum dots
- rev responsive element
- superconducting quantum interference devices

REFERENCES

Adekoya, J. A., Ogunniran, K. O., Siyanbola, T. O., Dare, E. O., & Revaprasadu, N., (2018). Band structure, morphology, functionality, and size-dependent properties of metal nanoparticles. In: Seehra, M. S. S., & Bristow, A. D., (eds.), *Nanoscale Effects and Applications*. Intech Open.

Afsahi, S., Lerner, M. B., Goldstein, J. M., Lee, J., Tang, X., Bagarozzi, D. A., Pan, D., et al., (2018). Novel graphene-based biosensor for early detection of zika virus infection. *Biosens. Bioelectron., 100*, 85–88.

Agarwal, S. K., (2005). *Bioelectronics*. New Delhi: APH Publishing Corporation.

Aldewachi, H., Aldewachi, H., Chalati, T., Woodroofe, M. N., Bricklebank, N., Sharrack, B., & Gardiner, P., (2017). Gold nanoparticle-based colorimetric biosensors. *Nanoscale, 101*, 18–33.

Alterman, M., Sjobom, H., Safsten, P., Markgren, P. O., Danielson, U. H., Hamalainen, M., Lofas, S., et al., (2001). P1/P1′ Modified HIV protease inhibitors as tools in two new sensitive surface plasmon resonance biosensor screening assays. *European Journal of Pharmaceutical Sciences, 13*, 203–212.

Andreescu, S., & Marty, J. L., (2006). Twenty years research in cholinesterase biosensors: From basic research to practical applications. *Biomol. Eng., 23*, 1–15.

Andreescu, S., Fournier, D., & Marty, J. L., (2003). Development of highly sensitive sensor based on bioengineered acetylcholinesterase immobilized by affinity method. *Analytical Letters, 36*, 1865–1885.

Andreescu, S., Magearu, V., Lougarre, A., Fournier, D., & Marty, J. L., (2004). Immobilization of enzymes on screen-printed sensors via a histidine tail. application to the detection of pesticides using modified cholinesterase. *Analytical Letters, 34*, 529–540.

Arya, S. K., Prusty, A. K., Singh, S. P., Solanki, P. R., Pandey, M. K., Datta, M., & Malhotra, B. D., (2007). Cholesterol biosensor based on N-(2-aminoethyl)-3-aminopropyl-trime-thoxysilane self-assembled monolayer. *Anal. Biochem., 363*, 210–218.

Azamian, B. R., Davis, J. J., Coleman, K. S., Bagshaw, C. B., & Green, M. L., (2002). Bioelectrochemical single-walled carbon nanotubes. *Journal of the American Chemical Society, 124,* 12664, 12665.

Bahadır, E. B., & Sezgintürk, M. K., (2015). Applications of electrochemical immunosensors for early clinical diagnostics. *Talanta, 132,* 162–174.

Bahadır, E. B., & Sezgintürk, M. K., (2016). A review on impedimetric biosensors. *Artif Cells Nanomed. Biotechnol., 44,* 248–262.

Barredo, J. L., (2005). Microbial enzymes and biotransformations. *Methods in Biotechnology, 17.* Humana Press.

Bertók, T., Katrlík, J., Gemeiner, P., & Tkac, J., (2013). Electrochemical lectin based biosensors as a label-free tool in glycomics. *Mikrochim Acta, 180,* 1–13.

Bhalla, N., & Singh, N., (2016). Introduction to biosensors. *Essays Biochem., 60,* 1–8.

Bisht, V., Takashima, W., & Kaneto, K., (2005). An amperometric urea biosensor based on covalent immobilization of urease onto an electrochemically prepared copolymer poly (N-3-aminopropyl pyrrole-co-pyrrole) film. *Biomaterials, 26,* 3683–3690.

Bolincier, J., Ungerstedt, U., & Arner, P., (1992). Microdialysis measurement of the absolute glucose concentration in subcutaneous adipose tissue allowing glucose monitoring in diabetic patients. *Diabetologia, 35,* 1177–1780.

Bonnet, C., Andreescu, S., & Marty, J. L., (2003). Adsorption: An easy and efficient immobilization of acetylcholinesterase on screen-printed electrodes. *Analytica Chimica Acta, 481,* 209–211.

Cai, C., & Chen, J., (2004). Direct electron transfer of glucose oxidase promoted by carbon nanotubes. *Anal. Biochem., 332,* 75–83.

Cai, H., Xu, C., He, P., & Fang, Y., (2001). Colloid Au-enhanced DNA immobilization for the electrochemical detection of sequence-specific DNA. *Journal of Electroanalytical Chemistry, 510,* 78–85.

Cao, X., Cao, X., Guo, H., Li, T., Jie, Y., Wang, N., & Wang, Z. L., (2016). Piezotronic effect enhanced label-free detection of DNA using a Schottky-contacted ZnO nanowire biosensor. *ACS Nano, 10,* 8038–8044.

Cass, A. E., Davis, G., Francis, G. D., Hill, H. A. O., Aston, W. J., Higgins, I. J., Plotkin, E. V., et al., (1984). Ferrocene-mediated enzyme electrode for amperometric determination of glucose. *Analytical Chemistry, 56,* 667–671.

Chamorro-Garcia, A., & Merkoci, A., (2016). Nanobiosensors in diagnostics. *Nanobiomedicine (Rij), 3,* 1849543516663574.

Chauhan, N., Toru, M., Nair, D., & Kumar, S., (2017). Graphene based biosensors-accelerating medical diagnostics to new-dimensions. *Journal of Materials Research, 32,* 2860–2682.

Chemla, Y. R., Grossman, H. L., Poon, Y., McDermott, R., Stevens, R., Alper, M. D., & Clarke, J., (2000). Ultrasensitive magnetic biosensor for homogeneous immunoassay. *Proc. Natl. Acad. Sci. USA, 97,* 14268–14272.

Chen, M., Xiong, H., Wen, W., Zhang, X., Gu, H., & Wang, S., (2013). Electrochemical biosensors for the assay of DNA damage initiated by ferric ions catalyzed oxidation of dopamine in room temperature ionic liquid. *Electrochimica Acta, 114,* 265–270.

Chithrani, B. D., Ghazani, A. A., & Chan, W. C., (2006). Determining the size and shape dependence of gold nanoparticle uptake into mammalian cells. *Nano Lett., 6,* 662–628.

Clark, Jr. L. C., & Lyons, C., (1962). Electrode systems for continuous monitoring in cardiovascular surgery. *Ann. N.Y. Acad. Sci., 102,* 29–45.

Clarke, D., (1985). The development and application of biosensing devices for bioreactor monitoring and control. *Biosensors, 1*, 213–320.

Crumbliss, A. L., Perine, S. C., Stonehuerner, J., Tubergen, K. R., Zhao, J., Henkens, R. W., & O'Daly, J. P., (1992). Colloidal gold as a biocompatible immobilization matrix suitable for the fabrication of enzyme electrodes by electrodeposition. *Biotechnol. Bioeng., 40*, 483–490.

Cui, Y., & Lieber, C. M., (2001). Functional nanoscale electronic devices assembled using silicon nanowire building blocks. *Science, 291*, 851–853.

Cui, Y., Wei, Q., Park, H., & Lieber, C. M., (2001). Nanowire nano-sensors for highly sensitive and selective detection of biological and chemical species. *Science, 293*, 1289–1292.

Cullum, B. M., Griffin, G. D., Miller, G. H., & Vo-Dinh, T., (2000). Intracellular measurements in mammary carcinoma cells using fiber-optic nano-sensors. *Anal. Biochem., 277*, 25–32.

Curri, M. L., Agostiano, A., Leo, G., Mallardi, A., Cosma, P., & Della, M. M., (2002). Development of a novel enzyme/semiconductor nanoparticles system for biosensor application. *Materials Science and Engineering: C, 22*, 449–452.

Damborsky, P., Svitel, J., & Katrlik, J., (2016). Optical biosensors. *Essays Biochem., 60*, 91–100.

Danielsson, B., (1990). Calorimetric biosensors. *Journal of Biotechnology, 15*, 187–200.

Davis, J. J., Coleman, K. S., Azamian, B. R., Bagshaw, C. B., & Green, M. L., (2003). Chemical and biochemical sensing with modified single-walled carbon nanotubes. *Chemistry, 9*, 3732–3739.

De Volder, M. F., Tawfick, S. H., Baughman, R. H., & Hart, A. J., (2013). Carbon nanotubes: Present and future commercial applications. *Science, 339*, 535–539.

Del, V. M., & Bonanni, A., (2014). Impedimetric DNA biosensors based on nanomaterials. In: Tiwari, A., & Turner, A. P. F., (eds.), *Biosensors Nanotechnology* (pp. 81–110). Wiley-Scrivener.

Diaconu, I., Cristea, C., Hârceagă, V., Marrazza, G., Berindan-Neagoe, I., & Săndulescu, R., (2013). Electrochemical immunosensors in breast and ovarian cancer. *Clin. Chim. Acta, 425*, 128–138.

Dolatabadi, J. E. N., & De La Guardia, M., (2014). Nanomaterial-based electrochemical immunosensors as advanced diagnostic tools. *Anal. Methods, 6*, 3891–3900.

Dong, X. Y., Mi, X. N., Zhang, L., Liang, T. M., Xu, J. J., & Chen, H. Y., (2012). DNAzyme-functionalized Pt nanoparticles/carbon nanotubes for amplified sandwich electrochemical DNA analysis. *Biosens. Bioelectron., 38*, 337–341.

Drummond, T. G., Hill, M. G., & Barton, J. K., (2003). Electrochemical DNA sensors. *Nat. Biotechnol., 21*, 1192–1199.

Du, Y., Chen, C., Yin, J., Li, B., Zhou, M., Dong, S., & Wang, E., (2010). Solid-state probe based electrochemical aptasensor for cocaine: A potentially convenient, sensitive, repeatable, and integrated sensing platform for drugs. *Anal. Chem., 82*, 1556–1563.

Ekanayake, E. M., Preethichandra, D. M., & Kaneto, K., (2007). Polypyrrole nanotube array sensor for enhanced adsorption of glucose oxidase in glucose biosensors. *Biosens. Bioelectron., 23*, 107–113.

Esseghaier, C., Bergaoui, Y., Ben, F. H., Tlili, A., Helali, S., Ameur, S., & Abdelghani, A., (2008). Impedance spectroscopy on immobilized streptavidin horseradish peroxidase layer for biosensing. *Sensors and Actuators B: Chemical, 134*, 112–116.

Fägerstam, L. G., Frostell, Å., Karlsson, R., Kullman, M., Larsson, A., Malmqvist, M., & Butt, H., (1990). Detection of antigen-antibody interactions by surface plasmon resonance. Application to epitope mapping. *J. Mol. Recognit., 3*, 208–214.

Gäberlein, S., Spener, F., & Zaborosch, C., (2000). Microbial and cytoplasmic membrane-based potentiometric biosensors for direct determination of organophosphorus insecticides. *Appl. Microbiol. Biotechnol., 54*, 652–658.

Gao, X., Cui, Y., Levenson, R. M., Chung, L. W., & Nie, S., (2004). *In vivo* cancer targeting and imaging with semiconductor quantum dots. *Nat. Biotechnol., 22*, 969–976.

Giljohann, D. A., Seferos, D. S., Patel, P. C., Millstone, J. E., Rosi, N. L., & Mirkin, C. A., (2007). Oligonucleotide loading determines cellular uptake of DNA-modified gold nanoparticles. *Nano Lett., 7*, 3818–3821.

Giroud, F., Gorgy, K., Gondran, C., Cosnier, S., Pinacho, D. G., Marco, M. P., & Sánchez-Baeza, F. J., (2009). Impedimetric immunosensor based on a polypyrrole-antibiotic model film for the label-free picomolar detection of ciprofloxacin. *Anal. Chem., 81*, 8405–8409.

Grimm, J., Perez, J. M., Josephson, L., & Weissleder, R., (2004). Novel nanosensors for rapid analysis of telomerase activity. *Cancer Research, 64*, 639–643.

Guan, J. G., Miao, Y. Q., & Zhang, Q. J., (2004). Impedimetric biosensors. *Journal of Bioscience and Bioengineering, 97*, 219–226.

Guilbault, G. G., & Montalvo, J. G., (1970). Enzyme electrode for the substrate urea. *Journal of the American Chemical Society, 92*, 2533–2538.

Guo, X., (2012). Surface plasmon resonance-based biosensor technique: A review. *J. Biophotonics, 5*, 483–501.

Gwenin, C. D., Kalaji, M., Williams, P. A., & Jones, R. M., (2007). The orientationally controlled assembly of genetically modified enzymes in an amperometric biosensor. *Biosens. Bioelectron., 22*, 2869–2875.

Halliwell, C. M., Simon, E., Toh, C. S., Bartlett, P. N., & Cass, A. E., (2002). Immobilization of lactate dehydrogenase on poly(aniline)-poly(acrylate) and poly(aniline)-poly(vinyl sulphonate) films for use in a lactate biosensor. *Analytica Chimica Acta, 453*, 191–200.

Hamidi-Asl, E., Palchetti, I., Hasheminejad, E., & Mascini, M., (2013). A review on the electrochemical biosensors for determination of microRNAs. *Talanta, 115*, 74–83.

Harisinghani, M. G., Barentsz, J., Hahn, P. F., Deserno, W. M., Tabatabaei, S., Van, D. K. C. H., De La Rosette, J., & Weissleder, R., (2003). Noninvasive detection of clinically occult lymph-node metastases in prostate cancer. *N. Engl. J. Med., 348*, 2491–2499.

Haun, J. B., Devaraj, N. K., Hilderbrand, S. A., Lee, H., & Weissleder, R., (2010). Bioorthogonal chemistry amplifies nanoparticle binding and enhances the sensitivity of cell detection. *Nat. Nanotechnol., 5*, 660–665.

Haun, J. B., Yoon, T. J., Lee, H., & Weissleder, R., (2010). Magnetic nanoparticle biosensors. *Wiley Interdiscip Rev. Nanomed Nanobiotechnol., 2*, 291–304.

Holzinger, M., Le Goff, A., & Cosnier, S., (2014). Nanomaterials for biosensing applications: A review. *Front Chem., 2*, 63.

Hong, S. Y., Tobias, G., Al-Jamal, K. T., Ballesteros, B., Ali-Boucetta, H., Lozano-Perez, S., Nellist, P. D., et al., (2010). Filled and glycosylated carbon nanotubes for *in vivo* radioemitter localization and imaging. *Nat. Mater., 9*, 485–490.

Hrapovic, S., Liu, Y., Male, K. B., & Luong, J. H., (2004). Electrochemical biosensing platforms using platinum nanoparticles and carbon nanotubes. *Anal. Chem., 76*, 1083–1088.

Huang, Y., Dong, X., Liu, Y., Li, L. J., & Chen, P., (2011). Graphene-based biosensors for detection of bacteria and their metabolic activities. *Journal of Materials Chemistry, 21*, 12358.

Huang, Y., Zhang, W., Xiao, H., & Li, G., (2005). An electrochemical investigation of glucose oxidase at a Cds nanoparticles modified electrode. *Biosens. Bioelectron., 21*, 817–821.

Iijima, S., (1991). Helical microtubules of graphitic carbon. *Nature, 354*, 56–58.

Jagiello, K., Chomicz, B., Avramopoulos, A., Gajewicz, A., Mikolajczyk, A., Bonifassi, P., Papadopoulos, M. G., et al., (2016). Size-dependent electronic properties of nanomaterials: How this novel class of nanodescriptors supposed to be calculated? *Structural Chemistry, 28*, 635–643.

Janegitz, B. C., Silva, T. A., Wong, A., Ribovski, L., Vicentini, F. C., Sotomayor, M. D. P. T., & Fatibello-Filho, O., (2017). The application of graphene for in vitro and in vivo electrochemical biosensing. *Biosens. Bioelectron., 89*, 224–233.

Jung, J. H., Cheon, D. S., Liu, F., Lee, K. B., & Seo, T. S., (2010). A graphene oxide based immuno-biosensor for pathogen detection. *Angew. Chem. Int. Ed. Engl., 49*, 5708–5711.

Kabashin, A. V., Evans, P., Pastkovsky, S., Hendren, W., Wurtz, G. A., Atkinson, R., Pollard, R., et al., (2009). Plasmonic nanorod metamaterials for biosensing. *Nat. Mater., 8*, 867–871.

Kairdolf, B. A., Smith, A. M., Stokes, T. H., Wang, M. D., Young, A. N., & Nie, S., (2013). Semiconductor quantum dots for bioimaging and biodiagnostic applications. *Annu. Rev. Anal. Chem. (Palo Alto Calif), 6*, 143–162.

Kaisheva, A., Atanasov, P., Gamburzev, S., Dimcheva, N., & Iliev, I., (1992). Amperometric biosensor for glucose and lactate. *Sensors and Actuators B: Chemical, 8*, 53–57.

Kasry, A., Ardakani, A. A., Tulevski, G. S., Menges, B., Copel, M., & Vyklicky, L., (2012). Highly efficient fluorescence quenching with graphene. *The Journal of Physical Chemistry C, 116*, 2858–2862.

Katz, E., Willner, I., & Wang, J., (2004). Electroanalytical and bioelectroanalytical systems based on metal and semiconductor nanoparticles. *Electroanalysis, 16*, 19–44.

Khimji, I., Kelly, E. Y., Helwa, Y., Hoang, M., & Liu, J., (2013). Visual optical biosensors based on DNA-functionalized polyacrylamide hydrogels. *Methods, 64*, 292–298.

Kim, E. J., Lee, Y., Lee, J. E., & Gu, M. B., (2002). Application of recombinant fluorescent mammalian cells as a toxicity biosensor. *Water Science and Technology, 46*, 51–56.

Korkut, S., Keskinler, B., & Erhan, E., (2008). An amperometric biosensor based on multiwalled carbon nanotube-poly(pyrrole)-horseradish peroxidase nanobiocomposite film for determination of phenol derivatives. *Talanta, 76*, 1147–1152.

Krovi, S. A., Smith, D., & Nguyen, S. T., (2010). "Clickable" polymer nanoparticles: A modular scaffold for surface functionalization. *Chem. Commun. (Camb.), 46*, 5277–5279.

Kuila, T., Bose, S., Khanra, P., Mishra, A. K., Kim, N. H., & Lee, J. H., (2011). Recent advances in graphene-based biosensors. *Biosens. Bioelectron., 26*, 4637–4648.

Kulys, J., Higgins, I. J., & Bannister, J. V., (1992). Amperometric determination of phosphate ions by biosensor. *Biosensors and Bioelectronics, 7*, 187–191.

Kwon, S. J., & Bard, A. J., (2012). DNA analysis by application of Pt nanoparticle electrochemical amplification with single label response. *J. Am. Chem. Soc., 134*, 10777–10779.

Lad, U., Khokhar, S., & Kale, G. M., (2008). Electrochemical creatinine biosensors. *Anal. Chem., 80*, 7910–7917.

Lakard, B., Magnin, D., Deschaume, O., Vanlancker, G., Glinel, K., Demoustier-Champagne, S., Nysten, B., et al., (2011). Urea potentiometric enzymatic biosensor based on charged biopolymers and electrodeposited polyaniline. *Biosens. Bioelectron., 26*, 4139–4145.

Langer, J. J., Filipiak, M., Ke, J., Jasnowska, J., Włodarczak, J., & Buładowski, B., (2004). Polyaniline biosensor for choline determination. *Surface Science, 573*, 140–145.

Larsen, L. H., Kjaer, T., & Revsbech, N. P., (1997). A microscale No(3)(-) biosensor for environmental applications. *Anal. Chem., 69*, 3527–3531.

Lazerges, M., & Bedioui, F., (2013). Analysis of the evolution of the detection limits of electrochemical DNA biosensors. *Anal. Bioanal. Chem., 405*, 3705–3714.

Lee, H. J., & Yook, J. G., (2014). Recent research trends of radio-frequency biosensors for biomolecular detection. *Biosens. Bioelectron., 61*, 448–459.

Lei, J., & Ju, H., (2012). Signal amplification using functional nanomaterials for biosensing. *Chem. Soc. Rev., 41*, 2122–2134.

Li, G., Liao, J. M., Hu, G. Q., Ma, N. Z., & Wu, P. J., (2005). Study of carbon nanotube modified biosensor for monitoring total cholesterol in blood. *Biosens. Bioelectron., 20*, 2140–2144.

Lin, Y., Lu, F., Tu, Y., & Ren, Z., (2004). Glucose biosensors based on carbon nanotube nanoelectrode ensembles. *Nano Letters, 4*, 191–195.

Lubbers, D., & Opitz, N., (1975). The PCO_2/PO_2 optrode: A new probe for measuring PCO_2 and PO_2 of gases and liquids. *Z. Naturforsch C., 30*, 532–533.

Luo, X., Morrin, A., Killard, A. J., & Smyth, M. R., (2006). Application of nanoparticles in electrochemical sensors and biosensors. *Electroanalysis, 18*, 319–326.

Ma, F., Li, C., & Zhang, C., (2018). Development of quantum dot-based biosensors: Principles and applications. *Journal of Materials Chemistry B, 6*, 6173–6190.

MacKenzie, R., Auzelyte, V., Olliges, S., Spolenak, R., Solak, H. H., & Vörös, J., (2009). *Nanowire Development and Characterization for Applications in Biosensing* (pp. 143–173). Springer, Boston, MA.

Malhotra, B., & Ali, A., (2017). *Nanomaterials for Biosensors: Fundamentals and Applications*. Amsterdam, Netherlands: Elsevier,.

Malik, P., Katyal, V., Malik, V., Asatkar, A., Inwati, G., & Mukherjee, T. K., (2013). Nanobiosensors: Concepts and variations. *ISRN Nanomaterials*, 1–9.

Masson, J. F., (2017). Surface plasmon resonance clinical biosensors for medical diagnostics. *ACS Sens., 2*, 16–30.

Mathebe, N. G., Morrin, A., & Iwuoha, E. I., (2004). Electrochemistry and scanning electron microscopy of polyaniline/peroxidase-based biosensor. *Talanta, 64*, 115–120.

McRipley, M. A., & Linsenmeier, R. A., (1996). Fabrication of a mediated glucose oxidase recessed microelectrode for the amperometric determination of glucose. *Journal of Electroanalytical Chemistry, 414*, 235–246.

Meshram, B. D., Agrawal, A. K., Adil, S., Ranvir, S., & Sande, K. K., (2018). Biosensor and its application in food and dairy industry: A review. *International Journal of Current Microbiology and Applied Sciences, 7*, 3305–3324.

Mistry, K. K., Layek, K., Mahapatra, A., RoyChaudhuri, C., & Saha, H., (2014). A review on amperometric-type immunosensors based on screen-printed electrodes. *Analyst, 139*, 2289–2311.

Morales-Narváez, E., Baptista-Pires, L., Zamora-Gálvez, A., & Merkoçi, A., (2017). Graphene-based biosensors: Going simple. *Adv. Mater., 29*, 1604905.

Morrin, A., Ngamna, O., Killard, A. J., Moulton, S. E., Smyth, M. R., & Wallace, G. G., (2005). An amperometric enzyme biosensor fabricated from polyaniline nanoparticles. *Electroanalysis, 17*, 423–430.

Mulchandani, A., (2011). Microbial biosensors for organophosphate pesticides. *Appl. Biochem. Biotechnol., 165*, 687–699.

Nagiev, T. M., (2006). Enzymatic biosensors and their biomimetic analogs: Advanced analytical appliances. In: Nagiev, T. M., (ed.), *Coherent Synchronized Oxidation Reactions by Hydrogen Peroxide* (pp. 289–307). Amsterdam: Elsevier.

Navakul, K., Warakulwit, C., Yenchitsomanus, P. T., Panya, A., Lieberzeit, P. A., & Sangma, C., (2017). A novel method for dengue virus detection and antibody screening using a graphene-polymer based electrochemical biosensor. *Nanomedicine, 13*, 549–557.

Nilsson, J., Ståhl, S., Lundeberg, J., Uhlén, M., & Nygren, P. Å., (1997). Affinity fusion strategies for detection, purification, and immobilization of recombinant proteins. *Protein Expr.. Purif., 11*, 1–16.

Odenthal, K. J., & Gooding, J. J., (2007). An introduction to electrochemical DNA biosensors. *Analyst., 132*, 603–610.

Olaniran, A. O., Hiralal, L., & Pillay, B., (2011). Whole-cell bacterial biosensors for rapid and effective monitoring of heavy metals and inorganic pollutants in wastewater. *J. Environ. Monit., 13*, 2914–2920.

Patolsky, F., Weizmann, Y., & Willner, I., (2004). Long-range electrical contacting of redox enzymes by SWCNT connectors. *Angew. Chem. Int. Ed. Engl., 43*, 2113–2117.

Peña-Bahamonde, J., Nguyen, H. N., Fanourakis, S. K., & Rodrigues, D. F., (2018). Recent advances in graphene-based biosensor technology with applications in life sciences. *J. Nanobiotechnology, 16*, 75.

Peng, H. I., & Miller, B. L., (2011). Recent advancements in optical DNA biosensors: Exploiting the plasmonic effects of metal nanoparticles. *Analyst., 136*, 436–447.

Pickup, J. C., Hussain, F., Evans, N. D., & Sachedina, N., (2005). *In vivo* glucose monitoring: The clinical reality and the promise. *Biosens. Bioelectron., 20*, 1897–1902.

Pohanka, M., (2017). The piezoelectric biosensors: Principles and applications: A review. *International Journal of Electrochemical Science*, 496–506.

Ponomareva, O. N., Arlyapov, V. A., Alferov, V. A., & Reshetilov, A. N., (2011). Microbial biosensors for detection of biological oxygen demand: A review. *Appl. Biochem. Microbiol., 47*, 1–11.

Presnova, G. V., Rybcova, M. Y., & Egorov, A. M., (2009). Electrochemical biosensors based on horseradish peroxidase. *Russian Journal of General Chemistry, 78*, 2482–2488.

Pumera, M., (2011). Graphene in biosensing. *Materials Today, 14*, 308–315.

Purohit, H. J., (2003). Biosensors as molecular tools for use in bioremediation. *Journal of Cleaner Production, 11*, 293–301.

Rahman, M. A., Kwon, N. H., Won, M. S., Choe, E. S., & Shim, Y. B., (2005). Functionalized conducting polymer as an enzyme-immobilizing substrate: An amperometric glutamate microbiosensor for *in vivo* measurements. *Anal. Chem., 77*, 4854–4860.

Rahman, M. M., Shiddiky, M. J., Rahman, M. A., & Shim, Y. B., (2009). A lactate biosensor based on lactate dehydrogenase/nicotinamide adenine dinucleotide (oxidized form) immobilized on a conducting polymer/multiwall carbon nanotube composite film. *Anal. Biochem., 384*, 159–165.

Ramanathan, K., & Danielsson, B., (2001). Principles and applications of thermal biosensors. *Biosensors and Bioelectronics, 16*, 417–423.

Ramanathan, S., Patibandla, S., Bandyopadhyay, S., Edwards, J. D., & Anderson, J., (2006). Fluorescence and infrared spectroscopy of electrochemically self-assembled ZnO nanowires: Evidence of the quantum confined stark effect. *Journal of Materials Science: Materials in Electronics, 17*, 651–655.

Rao, C. N. R., Sood, A. E., Subrahmanyam, K. E., & Govindaraj, A., (2009). Graphene: The new two-dimensional nanomaterial. *Angew Chem. Int. Ed. Engl., 48*, 7752–7777.

Reshetilov, A. N., Iliasov, P. V., & Reshetilova, T. A., (2010). The microbial cell-based biosensors. In: Somerset, V. S., (ed.), *Intelligent and Biosensors*. Intech Open.

Richardson, J., Hawkins, P., & Luxton, R., (2001). The use of coated paramagnetic particles as a physical label in a magneto-immunoassay. *Biosensors and Bioelectronics, 16*, 989–993.

Rishpon, J., & Buchner, V., (2005). Chapter 8 electrochemical antibody-based sensors. *Comprehensive Analytical Chemistry, 44*, 329–373.

Rocha, S., & Teresa, A. P., (2014). Sensors and biosensors based on magnetic nanoparticles. *TrAC Trends in Analytical Chemistry, 62*, 28–36.

Rodriguez-Mozaz, S., De Alda, M. J. L., Marco, M. P., & Barceló, D., (2005). Biosensors for environmental monitoring a global perspective. *Talanta, 65*, 291–297.

Rodriguez-Mozaz, S., Marco, M. P., De Alda, M. L., & Barceló, D., (2004). Biosensors for environmental applications: Future development trends. *Pure and Applied Chemistry, 76*, 723–752.

Ronkainen, N. J., Halsall, H. B., & Heineman, W. R., (2010). Electrochemical biosensors. *Chem. Soc. Rev., 39*, 1747–1763.

Sagadevan, S., & Periasamy, M., (2014). Recent trends in nanobiosensors and their applications: A review. *Rev. Adv. Mater. Sci., 36*, 62–69.

Shaolin, M., & Huaiguo, X., (1996). Bioelectrochemical characteristics of glucose oxidase immobilized in a polyaniline film. *Sensors and Actuators B: Chemical, 31*, 155–160.

Shi, A., Wang, J., Han, X., Fang, X., & Zhang, Y., (2014). A sensitive electrochemical DNA biosensor based on gold nanomaterial and graphene amplified signal. *Sensors and Actuators B: Chemical, 200*, 206–212.

Shi, S., Wang, X., Sun, W., Wang, X., Yao, T., & Ji, L., (2013). Label-free fluorescent DNA biosensors based on metallointercalators and nanomaterials. *Methods, 64*, 305–314.

Shin, H., (2011). Genetically engineered microbial biosensors for in situ monitoring of environmental pollution. *Appl. Microbiol. Biotechnol., 89*, 867–877.

Shirale, D. J., Bangar, M. A., Park, M., Yates, M. V., Chen, W., Myung, N. V., & Mulchandani, A., (2010). Label-free chemiresistive immunosensors for viruses. *Environ. Sci. Technol., 44*, 9030–9035.

Sireesha, M., Jagadeesh, B. V., Kranthi, K. A. S., & Ramakrishna, S., (2018). A review on carbon nanotubes in biosensor devices and their applications in medicine. *Nanocomposites, 4*, 36–57.

Song, W., Li, H., Liang, H., Qiang, W., & Xu, D., (2014). Disposable electrochemical aptasensor array by using in situ DNA hybridization inducing silver nanoparticles aggregate for signal amplification. *Anal. Chem., 86*, 2775–2783.

Sotiropoulou, S., Gavalas, V., Vamvakaki, V., & Chaniotakis, N. A., (2003). Novel carbon materials in biosensor systems. *Biosensors and Bioelectronics, 18*, 211–315.

Stern, E., Klemic, J. F., Routenberg, D. A., Wyrembak, P. N., Turner-Evans, D. B., Hamilton, A. D., LaVan, D. A., et al., (2007). Label-free immunodetection with CMOS-compatible semiconducting nanowires. *Nature, 445*, 519–522.

Tilmaciu, C. M., & Morris, M. C., (2015). Carbon nanotube biosensors. *Front Chem., 3*, 59.

Trojanowicz, M., (2002). Determination of pesticides using electrochemical enzymatic biosensors. *Electroanalysis, 14*, 1311–1328.

Trojanowicz, M., (2014). Enantioselective electrochemical sensors and biosensors: A mini-review. *Electrochemistry Communications, 38*, 47–52.

Turner, A. P. F., Karube, I., & Wilson, G. S., (1987). *Biosensors Fundamentals and Applications*. Oxford, New York: Oxford University Press.

Veiseh, O., Gunn, J. W., & Zhang, M., (2010). Design and fabrication of magnetic nanoparticles for targeted drug delivery and imaging. *Adv. Drug Deliv. Rev., 62*, 284–304.

Villalonga, R., Fujii, A., Shinohara, H., Tachibana, S., & Asano, Y., (2008). Covalent immobilization of phenylalanine dehydrogenase on cellulose membrane for biosensor construction. *Sensors and Actuators B: Chemical, 129*, 195–199.

Wang, C., Tan, X., Chen, S., Yuan, R., Hu, F., Yuan, D., & Xiang, Y., (2012). Highly-sensitive cholesterol biosensor based on platinum-gold hybrid functionalized ZnO nanorods. *Talanta, 94*, 263–270.

Wang, H., & Shaolin, M., (1999). Bioelectrochemical characteristics of cholesterol oxidase immobilized in a polyaniline film. *Sensors and Actuators B: Chemical, 56*, 22–30.

Wang, J., & Musameh, M., (2005). Carbon-nanotubes doped polypyrrole glucose biosensor. *Analytica Chimica Acta, 539*, 209–213.

Wang, J., (2002). Electrochemical nucleic acid biosensors. *Analytica Chimica Acta, 469*, 63–71.

Wang, J., (2003). Nanoparticle-based electrochemical DNA detection. *Analytica Chimica Acta, 500*, 247–257.

Wang, J., Liu, G., Polsky, R., & Merkoçi, A., (2002). Electrochemical stripping detection of DNA hybridization based on cadmium sulfide nanoparticle tags. *Electrochemistry Communications, 4*, 722–726.

Wang, J., Rivas, G., Cai, X., Palecek, E., Nielsen, P., Shiraishi, H., Dontha, N., et al., (1997). DNA Electrochemical biosensors for environmental monitoring: A review. *Analytica Chimica Acta, 347*, 1–8.

Wang, J., Wang, L., Di, J., & Tu, Y., (2009). Electrodeposition of gold nanoparticles on indium/tin oxide electrode for fabrication of a disposable hydrogen peroxide biosensor. *Talanta, 77*, 1454–1459.

Wang, Z., & Dai, Z., (2015). Carbon nanomaterial-based electrochemical biosensors: An overview. *Nanoscale, 7*, 6420–6431.

Wang, Z., Luo, X., Wan, Q., Wu, K., & Yang, N., (2014). versatile matrix for constructing enzyme-based biosensors. *ACS Applied Materials and Interfaces, 6*, 17296–17305.

Wang, Z., Zhang, J., Ekman, J. M., Kenis, P. J., & Lu, Y., (2010). DNA-mediated control of metal nanoparticle shape: One-pot synthesis and cellular uptake of highly stable and functional gold nanoflowers. *Nano Lett., 10*, 1886–1891.

Wegner, K. D., & Hildebrandt, N., (2015). Quantum dots: Bright and versatile *in vitro* and *in vivo* fluorescence imaging biosensors. *Chem. Soc. Rev., 44*, 4792–4834.

Wollenberger, U., Schubert, F., & Scheller, F. W., (1992). Biosensor for sensitive phosphate detection. *Sensors and Actuators B: Chemical, 7*, 412–415.

Xu, L., Zhu, Y., Tang, L., Yang, X., & Li, C., (2007). Biosensor based on self-assembling glucose oxidase and dendrimer-encapsulated Pt nanoparticles on carbon nanotubes for glucose detection. *Electroanalysis, 19*, 717–722.

Xu, X., Liu, S., & Ju, H., (2003). A novel hydrogen peroxide sensor via the direct electrochemistry of horseradish peroxidase immobilized on colloidal gold modified screen-printed electrode. *Sensors, 3,* 350–560.

Xu, Y., & Wang, E., (2012). Electrochemical biosensors based on magnetic micro/ nanoparticles. *Electrochimica Acta, 84,* 62–73.

Yang, C. H., Kuo, L. S., Chen, P. H., Yang, C. R., & Tsai, Z. M., (2012). Development of a multilayered polymeric DNA biosensor using radiofrequency technology with gold and magnetic nanoparticles. *Biosens. Bioelectron., 31,* 349–356.

Yang, N., Chen, X., Ren, T., Zhang, P., & Yang, D., (2015). Carbon nanotube-based biosensors. *Sensors and Actuators B: Chemical, 207,* 690–715.

Yao, D., Vlessidis, A. G., & Evmiridis, N. P., (2002). Development of an Interference-free chemiluminescence method for monitoring acetylcholine and choline based on immobilized enzymes. *Analytica Chimica Acta, 462,* 199–208.

Yu, X., (2003). Peroxidase activity of enzymes bound to the ends of single-wall carbon nanotube forest electrodes. *Electrochemistry Communications, 5,* 408–411.

Yu, X., Yang, J., & Chai, Q., (2016). Applications of gold nanoparticles in biosensors. *Nano LIFE, 06,* 1642001.

Zeng, S., Yong, K. T., Roy, I., Dinh, X. Q., Yu, X., & Luan, F., (2011). A review on functionalized gold nanoparticles for biosensing applications. *Plasmonics, 6,* 491–506.

Zhai, J., Cui, H., & Yang, R., (1997). DNA based biosensors. *Biotechnology Advances, 15,* 43–58.

Zhang, B., Qiao, M., Liu, Y., Zheng, Y., Zhu, Y., & Paton, G. I., (2013). Application of microbial biosensors to complement geochemical characterization: A case study in Northern China. *Water Air Soil Pollut., 224,* 1–16.

Zhang, C. Y., & Johnson, L. W., (2006). Quantum-dot-based nanosensor for RRE IIB RNA-rev peptide interaction assay. *J. Am. Chem. Soc, 128,* 5324–5325.

Zhang, J., & Cass, A. E. G., (2000). Electrochemical analysis of immobilized chemical and genetic biotinylated alkaline phosphatase. *Analytica Chimica Acta, 408,* 241–247.

Zhao, J., O'daly, J. P., Henkens, R. W., Stonehuerner, J., & Crumbliss, A. L., (1996). A xanthine oxidase/colloidal gold enzyme electrode for amperometric biosensor applications. *Biosensors and Bioelectronics, 11,* 493–502.

Zhao, W. W., Xu, J. J., & Chen, H. Y., (2014). Photoelectrochemical DNA biosensors. *Chem. Rev., 114,* 7421–7441.

Zhao, Y. D., Zhang, W. D., Chen, H., Luo, Q. M., & Li, S. F. Y., (2002). Direct electrochemistry of horseradish peroxidase at carbon nanotube powder microelectrode. *Sensors and Actuators B: Chemical, 87,* 168–172.

Zhu, L., Yang, R., Zhai, J., & Tian, C., (2007). Bienzymatic glucose biosensor based on co-immobilization of peroxidase and glucose oxidase on a carbon nanotubes electrode. *Biosens. Bioelectron, 23,* 528–535.

Zhu, N., Zhang, A., He, P., & Fang, Y., (2003). Cadmium sulfide nanocluster-based electrochemical stripping detection of DNA hybridization. *The Analyst, 128,* 260–264.

CHAPTER 3

Photonic Crystal Cavity-Based Sensors and Their Potential Applications

THAN SINGH SAINI,[1] AJEET KUMAR,[2] and
RAVINDRA KUMAR SINHA[2,3]

[1]*Optical Functional Materials Laboratory, Toyota Technological Institute, Nagoya–468-8511, Japan, E-mail: tsinghdph@gmail.com*

[2]*TIFAC-Center of Relevance and Excellence in Fiber Optics and Optical Communication, Department of Applied Physics, Delhi Technological University, Delhi–110042, India*

[3]*CSIR-Central Scientific Instrument Organization, Chandigarh–160030, India*

ABSTRACT

The sensor is a device which is used to detect any physical and chemical property of the sample. Recently, optical sensing has gained much credit in different fields including bio-medical, military, environmental monitoring, and industrial process control. Photonic crystals comprise the periodic arrangement of the dielectric pattern and have the competency of guiding and controlling light at the scale of the optical wavelength. During the past several years, photonic crystal sensors have been a most significant research field for the detection of biochemical interactions leveraging electrochemical, optical, electrical, and calorimetric transducing systems. This chapter covers the photonic crystal cavity (PCC)-based sensors and their potential applications in different sorts of sensing including refractive index (RI), biochemical, and gas sensing. The details of the geometrical structure, specific measurement principle, and sensing properties are presented. It is conceivable to get miniature and highly sensitive optical sensors because of the ultra-compact size, exceptional resonant properties, and tractability in the structural design of a PCC. Finally, the crucial difficulties and new directions of photonic crystal cavities for sensing applications are discussed.

3.1   INTRODUCTION

The sensor is a device which is used to detect any physical and chemical properties of the sample. The optical sensing has gained much credit in different fields, including bio-medical, military, environmental monitoring, and industrial process control. Photonic crystals are the periodic arrangement of the dielectric structures (1D, 2D, or 3D) and have the competency of guiding and manipulating light at the subwavelength scale (Joannopoulos et al., 1995; Noda et al., 2000; Yablonovitch, 1987). In the case of three-dimensional photonic crystals with a bandgap, certain frequencies of the light are prohibited from propagating, which is the characteristic to makes them the ultimate devices to control the light. The spontaneous emission of the light can be rigorously forbidden in photonic crystals with the electromagnetic (EM) bandgap which overlaps the electronic band edge (Yablonovitch, 1987). The light photons can be localized in disordered dielectric media (John, 1987). Another fascinating characteristic of the photonic crystals is that the photons can be stored or slowed down by adding an embedded microcavity (Vahala, 2003). Additionally, photonic crystals are suitable to 'mold the flow of light' (Joannopoulos, 1995). In our everyday life, the photonic crystals play a very important role to improve our lives. One of the practical examples of the photonic crystal is the anti-reflective coating on spectacle lenses. The coating on the top surface of the lenses which reduces the reflection is due to the 1-dimensional photonic crystals, generally known as an anti-reflective coating or anti-glare coatings. Anti-reflective coatings improve the vision, make glasses look better, and cause less strain to the eyes. When anti-reflective coating put on the lenses of a camera, it helps in taking great images. Such anti-reflective coatings can be engineered for various other applications, where other parts of the spectrum are required to be transmitted, compared to the transmission of just visible spectrum in the glasses. The photonic crystal fibers are the 2-dimensional photonic crystals which are being used widely in various modern applications. The transverse cross-section of a photonic crystal fiber composed of several periodically placed, closely spaced air holes. The cross-sectional plane is the periodic structures in both the direction. The perpendicular to the plane could run for several meters, and the structure does not change longitudinally. Hence, such a structure is called a 2-dimensional photonic crystal.

A very interesting application of the photonic crystal is to increase the efficiency of incandescent bulbs. An incandescent bulb works on the principle of the restive heating of the tungsten filament sealed inside a glass bulb. The efficiency of the incandescent bulb is very low (2.2%) and most of the energy is wasted. For example, an average 110 W incandescent bulb gives approximately 1300 to 1400 Lumens. This means incandescent bulb provides about 12 Lumens of light per watt. However, the fluorescent lamps can emit approximately 60 Lumens, and some LEDs (light-emitting diodes) can emit up to 150 Lumens per watt. To increase the efficiency of the incandescent bulb, photonic crystal coating can be done on the surface of the bulb, which bounces the infrared radiations back towards the filament of the bulb and let's only light escape out. Using the coating of photonic crystal on the bulb surface, the efficiency can be increased to 40%, which is quite huge and very comparable to efficiency obtained using the best LEDs. Apart from the above-mentioned applications, photonic crystals are very applicable for sensing applications. During the past several years, photonic crystal sensors have been a most significant research topic for the recognition of biochemical interactions leveraging optical, electrical, electrochemical, and calorimetric transducing systems. The light can be strongly confined in the photonic crystal cavities which are finding potential applications in several areas of the physics and engineering, comprising photonic chips, coherent electron-photon interactions, nonlinear optics, and quantum information processing (Noda et al., 2000, b; Khitrova et al., 1999; Painter et al., 1999; Spillane et al., 2002; Michler et al., 2000; Song et al., 2003). The quality factor (Q) of the cavity is a dimensionless parameter which provides the connection between the energy dissipation and stored energy per cycle.

In the case of the cavity materials with no absorption, Q-value can be calculated by the reflection losses at the boundary between the interior and exterior of the photonic crystal cavity (PCC). In general, for light confinement, the phenomena of the total internal reflection (TIR) and the Bragg reflection are used. In the case of the larger cavity (when cavity size is bigger than the wavelength of the light), a very high Q can be achieved (Armani et al., 2003; Vernooy et al., 1998). In this case, when the size of the cavity is considerably larger than the operating wavelength, the behavior of light confined in the cavity obeys the theory of ray optics, and each ray of light reflected at the interface can be designed to fulfill the conditions of TIR or Bragg reflection. However, in the case of smaller cavities (cavity size is comparable or less than the wavelength of light), deviance from the ray optics becomes thoughtful and Q is significantly reduced. The confinement of light in the small cavity containing various plane wave components with wave vectors (k) of several magnitudes and the directions owing to the localization of the light. As it is challenging to design all such plane wave components to follow TIR or Bragg reflection conditions, photonic crystal nanocavities with the high Q values are very important (Akahane et al., 2003). To resolve this problem, one of the best approaches is the addition of Bragg reflection effect in manifold directions. The photonic structures with 2D or 3D periodic variations in the refractive indices on the scale of the wavelength of light are essential for such extension. For the 3D photonic crystals, Bragg reflection conditions can be satisfied for all the propagation directions of the light in a definite range of frequency, known as the photonic bandgap. The defect or disorder created into the 3D photonic crystal would become a crucial photonic crystal nano-cavity with large Q value. The strong confinement and high Q gives rise to an optical mode with the resonant wavelength, which is very sensitive to the local changes in their surrounding medium and hence make PCCs a proficient building block for application of highly sensitive and ultra-compact optical sensing devices. However, the fabrication of 3-D photonic crystals with strong confinement of light is very difficult. The cavity surrounded by the 2-D photonic crystal is considered a practical solution. Within the 2-D photonic crystal structures, the cavity can be designed by hosting point defects in the arranged lattice. The PCC exhibits very strong special and temporal confinement of light and high Q (Lalanne et al., 2008). There is a very strong interaction between the material and the optical field within the PCC. The enhancement in the interaction effect provides the PCC mode with a resonating wavelength which is very sensitive to the indigenous variations in its neighboring medium and builds PCC a capable candidate for highly sensitive optical sensors (Chakravarty et al., 2014). The active sensing region of the PCC is typically micrometer in size which supplies an unconventional sensing platform for real-time observation with the smart-design. However, there are some vital problems in the practical use of the PCC as a sensor. The difficulty in efficiently coupling of the light from a traditional single-mode optical fiber into PCC device is one of the major challenges for the practical applications of PCC (Zou et al., 2014). The most common method to decrease the coupling loss is to introduce photonic crystal waveguides on both sides of the PCC (Yang et al., 2013). The light is firstly radiated from the conventional single-mode fiber to the photonic crystal waveguide and then transmitted through the photonic crystal waveguide to PCC. The coupling loss, in general, can be significantly diminished by a precise lineup of the traditional fiber with the photonic crystal device through the accurate designing of the coupling interface and an adjustable mechanical device. The second difficulty is the thermal dependent refractive index (RI) of the silicon. The resonant wavelength of the silicon-based photonic crystal sensors depends on the external temperature (Chang et al., 2012). In practical applications, to exclude the undesired variations, a precision temperature controller is required, which increase the size and budget of the PCC sensor. In this direction, Karnutsch et al. reported a temperature-insensitive PCC sensor. The sensor was based on optofluidic technology (2009). Nevertheless, the operation of the optofluidic infiltrated PCC may also reduce the tractability of the PCC in structural design. Another difficulty in the PCC based sensor is the stability of resonant wavelength against fabrication errors. Currently, using the state-of-the-art fabrication technology, we can control the position of air hole by 1 nm and the size of the air holes by 2–4 nm in the photonic crystals (Faolain et al., 2007; Beggs et al., 2008). The Q value of the PCC is significantly reduced even at 1 nm error introduced in the radius of the air holes (Hagina et al., 2009).

As illustrated in Figure 3.1, the 2D photonic crystal cavities may be of various kind including (a) H0 cavity; (b) L4 cavity; (c) ring cavity; (d) shoulder-coupled photonic cavity. In 2D photonic crystals cavities with thickness of the order of the wavelength of light, the optical confinement can be achieved in both the plane and vertical directions (Noda et al., 2000b; Song et al., 2003).

In this chapter, an impression of the PCCs based optical sensors is provided. The rest of the chapter is organized as follows: In Section 3.2, the photonic crystal structures and their fabrication methods are described. Section 3.3 provides the potential applications of PCs in different fields. The principle of sensing with PCCs is provided in Section 3.4. The detailed study of a bi-periodic photonic crystal waveguide structure is given for optofluidic-gas sensing application in Section 3.5. The conclusion is provided in Section 3.6.

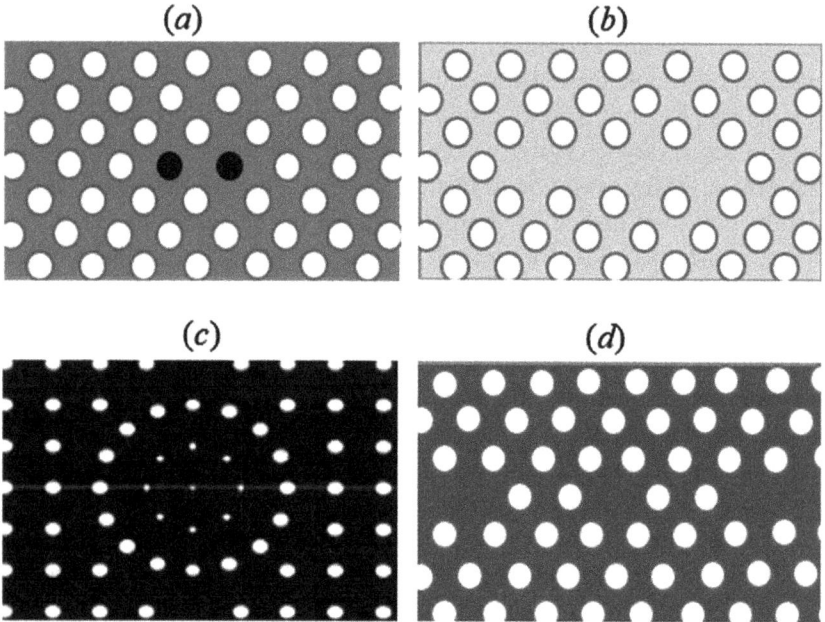

FIGURE 3.1 Various kind of photonic crystal cavities: (a) two air holes are replaced by high index rods (H0 cavity); (b) four missing air holes (L4 cavity); (c) ring cavity; (d) shoulder-coupled photonic cavity.

3.2 PHOTONIC CRYSTAL STRUCTURES AND THEIR FABRICATION METHODS

Photonic crystals are the periodic structures in 1-, 2-, and 3-dimensions with the periodicity of the order of the wavelength of light. In the traditional crystal structures, there is a periodic arrangement of the atoms or molecules. The structure of the photonic crystals is also similar, but in place of an atom, there are several 1,000 atoms. Photonic crystals would reflect certain wavelengths and let some other wavelengths pass through. This would make them appear of a certain color corresponding to the reflected wavelength. The energy associated with this certain wavelength which is prevented from being propagated through the crystal is called the photonic bandgap. Also, an important thing to remember is that photonic crystals may appear differently colored from different angles due to a directional band gap this is mostly a property of 2D photonic crystals. In the simplest type of the photonic crystal, there is a hexagonal pattern of air holes in the cross-section. The central air hole is missing to form the core. In the core the light guides. The core is a single vacancy defect in the crystals. Nature provides us with various kinds of photonic crystal nanostructured surfaces. The dazzling color of the feathers of butterfly and peacock feathers, *Eupholus magnificus* insect, sea mouse, and opals are due to the special geometrical preparation on their surfaces, where the broadband light reflects and illuminates through the photonic structures (Kinoshita et al., 2002; Zi et al., 2003; Pouya et al., 2011; McPhedran et al., 2003). The photonic crystal structure can be fabricated in 1-D, 2-D, and 3-D orientations using the diverse range of materials including silicon, glass, polymers, colloids, and silk (Vahala, 2003; Russel, 2003; Winn et al., 1998; Pacholski, 2013; Jamois et al., 2003; Freeman et al., 2008; Edrington et al., 2011; Gonzalez-Urbina et al., 2012; MacLeod and Rosei, 2013; Kim et al., 2012; Diao et al., 2013). The various fabrication techniques of the photonic crystals are provided in subsections.

3.2.1 COLLOIDAL SELF-ASSEMBLY METHOD

The self-assembly method is the broadly used method to produce ordered structures of the colloidal particles. The colloidal particles are arranged by engineering the intercolloid potential. In this technique, the colloids consist of silica, polymers, or polystyrene are relocated from the solution and self-assembled using evaporation, spin-coating, sedimentation, or vertical deposition on a surface to create photonic crystal structures that impersonate rainbow-like colors (Kang et al., 2008; Rogach et al., 2000; Liu et al., 2008; Zhang et al., 2009; Norris et al., 2004). Gravity sedimentation of colloids from dispersions and the lateral assembly of colloidal particles by an alternating electric field are some other techniques to achieve similar kinds of self-assembled 2D crystal layers (Miguez et al., 1998; Xie et al., 2008). The self-assembled colloidal spheres are used to make artificial opals which have a lot of research attention as photonic crystals, as the components of solar cells, light sources as well as in the field of plasmonics, and chemical sensors. Xu et al. provided an extensive review of the colloidal self-assembly method and distinctive applications of the colloidal self-assembly methods in the biological and optics and fields (Xu et al., 2016). In the surface evaporation-induced self-assembly, the colloidal crystals are prepared. The colloidal suspension is put on the clean surface of the substrate then the colloidal particles are self-assembled into the 2-D or 3-D close-packed colloidal crystals through the regulated pressure, humidity, temperature, and other circumstances. Several typical self-assembly based methods including spin coating, interface, physical templet, EM induced, and self-assembly is driven by noncovalent interactions (Xu et al., 2016). Here in this chapter, the physical templet self-assembly process is provided in subsections.

3.2.1.1   PHYSICAL TEMPLET SELF-ASSEMBLY

The physical templates with high accuracy can be made-up by photolithography, electronic etching, reactive ion etching, and focused ion beam etching techniques. Lin and coworkers have explored the self-assembly of the colloidal spheres and demonstrated the various type of 2-D self-assembly photonic structures by merging entropic depletion and patterned template (Lin et al., 2000). The period and the well-defined shape of a patterned nanoparticle film can be organized by the interferometric lithography. The thickness of the film of the nanoparticles (NPs) can be tuned using the spin coating. Dai and co-workers have demonstrated patterned template self-assembly arranged by photolithography of Ferrimagnetic NPs into pillars or ring assemblies over a large area (>1 cm^2) by spin coating, as illustrated in Figures 3.2 and 3.3 (Dai et al., 2013). Such an approach enables large production rate self-assembly for the future cutting-edge photonic device creation and can also be used for other nanoparticle systems. The self-assembly of the NPs into multifarious geometries can be obtained by a least set of the post guiding topographies patterned of the substrate.

3.2.2   SILICONE METHOD

In the silicone method, first of all, the glass slides (i.e., substrate) is put in the plasma cleaner for approximately 5 minutes. The aqueous dispersions of PB beads are placed on the glass slides. Then the liquid film is covered with the silicone liquid and the sample is placed on the hot plate until the water is evaporated. After that, the liquid silicone is removed by Kim-Wipe. Now, the crystal is to put in the elastomer PDMS matrix. PDMS fills the voids, expanding or contracting depending on the environmental change.

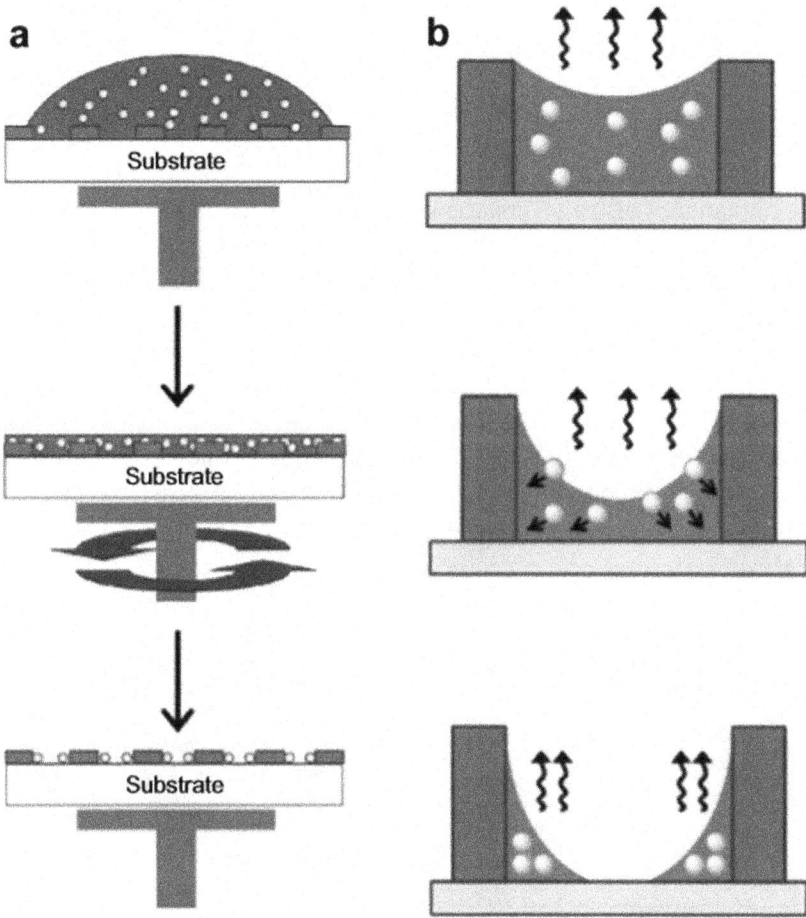

FIGURE 3.2 (a) Representative sketch of the evaporation self-assembly method on the pattern substrates during spin-coating. (b) The illustrative figure of the single hole which demonstrations the details of evaporation.

Source: Reproduced with permission from: Dai et al. (2013). © American Chemical Society.

3.2.3 LITHOGRAPHIC FABRICATION TECHNIQUES

3.2.3.1 ELECTRON-BEAM LITHOGRAPHY

Electron-beam lithography is mostly used method for the prototype and research purposes. In the electron-beam lithography, the structures are inscribed directly into the photoresist using a focused beam of electrons (Ampere et al., 2003; Broers et al., 1996; Vieu et al., 2000). The elementary idea is to etch the cross-section of the photonic crystal pattern onto the substrate and fill the etched holes with the silica and then deposit an additional layer of the substrate. This process recurs for the individually anticipated cross-section of the photonic crystal pattern. Afterward the desired number of the layers, the silica is dissolved, leaving the photonic crystal structure which has a photonic bandgap. This technique is capable of defining extremely small features. The advantages of this technique are that since an individual hole must be obtained chronologically, it is natural to deliberately host the defects into the design by simply neglecting to etch a certain hole on a specific level. This process, however, is very costly and slow because everything is written serially. Therefore, electron-beam lithography is not suitable for mass production. The main benefit of electron-beam lithography is that it can draw customize patterns (direct-write) with <10 nm resolution by careful optimization of processes (Vieu et al., 2000).

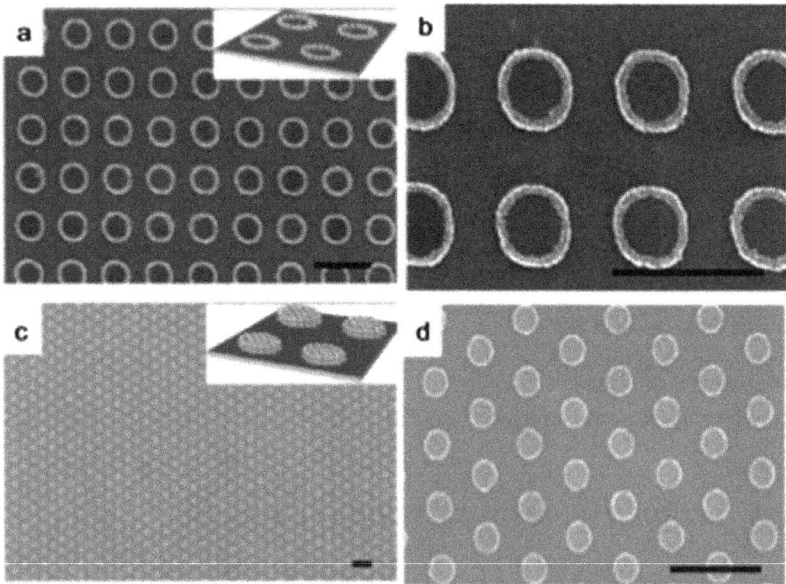

FIGURE 3.3 The SEM images of nano-rings (a, b) and nano-pillars; (c, d) after removing the templating photoresist. All scale bars are 1 μm.

Source: Reproduced with permission from: Dai et al. (2013). © American Chemical Society.

3.2.3.2   DEEP UV LITHOGRAPHY

Deep ultraviolet (UV) lithography is the extension of the optical lithography into the deep UV wavelengths range (248 nm or less) (Bogaerts et al., 2002). This technique offers high resolution as well as the speed essential for the mass production of the photonic integrated circuits. In this technique, a silicon-on-insulator (SOI) wafer is coated with the resist. The resist is prebaked and NFC antireflective coating is spun on the top of it. The wafer is illuminated in the steeper and then post-exposure bake. After the development, the wafer is prepared for etching. For mass production, the parallel process that can print several patterns, is needed. Conventional optical lithography has been the pillar for this purpose, but optical diffraction is its limitation. For photonic crystal structures, optical lithography enforces a limit on the periodicity of the structure. Therefore, the new type of optical lithography uses excimer lasers (wavelengths lie in deep UV). Using UV light, it is feasible to fabricate photonic structures of the dimensions below 100 nm. The smallest period of the photonic crystal structure that can be fabricated is demarcated as the ratio of operating wavelength to the numerical aperture of the lens system used. Using the lens system with a numerical aperture of 0.6 or more and 248 nm UV laser, the period is approximately 400 nm.

3.2.3.3   NANOIMPRINT LITHOGRAPHY

In nanoimprint lithography, a lithographic configuration is primarily manufactured using a deep UV or electron-beam lithography on a master mold that can be simply reassigned to the daughter reproductions. The principle of the nanoimprint lithography is based on the mechanical modification of the polymer resist using the template (stamp or mold) containing the nano/micropattern in a UV curing or thermos-mechanical process. Nanoimprinting lithography does not need multifarious and overpriced optics and light sources for creating the images. This technique is the fast, modest, and accessible pattern relocation technique alternative to electron-beam lithography (Kouba et al., 2006). The nanoimprinting lithography provides micro to nanometer scale patterns with the high resolution, high production rate, and the small cost. Since the direct mechanical deformation of resist takes place in the nanoimprinting lithography process, one can obtain the resolution beyond the diffraction limit that is encountered in conventional methods. However, the most important challenges of nanoimprinting lithography are the 1×mask/template fabrication and alignment. The eventual resolution of the patterns fabricated by nanoimprinting lithography is determined by the resolution of the features on the template surface. The discrete features of nanoimprinting lithography are the direct mechanical deformation of the resist and the contact nature of the process. In comparison to other lithography techniques, the particular advantage of nanoimprinting lithography technique is the ability of large-area fabrication and the complex 3-D micro/nanostructures with high production rate and low cost. In recent years, a lot of new nanoimprint lithography process including laser-assisted direct imprint, soft UV-nanoimprint lithography, electrical field, chemical nanoimprint, assisted nanoimprinting, etc., have been investigated.

3.3   PHOTONIC CRYSTALS FOR POTENTIAL SENSING APPLICATIONS

3.3.1   TELEMEDICINE

It is an enormous requirement for the manageable, robust, economical, and easy-to-use virus/illness analysis and prediction observing platforms to share the health confirmation at the point-of-living which includes clinical and home settings. Current development in digital health technologies has upgraded drug management and custom-made medication. Nowadays, smartphones with the high-resolution cameras are being used in the medical diagnostics and healthcare applications including imaging, cell counting from the whole body, and immunoassay testing (Yetisen et al., 2014; Zhang et al., 2016; Inan et al., 2017; Baday et al., 2015; Hu et al., 2016). For example: a 1-D photonic crystal slab can be integrated with the smartphone to measure the concentration of immunoglobulin gamma (IgG) molecules. The smartphone has been engaged not only as a reader for the microfluidic analyzes but also as an analyzer for physiological indexes. It is reported that a transportable imaging magnetic raising system white and red blood cells can be recognized and the cell numbers can be computed without using any labels (Baday et al., 2015). The leading causes of death in the world are due to cardiovascular diseases. About four in every five deaths happen in the middle and low-income countries. The cardiovascular diseases are escapable and curable and chiefly dependent on the timely and effective interventions such as therapeutic monitoring, prognosis, and diagnosis. However, in the present situation, these interventions offer very high-cost and in general lacking in middle and low-income countries. Recently, the smartphone-based readout for microfluidic assays has been reported and shown that a smartphone can be used for cardiovascular diseases (Hu et al., 2016). In the future, it is expected that a smartphone integrated with other devices can be capable of examining diseases, functioning blood tests, and imaging.

3.3.2 MICROFLUIDICS

Microfluidic technology integrated with photonic crystals is emerging as powerful bio-sensing diagnostic tools (Xiao and Mortensen, 2006; Fan and White, 2011). In the bio-sensing devices, microfluidic technology provides significant benefits. Some of them include inexpensive materials (glass, polymers, and papers) to fabricate the microfluidic channels, the capability to control low sample volume, flexibility in the production of multiple channels to permit multiplexed testing platforms, and easiness in the integration with the optical platforms (Schudel et al., 2009; Yetisen et al., 2013; Wang et al., 2014). Using the nano-replica molding process, polymer microfluidic channels with united label-free photonic crystal biosensors has been made-up (Choi and Cunningham, 2007). This system was established by measuring the kinetic binding interaction of protein A with IgG molecules.

3.3.3 SMART MATERIALS

Smart materials of advanced materials including carbon nanotubes (CNTs), graphene (GN), and polyinonic liquids are the multifunctional materials which can regulate their physical or chemical possessions, characteristically reversibly, against external stimuli such as electrical field, temperature, magnetic field, pH, and the light (Mastronardi et al., 2014; Verma et al., 2016). Numerous functionalities can be obtained in miniaturized devices using the smart materials that respond to the changes in their ambiances. Such multifunctional materials incorporated into the photonic crystal structures are most capable of highly sensitive, reliable, and rapid biosensing applications and drug delivery. For example, piezoelectric advanced materials can sense and monitor vibrational energy and reply by producing electrical energy to the power devices (Anton and Sodano, 2007; Pan et al., 2011).

Some smart materials are being industrialized that can change their shape with respect to stress, temperature, and magnetic field fluctuations. Photonic crystal incorporated in hydrogel materials (i.e., 3-D nanostructured polymers which mostly consist of water) provides either qualitative detection of bio target concentrations or quantitative spectral responses (Yetisen et al., 2014). A reusable optical glucose nano-sensor relevant to clinical purposes has been developed with high accuracy (Yetisen et al., 2014). Hydrogel materials can be responsible for external stimulation such as the interaction between antigen-antibody, pH, and temperature (Kang et al., 2008; Fenzl et al., 2013; Chiappelli et al., 2012; Yetisen et al., 2016; Cai et al., 2016; Yang et al., 2008). To fabricate photonic structures, the hydrogels can also be used in amalgamation with another material including GN or CNTs. A Se-doped MoS_2 nanosheet can improve hydrogen evolution reaction (Ren et al., 2015). Beta-glucan in oats can be determined by hosting GN oxide hydrogels in 1-D photonic crystals with a polyaniline defect layer (Ren et al., 2015b). GN-based 1-D photonic crystal can be used as an encouraging replacement of the metallic thin film as a sensor head for the application of future biosensing (Sreekanth et al., 2013). Additionally, CNTs incorporated onto the photonic crystal structures provide a photonic bandgap in the visible region of the EM structure. The multifunctional or smart materials have been extensively studied for potential applications in biosensing because of the unique properties of each material.

3.3.4   WEARABLE AND FLEXIBLE SENSORS

Nowadays, for the real-time and continuous observation of the physiological parameters and the health status of any individuals, wearable sensors and the smart materials have attracted a lot of attention (Tao et al., 2012; Olguin et al., 2009; Appelboom et al., 2014; Luo et al., 2014; Yao et al., 2014; Vilela et al., 2016). The physiological parameters include heart rate, blood oxygen level, skin temperature, and sweat glucose. A wearable sweat pH and skin temperature sensing system with a wireless interface and the body coupling via a smart textile has been presented (Caldara et al., 2013). Such wearable sensors can be used to the high risks patients for the observation of the hydration in a home-care environment. A wide range of the wearable bio and electrochemical sensors have been reported for immediate non-invasive observing of electrolytes and metabolites in the breath, sweat, tears, and saliva as indicators of the status of health of the human (Bandodkar and Wang, 2014; Matzeu et al., 2016). Non-invasive biosensors and electrochemical sensors find substantial use in an extensive range of potential personal health monitoring, sport, and military applications.

3.3.5 METAMATERIALS

The optical technology-based biosensors offer noteworthy openings in the field of biomedical research and clinical diagnostics for the revealing very small number of molecules present in the highly diluted solutions. The metamaterials based photonic crystal structures have remains a great interest for potential applications including biosensing and imaging (Ahmed et al., 2016; Aristov et al., 2016; Sreekanth et al., 2016; Parimi et al., 2003). An extremely high sensitivity (>2600 nm/RIU) can be obtained using 3-D plasmon crystal metamaterials (Aristov et al., 2016). A hyperbolic metamaterial-based miniaturized plasmonic biosensor with 16 alternating layer of Al_2O_3 and gold layers has been reported (Sreekanth et al., 2016). This one-dimensional multilayer photonic structure support plasmon modes for a broadband spectral range from visible to the near-infrared range with the sensitivity of 30000 nm/RIU and figure of merit (FOM) of 590 (Sreekanth et al., 2016). Such highly sensitive sensors have a potential milestone in the development of plasmonic biosensing technology. The unique feature of imaging can be obtained using a flat lens based on negative refraction in a photonic crystalline material (Parimi et al., 2003). Such features of the photonic crystals are based on their design with the proper dispersion profile to obtained negative refraction for the wide range of angles (Luo et al., 2002). Metamaterial-based biosensing provides label-free detection with high sensitivity. The integration of the photonic crystal structure with the emerging technologies is capable of biosensing applications with higher sensitivity at the point-of-care due to flexible, compact, and easy-to-use platforms.

3.4   PRINCIPLE OF SENSING WITH PHOTONIC CRYSTAL CAVITY (PCC)

For evaluation of the ability of any gas sensor, the detection limit and the sensitivity are two important parameters. The sensitivity of the sensor is demarcated as the ratio of the shift in resonance wavelength ($\Delta\lambda$) to the alteration in the gas concentration (ΔC) and represented as:

$$S = \frac{\Delta\lambda}{\Delta C} = \frac{\Delta\lambda}{\Delta n} \times \frac{\Delta n}{\Delta C} = S_n \times S_c \qquad (1)$$

where; S indicates the sensitivity, S_n denotes the shift in wavelength due to RI variation, and S_C represents the variation in RI due to the variation in the concentration of gas. The detection limit (D) of any gas sensor is defined as the minimum detectable variations of the concentration by any sensor, and can be expressed as the following relation:

$$D = \frac{\Delta\lambda_{min}}{S} = \frac{\lambda/Q}{S_n \times S_c} \qquad (2)$$

where; $\Delta\lambda_{min} = \lambda/Q$ signifies the minimum shift in the wavelength which can be detected by the sensor and equal to the linewidth of the resonant peak, λ indicates the central resonant wavelength of the output spectrum, and Q represents the quality factor of the PCC. Then Eqn. (2) indicates that the smaller value of D can be achieved by increasing the S_n and Q. The Transmittance (T) is also one of the important parameters of any PCC structure. The transmittance of any PCC governs the measurement precision of the sensing system in applied applications. If the coupling losses between PCC and the single-mode fibers are considered, the transmittance will be decreased. For the output signal less than 10%, there is a chance of embedding it in the background noise and the decrement in the detection precision of the sensing system. Also, the coupling losses are typically more than 30%. Therefore, the theoretical value of the transmittance should be more than 40%. For any sensor, if the value of ($S_n \times Q$) is larger, the sensing capability of the sensing system is better.

3.5   PHOTONIC CRYSTAL CAVITY (PCC)-BASED OPTICAL SENSORS

3.5.1   *PHOTONIC CRYSTAL MICROCAVITY FOR METHANE (CH$_4$) SENSING*

Methane (CH$_4$) gas is an inflammable gas with an enormously low volatile limit of 5% in the air. Methane gas conveys a noteworthy explosion hazard in coal mines and it is responsible for the greenhouse effect and global warming in the atmosphere. Therefore, it is very essential to create a high-sensitive gas sensor for precise measurement of the concentration of methane gas to ensure the level of methane gas below the safety limit in the environment. To improve the sensitivity of low concentration gases, the interaction time of the light and gases can be radically enhanced by an optical resonator. During the previous several years, plentiful gas sensors which are based on the microresonators such as photonic crystal resonant microcavity, whispering gallery mode sensors, and surface plasmon resonance (SPR) have been reported. The photonic crystal microcavity based sensors have fascinated the most attention in the recent year. A PCC exhibiting strong field confinement and high-quality factor can be shaped by hosting point defects in the periodic dielectric lattices. For the housing gas analysis, the air holes in the periodic microstructure are the natural candidate. There will be a change in the RI of the air holes with the variation in the concentration of infiltrated gas. Therefore, the resonant wavelength of the PCC will be shift from its actual resonant wavelength. A highly sensitive, miniaturized, and high precision methane gas sensor has been demonstrated using a cryptophane-E-infiltrated photonic crystal microcavity (Zhang et al., 2015). The proposed experimental setup and the representation diagram of the photonic crystal microcavity based sensor is illustrated in Figures 3.4(a) and (b), respectively. The cryptophane-E RI changes only with the deviation in the concentration of methane gas according to the relation, $n = 1.448–0.46$ C; (where n is the RI of cryptophane-E at its particular concentration C). As illustrated in Figure 3.4(b), a photonic crystal microcavity structure is designed on the SOI platform. The lattice constant, $a = 351$ nm, radius of the bulk air holes, $r = 0.3 \times a$, the thickness of the photonic crystal slab, $r = 0.6 \times a$. The photonic crystal microcavity is formed by growing a central defected holes with radii of r_1 (= 0.45 × a). Additionally, some air holes from the central row along the x-direction have symmetrically removed to improve the coupling efficiency between the ridge waveguide and the photonic crystal microcavity. The length of the central photonic crystal waveguide is denoted by L. The principle of sensing is based on the shift in the resonant wavelength with the variations in the methane gas concentration.

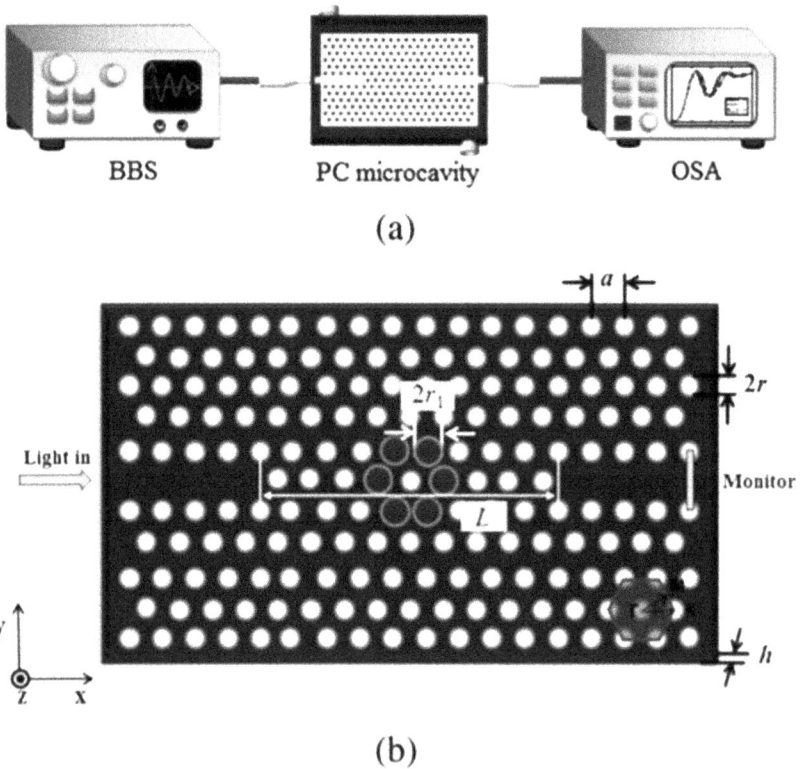

(a)

(b)

FIGURE 3.4   (a) The schematic of the methane gas sensor that is based on cryptophane-E infiltrated photonic crystal microcavity; and (b) the detailed configuration of cryptophane-E infiltrated photonic crystal microcavity.

Source: Reproduced with permission from: Zhang, Zhao, and Wanga (2015). © Elsevier.

To investigate the sensing concert of the photonic crystal microcavity based CH_4 gas sensor, the transmission spectra for various refractive indices of the defected holes was simulated. The simulated normalized transmission spectra of the photonic crystal microcavity are depicted in Figure 3.5(a) for numerous refractive indices of defected holes ranging from 1.40 to 1.45 with an increment of $\Delta n = 0.01$. Moreover, the distinction inclinations of the resonant wavelength and the Q value with the variation the RI are illustrated in Figure 3.5(b). The transmission characteristics of the photonic crystal microcavity reach up to 84.5%, which indicates that the propagation loss of the photonic crystal microcavity is insignificant. As depicted from Figure 3.5(b) that the resonating wavelength shifts towards the higher wavelength on increasing the RI of the defected holes increases. The magnitude of the transmittance remains unaltered within the whole series of the RI deviations. The variation in the RI of the air holes under the effect of a certain concentration of the CH_4 gas will impact on the effective RI of the waveguide and the photonic band structure because of the change of RI modification between Si substrate and the air holes. Both the effects, including the change in photonic band structure and the change in the effective RI of the waveguide, lead to a shift in the resonating wavelength in the same direction. For this photonic crystal microcavity structure, the increment in the RI of the air holes leads to a redshift of the resonant wavelength. The Q factor maintains its stability and does not degrade significantly on increasing the RI of the holes. For this photonic crystal microcavity-based gas sensor, the calculated refractive index sensitivity (RIS) S_n and the Q factor are about 135.65 nm/RIU and around 6203, respectively. Such a gas sensor establishes the opportunity of the cryptophane-E infiltrated photonic crystal microcavity for the potential application of CH_4 gas sensing.

3.5.2 PHOTONIC CRYSTAL BI-PERIODIC WAVEGUIDE FOR OPTOFLUIDIC-GAS SENSOR

The RI based optical sensors can be realized using the micro-rings, Mach-Zehnder interferometers, directional couplers, and photonic crystals. The photonic crystal provides a better platform for the realization of RI optical sensors because it offers a very low loss and high Q resonant cavity. A PCC-based bi-periodic waveguide structure was proposed for optofluidic-gas sensing (Kumar et al., 2015).

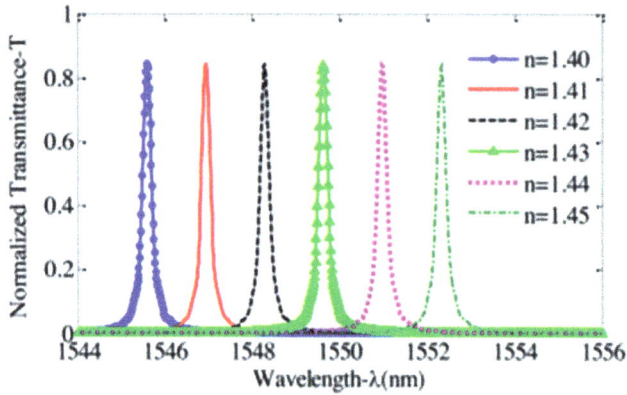

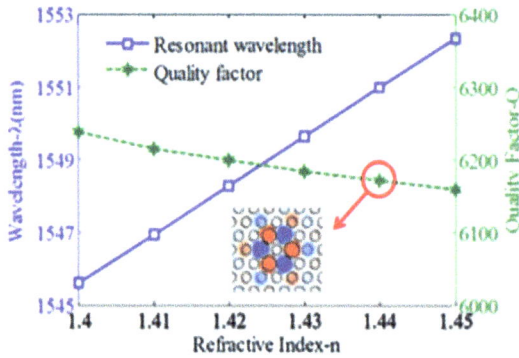

FIGURE 3.5 (a) The transmission spectrum of the photonic crystal microcavity with various infiltrated refractive indices. (b) Resonant wavelength and quality factor of photonic crystal microcavity (r1 = 0.45a, L = 9a) when the RI varying from 1.40 to 1.45 with the increment of $\Delta n = 0.01$.

Source: Reproduced with permission from: Zhang, Zhao, and Wanga (2015). © Elsevier.

3.5.2.1   SENSOR DESIGN

The schematic of the PCC-based sensor is shown in Figure 3.6. The structure of the sensor consists of a 2-dimensional waveguide with a triangular lattice of circular air holes. The importance of triangular lattice pattern of the air holes in the photonic crystal is that it provides large transverse electric (TE) bandgap and can be integrated along with other optoelectronic devices (Jamols et al., 2002). As shown in Figure 3.6, arrays of the air holes are arranged in a triangular lattice pattern in silicon substrate. The original photonic crystal consists of a finite array of 17×15 air holes on a silicon (Si: n = 3.5) substrate. The lattice periodicity is considered as '*a* (*a* = 428 nm).' A waveguide is fashioned by eradicating one row of air holes along the Γ-K direction. In order to form an array of super cavities, the radii of the air holes just next to waveguide sides are modulated at the alternate position. As illustrated in Figure 3.7, each super cavity possesses three air holes with a central air hole radius modulated. The size of the central air hole is kept larger than that of the other holes. The periodicity of the air holes in a single line of either side of the waveguide is considered as '*a'* (*a'* = 856 nm)' and thus creating a bi-periodic photonic crystal waveguide structure. In this way, the photonic crystal structure consists of two different sizes of the air holes of the radii of $R_1 = 0.35 \times a$ and $R_2 = 0.4 \times a$ with a lattice constant of *a* = 428 nm. In order to get a resonant mode in the photonic crystal structure, the radius of larger air holes, R_2 has been optimized. The light is coupled to the photonic crystal waveguide at one end and its transmission spectrum is obtained at the other end of the photonic crystal waveguide. The resonance wavelength of the mode supported by the cavity depends upon the local RI in the vicinity of the cavity and the structural parameters. If all the holes of the super cavities have been filled with an analyte, there is a variation in the local RI of the super cavities which shifts the resonance wavelength. The amount of the wavelength shift divided by the variation in RI provides the sensitivity of the device. The change in the resonance wavelength is given by the relation:

$$\Delta\lambda = \lambda_0 \frac{\Delta n}{n_0} \tag{3}$$

where; Δn represents the change in the RI of super cavities, *n* provides the initial RI of the super cavities, λ indicates the initial resonating wavelength, and $\Delta\lambda$ is the change in resonating wavelength when *n* changes to n+ Δn.

3.5.2.2   SIMULATION RESULTS

The numerical analysis was performed using a finite difference time domain method (FDTD). First of all, the resonant mode of super-cavity was simulated. After that, the size of the bigger holes (with radius R_2 in Figure 3.7) was varied to obtained resonant mode. It has been found

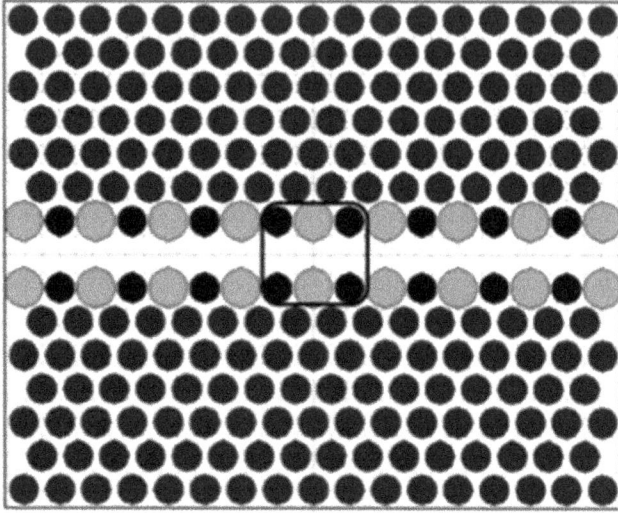

FIGURE 3.6   Schematic of the photonic crystal cavity RI and gas sensor.
Source: Reproduced with permission from: Kumar, Saini, and Sinha (2015). © Elsevier.

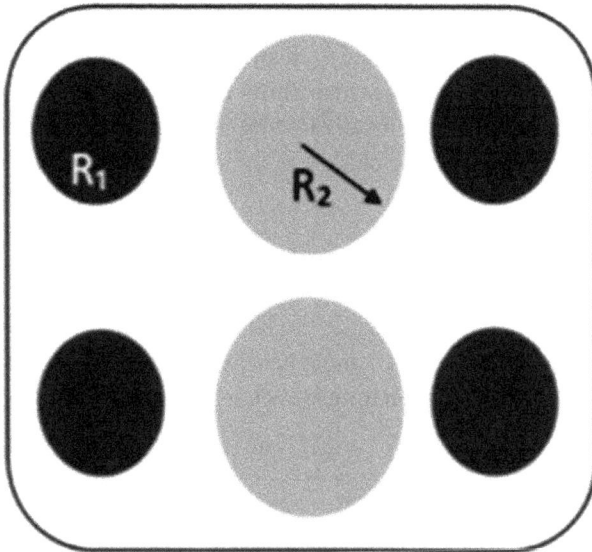

FIGURE 3.7   The super cavity which has been formed by changing the radius of one middle air hole on each side of the waveguide region.
Source: Reproduced with permission from: Kumar, Saini, and Sinha (2015). © Elsevier.

that the resonant mode can be excited when $R_2 = 0.4 \times a$ at the resonant wavelength of 1550 nm. In order to form the array of supercities along the waveguide structure, alternate air holes were modified with $R_2 = 0.4 \times a$. The simulated transmission spectrum for the bi-periodic waveguide structure is found to have a Lorentzian response with maximum transmission of 91.74%. It was found that the bi-periodic waveguide structure only allows the resonance wavelength to pass through the waveguide and reflects the other wavelengths. Figure 3.8 illustrates the magnetic field distribution for the sensor at the resonance wavelength of 1550 nm. The principle involved in the RI sensing is based on the shift of the resonant wavelength of supercavities. When infiltrated with gases or liquids, the super cavity can be used as a local sensor. Based on the RI of the gases or liquids, there would be corresponding resonant wavelengths. In the analysis, two schemes were employed to carry out the investigation of the bi-periodic sensor. In the first scheme, the refractive indices of all the holes in the super cavity were varied while, in the second case, refractive indices of the holes at the alternate position were varied.

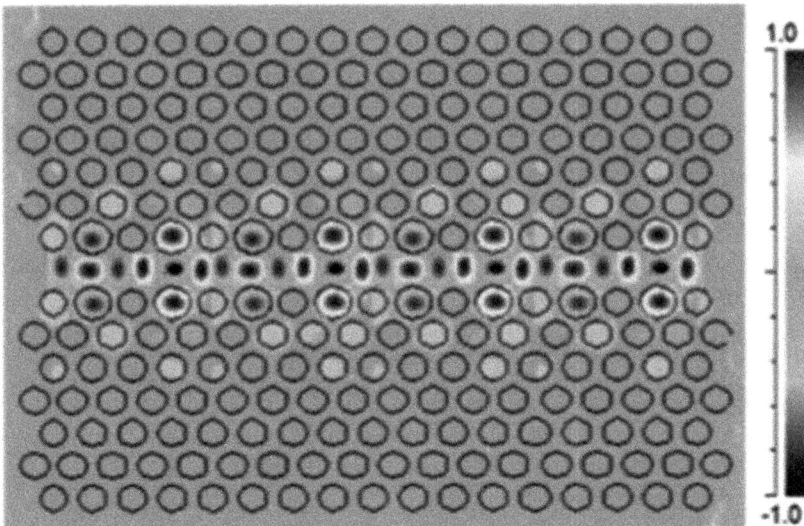

FIGURE 3.8   The distribution of the magnetic field in bi-periodic sensor at the resonance wavelength of 1550 nm.

Source: Reproduced with permission from: Kumar, Saini, and Sinha (2015). © Elsevier.

3.5.2.2.1   Case I: When All the Air Holes of Supercavities Have Been Filled with Analyte

The resonance wavelength of the mode supported by the cavity depends upon the local RI in the vicinity of the cavity and geometric parameters of the structure. In the first case, when all the air holes of the super cavity were filled with an analyte, there is a net alteration in the local RI of the super cavity which is responsible for the change in resonant wavelength. The shift in the resonant wavelength is according to the Eqn. (1). As illustrated in Figure 3.9, the simulated results show that the shift in the resonance wavelength is obtained approximately 0.061 nm for $\Delta n = 0.0001$. The calculated sensitivity is 610 nm/RIU. Even at the smallest change in the RI of the order of 10^{-4} leading to the high sensitivity of the structure. Such high sensitivity is suitable for gas sensing applications. The change in the resonant wavelength shift [i.e., $\Delta\lambda=\lambda(n)-\lambda(air)$] as the function of the ambient RI is illustrated in Figure 3.10. The calculated wavelength shift is 61 pm for $\Delta n = 10^{-4}$ with the detection limit of 1.002.

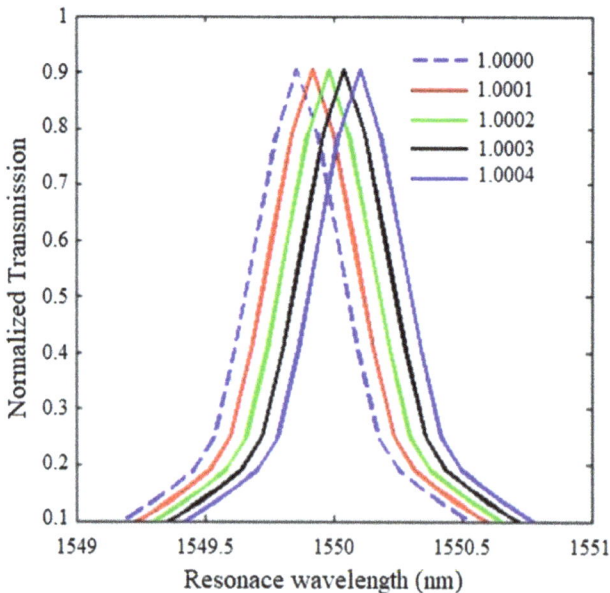

FIGURE 3.9   Normalized transmission spectra of the sensor with five different refractive indices of supercavities.

Source: Reproduced with permission from: Kumar, Saini, and Sinha (2015). © Elsevier.

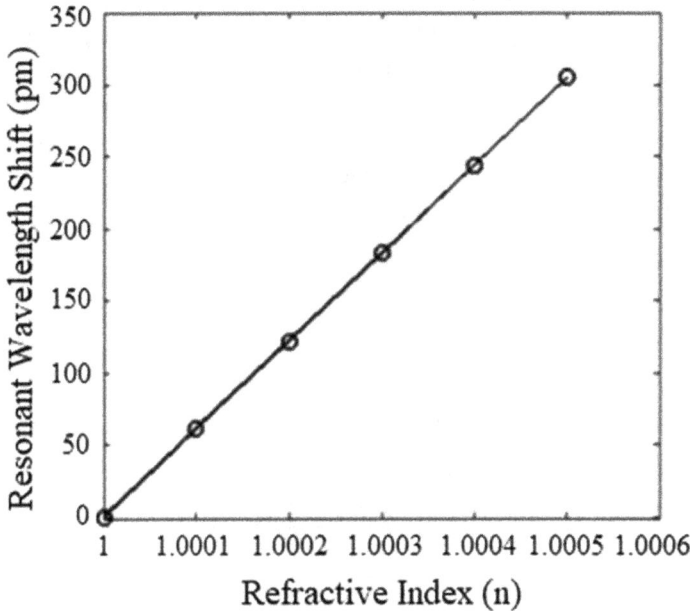

FIGURE 3.10 Resonant wavelength shift with the ambient refractive index.
Source: Reproduced with permission from: Kumar, Saini, and Sinha (2015). © Elsevier.

3.5.2.2.2 *Case II: When Only Larger Air Holes of Supercavities Have Been Filled with Analyte*

In the second scheme, in spite of filling all the air holes of supercities only larger air holes at the alternate position were infiltrated with the analyte. The principle is the same in this case also; there is a change in the local RI of the supercavities which is responsible for shifts the resonant wavelength. The simulation results show that the sensitivity is decreased dramatically in this case. As shown in Figure 3.11, the resonant wavelength shifts up to 0.3 nm for the change in RI $\Delta\lambda = 0.001$ with a wider spectral range of 1.0 to 1.5. The sensor sensitivity is 300 nm/RIU. Figure 3.12 illustrates the variation in the shift of the resonant wavelength as a function of the ambient RI. The shift in the wavelength is 0.3 nm for $\Delta\lambda = 0.001$ with RI range of 1.0 to 1.5. For better sensitivity of the photonic crystal waveguide sensor based on dispersive properties of the waveguide, the filling fraction of the holes filled with the analyte must be larger. But in this case, by merely filling in larger holes, sensitivity of 300 nm/RIU is obtained, which in turn means the requirement of the smaller volume of an analyte over conventional waveguide-based sensors. Also, the photonic crystal structure with supercavities is extra sensitive to the variation in RI. When these supercavities are arranged to form a complete waveguide, there is no coupling loss from the waveguide to the cavity, thus offering a wider measurement range of refractive sensing.

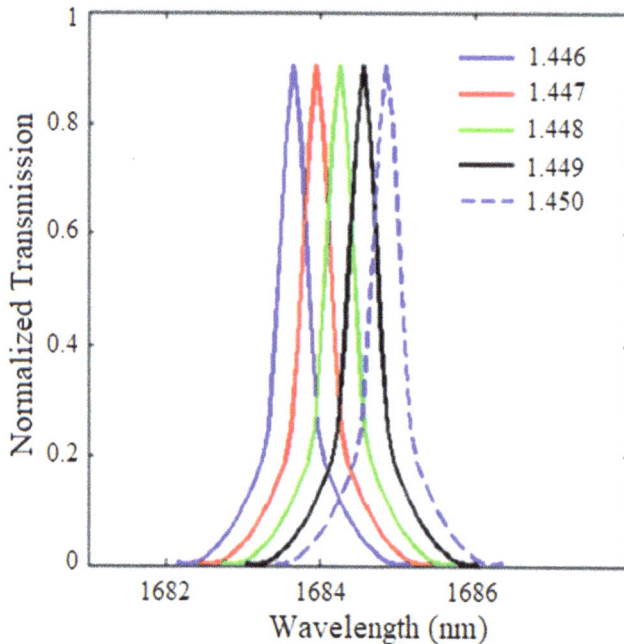

FIGURE 3.11   Transmission spectra for the sensor with different refractive indices.
Source: Reproduced with permission from: Kumar, Saini, and Sinha (2015). © Elsevier.

3.5.3   REFRACTIVE INDEX (RI) SENSOR BUILT ON MULTI-SLOT PHOTONIC CRYSTAL CAVITIES

The PCC offers the robust field confinement, long photon lifetime, and responsible for optical mode with a resonant wavelength which is extremely profound to the RI perturbation endorsed to the medium that infiltrated in the air holes of the PCC. Resultantly, PCC permits us to contrivance many RI sensors. A circular photonic crystal (CPC) highly

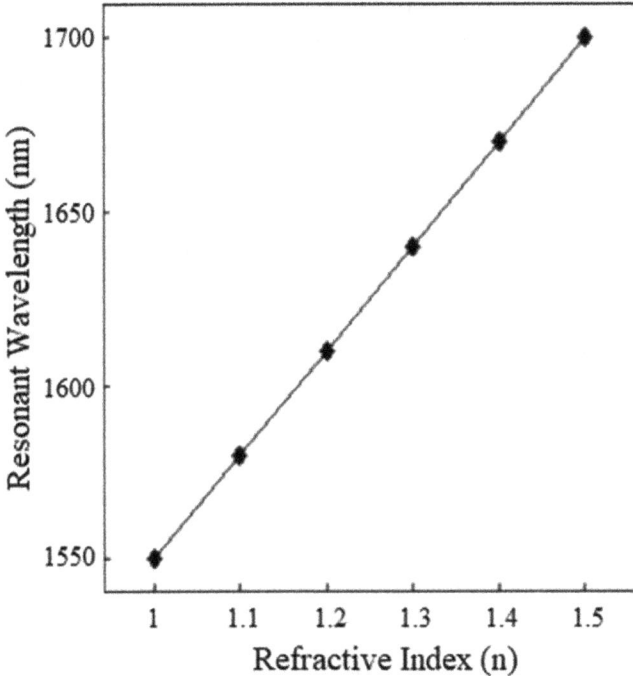

FIGURE 3.12   Resonant wavelength with refractive index.
Source: Reproduced with permission from: Kumar, Saini, and Sinha (2015). © Elsevier.

sensitive sensor device with good quality factor was proposed for RI sensing (Ge et al., 2018). The numerical investigation of a highly sensitive RI biosensor has been carried out based on Fano resonance in a PCC on a silicon chip (Peng et al., 2018). It is to be noted that the employment of the materials with low loss and optimization of the fabrication process, can improve the spectral performance of the Fano resonance. Recently, a design, fabrication, and characterization of a multi-slot PCC-based sensor were reported on the silicon on insulator platform for lab-on-a-chip applications (Xu et al., 2019). The schematic representation of a multi-slot PCC-based sensor is shown in Figures 3.13(a) and (b). The sensor possesses a 1-dimensional PCC which is uniformly divided with the four nanogaps in the y-direction. The PCC consists of the amalgamation of the weak mode confinement field and an extremely confined electric field in the slot region, because of the decrement in the RI of the multi-slot system. Both of the field subsidies a strong overlap of the optical field along with the analyte. The upper view of the multi-slot PCC is illustrated in Figure 3.13(b). As shown in Figure 3.13(b), a, b, and s indicate the period (in the x-direction), longitudinal length of individually post (y-direction), and the gap between the neighboring posts, respectively. The scattering effect perpendicular to the surface PCC should be reduced to obtain high Q. The sensitivity of the sensor was dramatically enhanced by optimizing the photonic crystal structure for distribution of most of the light in the lower index region. The distribution of the electric field from both the top and the side orientation while keeping the center of the cavity in the middle is depicted in Figures 3.13(c) and (d), respectively. Finally, the simulated band structure of the periodic multi-slot post cell is shown in Figure 3.13(e). To fabricate the sensing device, a pattern was demarcated using the direct writing 100 keV electron-beam lithography (JEOL JBX-6300FS) using a positive ZEP-520A resists. An anisotropic inductively coupled plasma process was employed to transfer the pattern onto the underlying silicon layer. A designed grating coupler for TE polarization is used to characterize the multi-slot PCC. The device is probed by means of an optical fiber arrangement.

To see the performance of the fabricated multi-slot PCC sensing device, the NaCl solutions of various concentrations varying from 0% to 5% with the step of 1% were prepared. The multi-slot PCC sensor was allowed to immerse in NaCl solution and the transmission spectrum of the device was measured. To minimize the impact of external thermal noise and drift for the duration of the optical measurement, the temperature of the test stage was kept constant at 20C with a thermoelectric controller. The measured transmission spectra are shown in Figure 3.14(a) when the sensing device is submerged in the NaCl solutions with various concentrations. It is very clear that the resonant wavelength rises with the concentration of the NaCl solution. To remove the residuals after individual measurement, the device was washed with the sanitized water and agitated on a 90°C hot plate for 10 minutes. The dependence of the resonant wavelength shifts on the refractive indices corresponding to each concentration is shown in Figure 3.14(b). The resonant wavelength shifts and the RI show a linear relation. As illustrated in Figure 3.14(b), the RIS ($S = \Delta\lambda/\Delta n$) of the PCC sensor is 586 nm/RIU obtained by linear fitting of the experimental data. The Q value estimated from the fit data with numerous refractive indices and found between the ranges of 3500 to 4200. This compact multi-slot PCC based sensing device can be integrated with the microfluidic channels and has the robust potential for the lab-on-chip demonstrations.

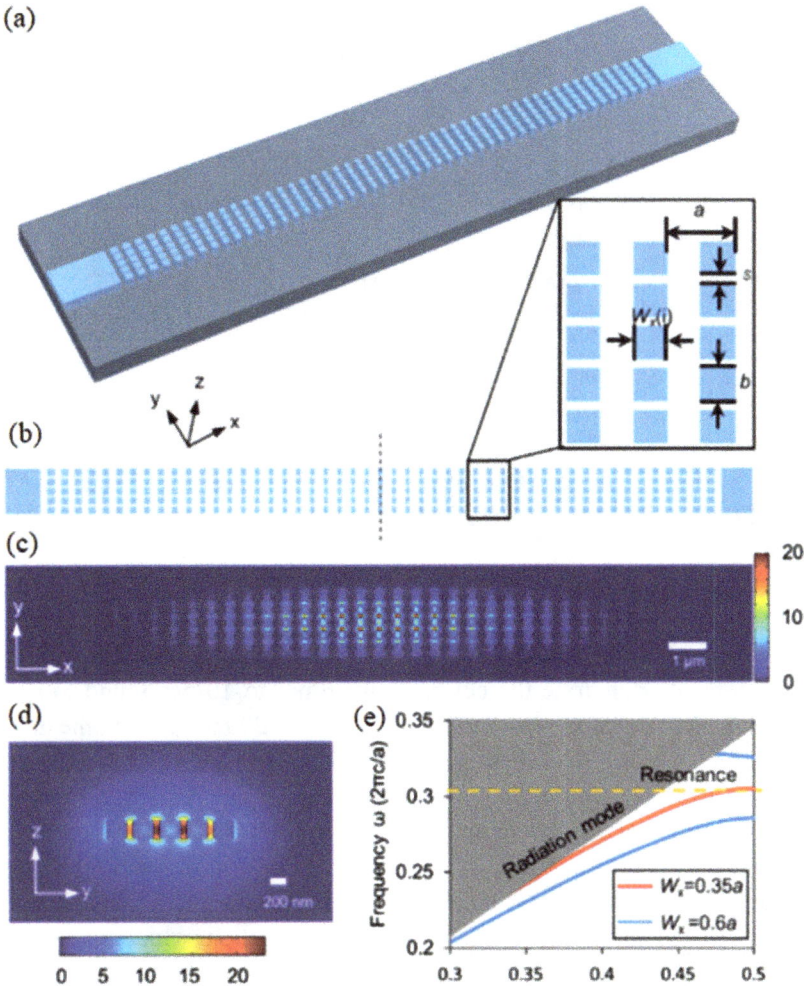

FIGURE 3.13 (a) The schematics of the Si multi-slot PCC sensing device; (b) the top view of the multi-slot PCC device; inset: zoom-in view of the framed portion; (c) distribution of the electric field from top; (d) distribution of the electric field from the side taken at the center of the cavity; (e) simulated band structure of periodic multi-slot post cell (shown in the inset) with $W_x = 0.35a$, and $W_x = 0.6a$. The yellow dashed line indicates the resonant frequency. The gray region indicates the light cone of the water.

Source: Reproduced with permission from: Xu et al. (2019).

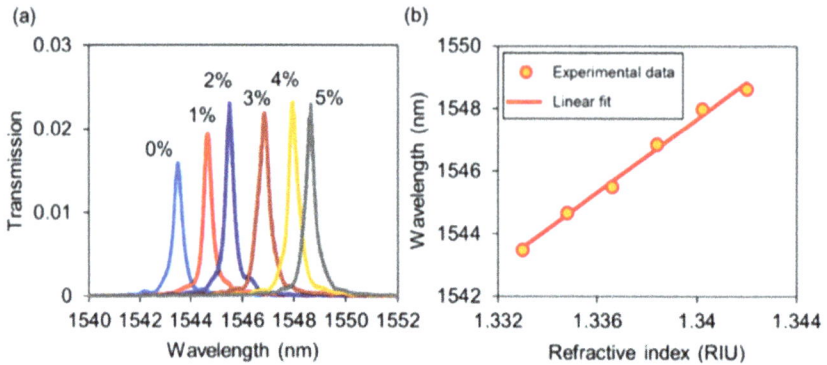

FIGURE 3.14 (a) The measured transmission responses of the multi-slot PCC immersed in the aqueous NaCl solution with different concentrations; (b) the variations of the resonant wavelength of the PCC sensor as a function of the background refractive index.

Source: Reproduced with permission from: Xu et al. (2019).

3.5.4 DETECTING SINGLE GOLD NANOPARTICLES (AUNPS) USING PHOTONIC CRYSTAL NANOBEAM CAVITIES

The applications of the NPs are growing in various fields including healthcare, sensing, and energy. For example, gold nanoparticles (AuNPs) exhibit critical efficiency dependence on their sizes. The AuNP with 2 nm to 6 nm diameters can penetrate the cell nucleus, 6 nm to 10 nm found to prefer peri-nuclear localization, and those of 100 nm to 200 nm exhibit the utmost probability for long circulation inside the body. It has been found that the existing optical techniques including UV-Vis. Spectrometry or dynamic light scattering (DLS) needs large sample volume and high concentration and suffers from less reliability when sizes go below 10 nm. On the other hand, a scanning/transmission electron microscope (TEM) needs a better laboratory atmosphere and serious sample preparation, which make its not appropriate for the frequent and fast analysis of the sample. Liang et al. demonstrated a photonic crystal nanobeam cavity with ultrahigh Q and small volume (Liang et al., 2015). The SOI platform was used to fabricate the photonic crystal nanobeam cavity by e-beam lithography and reactive ion etching techniques. The thickness of the oxide substrate and the device layer were measured as 2 μm and 220 nm, respectively. The nanobeam cavity consists of an array of rectangular gratings with 200 nm width of the silicon waveguide separated by 400 nm distance. The length of the waveguides varies from 220 nm to 240 nm from the middle of the nanobeam cavity towards both of its ends. The SU8 polymer pads also fabricated in a second e-beam lithography associated with the markers fabricated in the first e-beam lithography process. The SU8 pad transformed its mode to the Si waveguide mode and thus excited the cavity resonance mode. The scanning electron microscope (SEM) image (top view, *xy* plane) of the photonic crystal nanobeam cavity and the schematic of the experimental setup of the sensing system are shown in Figure 3.15. To see the performance of the photonic crystal nanobeam cavity, as illustrated in Figure 3.15(a), a tunable laser scanning from 1420 nm to 1520 nm was employed. A polarization controller was employed to launch the TE polarization mode. At the output, the transmitted light through the nanobeam cavity was coupled to the silicon waveguide and the SU8 pad, and finally, another tapered fiber was used to couple the light from the SU8 pad to the photodetector. The simulated electric file intensities in the middle cut of *xy*-plane and *xz*-plane are showing if Figures 3.15(c) and (d), respectively.

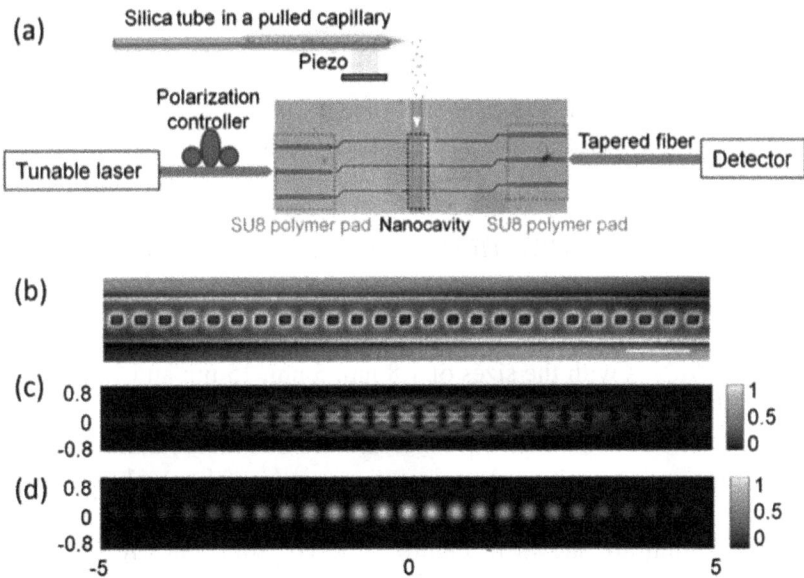

FIGURE 3.15 (a) The photonic crystal nanobeam sensing device and piezo spray setup; (b) scanning electron microscope image of the nanobeam cavity (top view, xy plane); (c) simulated electric field intensity in middle cut of the xy plane; and (d) simulated electric field intensity in middle cut of the xz plane.

Source: Reproduced with permission from: Liang and Quan (2015). © American Chemical Society.

The transmitted signal from the photonic crystal nano-beam cavity is illustrated in Figure 3.16. In Figure 3.16, the lower order cavity modes are excited in the longer wavelength range and have a high Q value. The Q of the fundamental mode was measured as high as 2.5×10^5. The Q value of all higher-order modes was measured to be in the range of 10^3–10^5.

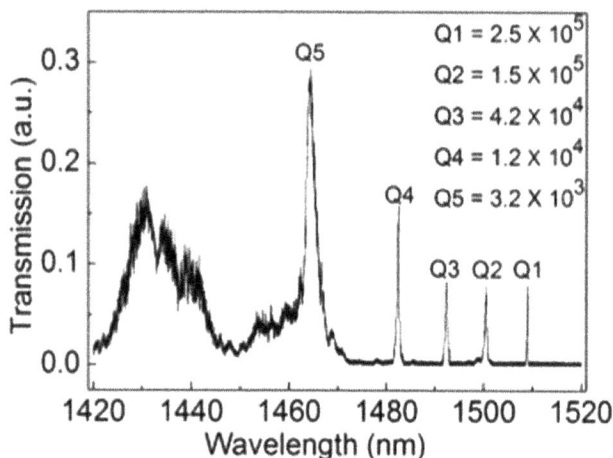

FIGURE 3.16 The resonance spectrum of the air-mode photonic crystal nano-beam cavity. *Source*: Reproduced with permission from: Liang and Quan (2015). © American Chemical Society.

3.5.4.1 SINGLE NANOPARTICLE DETECTION

The photonic crystal air-mode nano-beam cavity can be used to detect single AuNPs. To derive a micro-pipet, a piezoelectric actuator was used. The AuNPs with the sizes of 1.8 nm, 5 nm, 15 nm and 25 nm were deposited in the center of the nanocavity. The piezoelectric stage generates ultrasonic waves. Ultrasonic waves vibrate NPs into aerosols, subsequently evaporating and depositing them in a photonic crystal nano-beam cavity. The histograms of the resonances for the NPs of the sizes of 5 nm, 15 nm, and 25 nm are shown in Figure 3.17. The solid lines represent the fitting curves of a normal distribution of the counts. The signal-to-noise ratio (defined as the ratio of the shift of normal distribution center and the average of the half-width-half-maximum of the two normal distributions) was obtained as 15, 19, and 10 for the 5 nm, 15 nm, and 25 nm sizes of AuNPs, respectively. For the case of nanoparticle with 1.8 nm size, the two AuNPs were deposited into the nanocavity. The signal-to-noise ratio of the two events was 1.4 and 4.

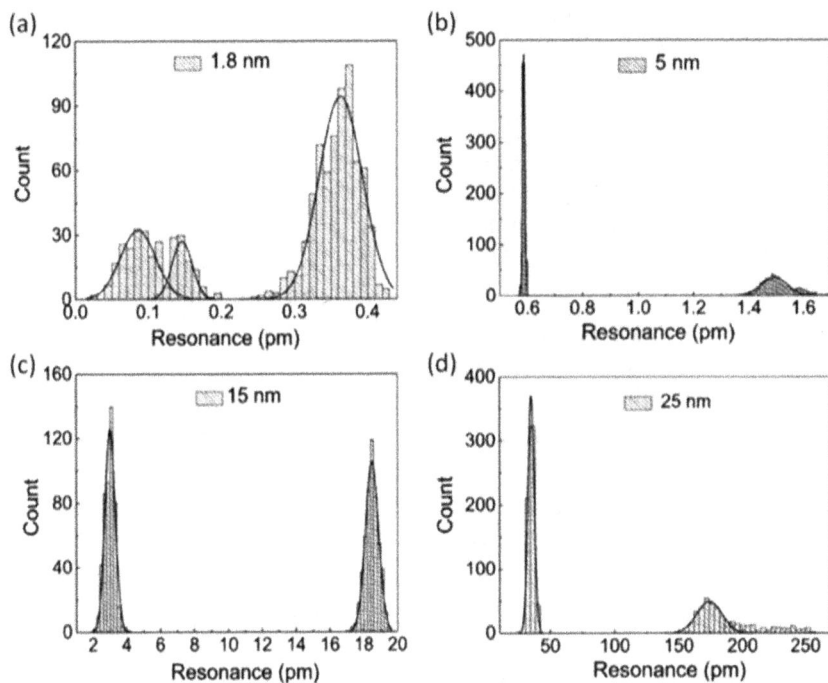

FIGURE 3.17 The histograms of the nanobeam cavity resonances: (a) for two nanoparticles of 1.8 nm size deposited into the nanocavity; (b) single nanoparticle of 5 nm size deposited into the nanocavity; (c) single nanoparticle of 15 nm size deposited into the nanocavity; (d) single nanoparticle of 25 nm size deposited into the nanocavity.

Source: Reproduced with permission from: Liang and Quan (2015). © American Chemical Society.

3.6 CHALLENGES AND THE FUTURE DIRECTIONS OF PHOTONIC CRYSTAL CAVITIES FOR SENSING APPLICATIONS

The PCC-based optical sensors have great potential and growing very rapidly. However, there exist several key challenges for their hands-on applications. Some of the key challenges include fabrication errors, influence by temperature, and difficulty in the coupling. The stability of the resonant wavelength of the PCC against errors in the fabrication process is the substantial factor. At the present stage of the fabrication technology of photonic crystals, the size and the position of the air holes can be controlled with the accuracy of 2–4 nm and 1 nm, respectively. The transmission characteristic of the bulk photonic crystal is limited by the fluctuations of the radii of air holes. Only 1% fluctuation in the hole radius may lead the large attenuations in the transmission. In this way, the fabrication errors in the cavity of photonic crystal will have a substantial influence on the resonant characteristics of the PCC.

One very important challenge is the coupling of the light from a traditional single-mode fiber into the PCC device. A conventional technique to decrease the coupling loss is to introduce photonic crystal waveguide on both of the sides of PCC. The light radiated from the traditional single-mode fiber to the photonic crystal waveguide and then transmitted through the photonic crystal waveguide to the PCC. However, again the typical waveguide dimensions (<1000 nm width and <500 nm thickness) are not suitable for coupling the light in/from the single-mode fiber which has the core diameter 8–10 μm. Secondly, the transmission principle of photonic crystal waveguide is photonic bandgap effect, which differs from the principle of transmission in the traditional single-mode optical fiber (i.e., TIR). Generally, the coupling loss can be significantly diminished by the precise aligning of the traditional optical fiber with the photonic crystal using a regulating mechanical device and appropriate manipulative of the coupling interface. The resonant characteristics of silicon PCC device are swayed by environment temperature due to the thermal dependence RI of silicon. To forbid the undesired deviations, meticulous temperature control system is needed, which will then increase the cost and the size of the PCC based sensors. The use of an appropriate thermo-optic liquid and proper design of the PCC, can minimize or eliminate the influence of environmental temperature. However, the use of an optofluidic liquid in the PCC cans diminution the tractability of PCC in structural design. In this way, the temperature effect is also a serious problem.

The Q value of the PCC plays a vital role in the sensing characteristic of sensors based on the PCC. The enhancement in Q value can be achieved by precise control of the position and the size of air holes with an order of nanometer. However, the precise control of both the position and size of the air holes with the order of nanometer is very difficult. Therefore, such precision necessary to get sophisticated and optimized structures ultimately becomes a restrictive factor in realizing very high Q PCCs. Additionally, the operating wavelength of PCC is located at a certain value that cannot be changed after fabrication, which also limits the application circumstances and further progress of PCC based sensors. Nowadays, the nanophotonics (manipulating photon at the scale of optical wavelength) can be integrated with the microfluidics (the control of fluids at the micron scale). The infiltrated fluids hold a wide range of refractive indices from 1.33 (water) to 1.50 (silica oil matching fluids), and above 1.8 for Cargille fluids. These fluids are particularly active in tuning the photonic crystal structure beyond that manageable through infiltration of the solid materials. Such combination provides the potential technology to develop high-sensitive optical sensors and offers a flexible means to write, tune or reconfigure photonic devices for a track of applications. In particular, PCCs can be favorably exploited within optofluidic architectures. The optofluidic infiltration technique offers the potential to realize tunable and reconfigurable PCCs without structural variation. It also gives the opportunity to create spatially programmable PCCs for the practical requirement. To realized multiple sensing locations, several sensor arrays based on cascaded PCCs can be gathered. The cascaded PCC can further advance the compactness and integration of PCC-based sensor. Slow-light is also a promising approach for optical signal and spatial compression of optical energy. The slow-light increase the time of light-matter interaction. Therefore, many nonlinear phenomena can be enhanced under the effect of slow-light which permits us to design scale down and highly sensitive photonic crystal devices. In the coupled photonic crystal waveguides, the slow-light subsidizes the enhanced sensitivity of the resonance modes. In this way, the slow-light is a promising method for improving the sensitivities of the PCC-based sensors.

3.7 CONCLUSIONS

In this chapter, the review on the PCC-based sensors has been provided for the various applications such as RI sensing, gas sensing, and bio-sensing. The photonic crystal cavities played a very significant role in optical sensing and provide significant industrial values. The principle of sensing by the PCC is provided. The photonic crystal microcavity-based methane gas sensor offers high RIS and the Q value of 135.65 nm/RIU and 6203, respectively. Such highly sensitive gas sensor establishes the probability of the cryptophane-E infiltrated photonic crystal microcavity for the potential application of CH_4 gas sensing. An analysis of a photonic crystal-based bi-periodic waveguide structure providing a platform for both gas and fluid sensing is presented. The photonic crystal structure is implemented by changing the periodicity of holes just next to the waveguide and introducing an array of super cavities along the length of the waveguide. The transmission spectrum of the bi-periodic waveguide structure is simulated using the FDTD. The structure allows the only resonant wavelength of the super cavity to pass through the photonic crystal waveguide and other wavelengths are strongly reflected. A Lorentzian response has been obtained for the waveguide instead of the dispersion curve obtained for conventional waveguides. The bi-periodic waveguide structure offers several advantages over the conventional waveguides or microcavity structures. The bi-periodic waveguide structure offers high sensitivity in the wider spectral range of RI sensing. The same structure can be used either as a gas sensor or a fluid sensor by selective infiltration of holes of the super cavity. Additionally, the sensor is operated at a resonant wavelength of 1550 nm and can be integrated with the other optoelectronic devices used in broadband optical communication systems. For the applications of gas sensing, the bi-periodic waveguide structure offers better sensitivity of 610 nm/RIU with the minimum detection limit of the order of 10^{-4}. In the case of the optofluidic sensor, the bi-periodic waveguide structure offers a sensitivity of 300 nm/RIU along with a wider measurement range RI from 1.0 to 1.5 and the minimum detection limit of 0.001. A highly sensitive multi-slot PCC based sensor was discussed for RI sensing. The reported RIS of the multi-slot PCC sensor was 586 nm/RIU. The value of the Q was found between the ranges of 3500 to 4200.

A high Q, ultra-small volume air-mode photonic crystal nano-beam cavity is introduced for single AuNP detection. The silicon nano-beam cavity in conjunction with electrospray/piezo spray can be a good research means for rapid and frequent size categorization of the NPs on the limited samples. In addition to this, an ultrahigh Q, ultra-small volume nano-beam cavity is possibly an ideal platform to increase the interaction between single atoms, molecules, and solid-state quantum emitters with photons. The accessibility of such PCC sensor with small size, high Q value, high sensitivity, and easy fabrication, paves the way for the on-chip multiplexed sensor arrays. The biosensors based on the photonic integrated circuit are ultimate candidates for the lab-on-a-chip applications because of their robustness, capability for miniaturization, great sensitivity, and perspective for multiplexing and the mass fabrication at a low cost.

KEYWORDS

- **carbon nanotubes**
- **deep ultraviolet**
- **immunoglobulin gamma**
- **methane**
- **photonic crystal cavity**
- **silicon-on-insulator**
- **total internal reflection**

REFERENCES

Ahmed, R., Rifat, A. A., Yetisen, A. K., Dai, Q., Yun, S. H., & Butt, H., (2016). *J. Appl. Phys., 119*, 113105.

Akahane, Y., Asano, T., Song, B. S., & Noda, S., (2003). High-Q photonic nanocavity in a two-dimensional photonic crystal. *Nature, 425*, 944–947.

Ampere, A. T., Kuan, C., Chen, C. D., & Ma, K. J., (2003). Electron beam lithography in nanoscale fabrication: Recent development. *IEEE Trans. Electron. Package. Manuf., 26*, 141–149.

Anton, S. R., & Sodano, S. A., (2007). A review of power harvesting using piezoelectric materials (2003–2006). *Smart Mater. Struct., 16*, R1–R21.

Appelboom, G., Camacho, E., Abraham, M. E., Bruce, S. S., Dumont, E. L., Zacharia, B. E., D'Amico, R., et al., (2014). Smart wearable body sensors for patient self-assessment and monitoring. *Arch. Public Health, 72*, 28.

Aristov, A. I., Manousidaki, M., Danilov, A., Terzaki, K., Fotakis, C., Farsari, M., & Kabashin, A. V., (2016). 3D plasmonic crystal metamaterials for ultra-sensitive biosensing. *Sci. Rep., 6*, 25380.

Armani, D. K., Kippenberg, T. J., Spillane, S. M., & Vahala, K. J., (2003). Ultra-high-Q toroid microcavity on a chip. *Nature, 421*, 925–928.

Baday, M., Calamak, S., Durmus, N. G., Davis, R. W., Steinmetz, L. M., & Demirci, U., (2015). Integrating cell phone imaging with magnetic levitation (i-LEV) for label-free blood analysis at the point-of-living. *Small, 12*, 1222–1229.

Bandodkar, A. J., & Wang, J., (2014). Non-invasive wearable electrochemical sensors: A review. *Trends Biotechnol., 32*, 363–371.

Beggs, D. M., O'Faolain, L., & Krauss, T. F., (2008). Accurate determination of the functional hole size in photonic crystal slabs using optical methods. *Photonics Nanostruct. Fundam. Appl., 6* (3/4), 213–218.

Bogaerts, W., Wiaux, V., Taillaert, D., Beckx, S., Luyssaert, B., Bienstman, P., & Baets, R., (2002). Fabrication of photonic crystals in silicon-on-insulator using 248-nm deep UV lithography. *IEEE J. Set. Top. Quant. Electron., 8*, 928–934.

Broers, A. N., Hoole, A. C. F., & Ryan, J. M., (1996). Electron beam lithography-resolution limits. *Microelectron. Engg., 32*, 131–142.

Cai, Z., Luck, L. A., Punihaole, D., Madura, J. D., & Asher, S. A., (2016). Photonic crystal protein hydrogel sensor materials enabled by conformationally induced volume phase transition. *Chem. Sci., 7*, 4557–4562.

Caldara, M., Colleoni, C., Guido, E., Rosace, G., Re, V., & Vitali, A., (2013). A wearable sensor platform to monitor sweat pH and skin temperature. In: *2013 IEEE International Conference on Body Sensor Networks, BSN* (pp. 1–6).

Chakravarty, S., Hosseini, A., Xu, X. C., Zhu, L., Zou, Y., & Chen, R. T., (2014). Analysis of ultra-high sensitivity configuration in chip-integrated photonic crystal microcavity bio-sensors. *Appl. Phys. Lett., 104*, 191109 (1–5).

Chang, Y., Jhu, Y., & Wu, C., (2012). Temperature dependence of defect mode in a defective photonic crystal. *Opt. Commun., 285*, 1501–1504.

Chiappelli, M. C., & Hayward, R. C., (2012). Photonic multilayer sensors from photo-cross linkable polymer films. *Adv. Mater., 24*, 6100–6104.

Choi, C. J., & Cunningham, B. T., (2007). A 96-well microplate incorporating a replica molded microfluidic network integrated with photonic crystal biosensors for high throughput kinetic biomolecular interaction analysis. *Lab Chip, 7*, 550–556.

Dai, Q., Frommer, J., Berman, D., Virwani, K., Blake, D., Cheng, J. Y., & Nelson, A., (2013). High-throughput directed self-assembly of core-shell ferrimagnetic nanoparticle arrays. *Langmuir, 29*, 7472–7477.

Diao, Y. Y., Liu, X. Y., Toh, G. W., Shi, L., & Zi, J., (2013). Multiple structural coloring of silk-fibroin photonic crystals and humidity-responsive color sensing. *Adv. Funct. Mater., 23*, 5373–5380.

Edrington, A. C., Urbas, A. M., Derege, P., Chen, C. X., Swager, T. M., Hadjichristidis, N., Xenidou, M., et al., (2001). Polymer-based photonic crystals. *Adv. Mater., 13*, 421–425.

Fan, X., & White, I. M., (2011). Optofluidic microsystems for chemical and biological analysis. *Nat. Photonics, 5*, 591–597.

Fenzl, C., Wilhelm, S., Hirsch, T., & Wolfbeis, O. S., (2013). Optical sensing of the ionic strength using photonic crystals in a hydrogel matrix. *ACS Appl. Mater. Interfaces, 5*, 173–178.

Freeman, D., Grillet, C., Lee, M. W., Smith, C. L. C., Ruan, Y., Rode, A., Krolikowska, M., et al., (2008). Chalcogenide glass photonic crystals. *Photonics Nanostruct. Fundam. Appl., 6*, 3–11.

Ge, R., Xie, J., Yan, B., Liu, E., Tan, W., & Liu, J., (2018). Refractive index sensor with high sensitivity based on circular photonic crystal. *J. Opt. Soc. Am. A, 35*, 992–997.

Gonzalez-Urbina, L., Baert, K., Kolaric, B., Perez-Moreno, J., & Clays, K., (2012). Linear and nonlinear optical properties of colloidal photonic crystals. *Chem. Rev., 112*, 2268–2285.

Hagina, H., Takahashi, Y., Tanaka, Y., Asano, T., & Noda, S., (2009). Effects of fluctuation in air hole radii and positions on optical characteristics in photonic crystal heterostructure nanocavities. *Phys. Rev. B: Condens. Matter, 79*, 085112 (1–8).

Hu, J., Cui, X., Gong, Y., Xu, X., Gao, B., Wen, T., Lu, T. J., & Xu, F., (2016). Portable microfluidic and smartphone-based devices for monitoring of cardiovascular diseases at the point of care. *Biotechnol. Adv., 34*, 305–320.

Inan, H., Poyraz, M., Inci, F., Lifson, M. A., Baday, M., Cunningham, B. T., & Demirci, U., (2017). Photonic crystals: Emerging biosensors and their promise for point-of-care applications. *Chem. Soc. Rev., 46*, 366.

Jamois, C., Wehrspohn, R. B., Andreani, L. C., Hermann, C., Hess, O., & Go Sele, U., (2003). Silicon-based two-dimensional photonic crystal waveguides. *Photonics Nanostruct. Fundam. Appl., 1*, 1–13.

Jamols, C., Wehrspohn, R., Schilling, J., Muller, F., Hillebrand, R., & Hergert, W., (2002). Silicon-based photonic crystal slabs: Two concepts. *IEEE J. Quantum Electron., 38*, 805–810.

Joannopoulos, J. D., Meade, R. D., & Winn, J. N., (1995). *Photonic Crystals-Molding the Flow of Light* (pp. 15, 16). Princeton University Press, Princeton, New Jersey.

John, S., (1987). Strong localization of photons in certain disordered dielectric superlattices. *Phys. Rev. Lett, 58*, 2486.

Kang, J. H., Moon, J. H., Lee, S. K., Park, S. G., Jang, S. G., Yang, S., & Yang, S. M., (2008). Thermoresponsive hydrogel photonic crystals by three-dimensional holographic lithography. *Adv. Mater., 20*, 3061–3065.

Karnutsch, C., Smith, C. L. C., Graham, A., Tomljenovic-Hanic, S., McPhedran, R., Eggleton, B. J., O'Faolain, L., et al., (2009). Temperature stabilization of optofluidic photonic crystal cavities. *Appl. Phys. Lett., 94*, 231114 (1–3).

Khitrova, G., Gibbs, H. M., Jahnke, F., Kira, M., & Koch, S. W., (1999). Nonlinear optics of normal-mode coupling semiconductor microcavities. *Rev. Mod. Phys., 71*, 1591–1639.

Kim, S., Mitropoulos, A. N., Spitzberg, J. D., Tao, H., Kaplan, D. L., & Omenetto, F. G., (2012). Silk inverse opals. *Nat. Photonics, 6*, 818–823.

Kinoshita, S., Yoshioka, S., & Kawagoe, K., (2002). Mechanisms of structural color in the Morpho butterfly: Cooperation of regularity and irregularity in an iridescent scale. *Proc. Biol. Sci., 269*, 1417–1421.

Kouba, J., Kubenz, M., Mai, A., Ropers, G., Eberhardt, W., & Loechel, B., (2006). Fabrication of Nanoimprint stamps for photonic crystals. *J. Phys.: Conf. Ser., 34*, 897–903.

Kumar, A., Saini, T. S., & Sinha, R. K., (2015). Design and analysis of photonic crystal biperiodic waveguide structure based optofluidic-gas sensor. *Optik-International Journal for Light and Electron Optics, 126*, 5172–5175.

Lalanne, P., Sauwan, C., & Hugonin, J. P., (2008). Photonic confinement in photonic crystal nanocavities. *Laser Photonics Rev., 2*, 514–526.

Liang, F., & Quan, Q., (2015). Detecting single gold nanoparticles (1.8 nm) with ultrahigh-Q air mode photonic crystal nanobeam cavities. *ACS Photon., 2*, 1692–1697.

Lin, K. H., Crocker, J. C., Prasad, V., Schofield, A., Weitz, D. A., Lubensky, T. C., & Yodh, A. G., (2000). Entropically driven colloidal crystallization on patterned surfaces. *Phys. Rev. Lett., 85*, 1770–1773.

Liu, K., Schmedake, T. A., & Tsu, R., (2008). A comparative study of colloidal silica spheres: Photonic crystals versus Bragg's law. *Phys. Letts. A, 372*, 4517–4520.

Luo, C., Johnson, S. G., Joannopoulos, J. D., & Pendry, J. B., (2002). All-angle negative refraction without negative effective index. *Phys. Rev. B, 65*, 201104.

Luo, N., Ding, J., Zhao, N., Leung, B. H. K., & Poon, C. C. Y., (2014). Mobile health: Design of flexible and stretchable electrophysiological sensors for wearable healthcare systems. In: *Proceedings-11th International Conference on Wearable and Implantable Body Sensor Networks, BSN* (pp. 87–91).

MacLeod, J., & Rosei, F., (2013). Photonic crystals: Sustainable sensors from silk. *Nat. Mater., 12*, 98–100.

Marlow, F., Sharifi, P., Brinkmann, R., & Mendive, C., (2009). Opals: Status and prospects. *Angew. Chem. Int. Ed., 48*, 6212–6233.

Mastronardi, E., Foster, A., Zhang, X., & DeRosa, M., (2014). Smart materials based on DNA aptamers: Taking aptasensing to the next level. *Sensors, 14*, 3156–3171.

Matzeu, G., Florea, L., & Diamond, D., (2015). Advances in wearable chemical sensor design for monitoring biological fluids. *Sens. Actuators B, 211*, 403–418.

McPhedran, R. C., Nicorovici, N. A., McKenzie, D. R., Rouse, G. W., Botten, L. C., Welch, V., Parker, A. R., et al., (2003). Structural colors through photonic crystals. *Phys. B, 338*, 182–185.

Michler, P., Kiraz, A., Becher, C., Schoenfeld, W. V., Petroff, P. M., Zhang, L., Hu, E., & Imamoglu, A., (2000). A quantum dot single-photon turnstile device. *Science, 290*, 2282–2285.

Miguez, H., Meseguer, F., Lopez, C., Blanco, A., Moya, J. S., Requena, J., Mifsud, A., & Fornes, V., (1998). Control of the photonic crystal properties of fcc-packed submicrometer SiO_2 spheres by sintering. *Adv. Mater., 10*, 480–483.

Noda, S., Chutinan, A., & Imada, M., (2000b). Trapping and emission of photons by a single defect in a photonic bandgap structure. *Nature, 407*, 608–610.

Noda, S., Tomoda, K., Yamamoto, N., & Chutinan, A., (2000). Full three-dimensional photonic bandgap crystals at near-infrared wavelengths. *Science, 289*, 604–606.

Norris, D. J., Arlinghaus, E. G., Meng, L., Heiny, R., & Scriven, L. E., (2004). Opaline photonic crystals: How does self-assembly work? *Adv. Mater., 16*, 1393–1399.

O'Faolain, L., White, T. P., O'Brien, D., Yuan, X., Settle, M. D., & Krauss, T. F., (2007). Dependence of extrinsic loss on group velocity in photonic crystal waveguides. *Opt. Express, 15*, 13129–13138.

Olguin, O., Gloor, P. A., & Pentland, A., (2009). Wearable sensors for pervasive healthcare management. *Proc. 3rd International Conference on Pervasive Computing Technologies for Healthcare* (pp. 1–4).

Pacholski, C., (2013). Photonic crystal sensors based on porous silicon. *Sensors, 13*, 4694–4713.

Painter, O., Lee, R. K., Scherer, A., Yariv, A., O'brien, J. D., Dapkus, P. D., & Kim, I., (1999). Two-dimensional photonic band-gap defect mode laser. *Science, 284*, 1819–1821.

Pan, C., Li, Z., Guo, W., Zhu, J., & Wang, Z. L., (2011). Fiber-Based hybrid nanogenerators for/as self-powered systems in biological liquid. *Angew. Chem. Int. Ed. Engl., 50*, 11192–11196.

Parimi, P. V., Lu, W. T., Vodo, P., & Sridhar, S., (2003). Imaging by flat lens using negative refraction. *Nature, 426*, 404.

Peng, F., Wang, Z., Yuan, G., Guan, L., & Peng, Z., (2018). High-sensitivity refractive index sensing based on Fano resonances in a photonic crystal cavity-coupled microring resonator. *IEEE Photonics Journal, 10*, 6600808.

Pouya, C., Stavenga, D. G., & Vukusic, P., (2011). Discovery of ordered and quasi-ordered photonic crystal structures in the scales of the beetle *Eupholus magnificus*. *Opt. Express, 19*, 11355–11364.

Ren, J., Xuan, Liu, C., Yao, C., Zhu, Y., Liu, X., & Ge, L., (2015b). Graphene oxide hydrogel improved sensitivity in one-dimensional photonic crystals for detection of beta-glucan. *RSC Adv., 5*, 77211–77216.

Ren, X., Ma, Q., Fan, H., Pang, L., Zhang, Y., Yao, Y., Rena, X., & Liu, S., (2015). A Se-doped MoS_2 nanosheet for improved hydrogen evolution reaction. *Chem. Commun., 51*, 15997–16000.

Rogach, A., Susha, A., Caruso, F., Sukhorukov, G., Kornowski, A., Kershaw, S., Mohwald, H., et al., (2000). Nano-and microengineering: 3-D colloidal photonic crystals prepared from sub-μm-sized polystyrene latex spheres pre-coated with luminescent polyelectrolyte/nanocrystal shells. *Adv. Mater., 12*, 333–337.

Russell, P., (2003). Photonic crystal fibers. *Science, 299*, 358–362.

Schudel, B. R., Choi, C. J., Cunningham, B. T., & Kenis, P. J. A., (2009). Microfluidic chip for combinatorial mixing and screening of assays. *Lab Chip, 9*, 1676–1680.

Song, B. S., Noda, S., & Asano, T., (2003). Photonic devices based on in-plane hetero photonic crystals. *Science, 300*, 1537.

Spillane, S. M., Kippenberg, T. J., & Vahala, K. J., (2002). Ultralow-threshold Raman laser using a spherical dielectric microcavity. *Nature, 415*, 621–623.

Sreekanth, K. V., Alapan, Y., ElKabbash, M., Ilker, E., Hinczewski, M., Gurkan, U. A., De Luca, A., & Strangi, G., (2016). Extreme sensitivity biosensing platform based on hyperbolic metamaterials. *Nat. Mater., 15*, 621–627.

Sreekanth, K. V., Zeng, S., Yong, K. T., & Yu, T., (2013). Sensitivity enhanced biosensor using graphene-based one-dimensional photonic crystal. *Sens. Actuators B, 182*, 424–428.

Tao, W., Liu, T., Zheng, R., & Feng, H., (2012). Gait analysis using wearable sensors. *Sensors, 12*, 2255–2283.

Vahala, K. J., (2003). Optical microcavities. *Nature, 424*, 15–26, 839–846.

Verma, R., Adhikary, R. R., & Banerjee, R., (2016). Smart material platforms for miniaturized devices: Implications in disease models and diagnostics. *Lab Chip, 16*, 1978–1992.

Vernooy, D. W., Ilchenko, V. S., Mabuchi, H., Streed, E. W., & Kimble, H. J., (1998). High-Q measurements of fused-silica microspheres in the near-infrared. *Opt. Lett., 23*, 247–249.

Vieu, C., Carcenac, F., Pepin, A., Chen, Y., Mejias, M., Lebib, A., Manin-Ferlazzo, L., et al., (2000). Electron beam lithography: Resolution limits and applications. *Applied Surface Science, 164*, 111–117.

Vilela, D., Romeo, A., & Sanchez, S., (2016). Flexible sensors for biomedical technology. *Lab Chip, 16*, 402–408.

Wang, S., Tasoglu, S., Chen, P. Z., Chen, M., Akbas, R., Wach, S., Ozdemir, C. I., et al., (2014). Micro-a-fluidics ELISA for rapid CD4 cell count at the point-of-care. *Sci. Rep., 4*, 3796.

Winn, J. N., Fink, Y., Fan, S., & Joannopoulos, J. D., (1998). Omnidirectional reflection from a one-dimensional photonic crystal. *Opt. Lett., 23*, 1573–1575.

Xiao, S., & Mortensen, N. A., (2006). Highly dispersive photonic band- gap-edge optofluidic biosensors. *J. Eur. Opt. Soc., 1*, 06026.

Xie, R., & Liu, X. Y., (2008). Electrically directed on-chip reversible patterning of two-dimensional tunable colloidal structures. *Adv. Funct. Mater., 18*, 802–809.

Xu, P., Zheng, J., Zhou, J., Chen, Y., Zou, C., & Majumdar, A., (2019). Multi-slot photonic crystal cavities for high-sensitivity refractive index sensing. *Opt. Express, 27*, 3609–3616.

Xu, Z., Wang, L., Fang, F., Fu, Y., & Yin, Z., (2016). A review on colloidal self-assembly and their applications. *Current Nanoscience, 12*, 725–746.

Yablonovitch, E., (1987). Inhibited spontaneous emission in solid-state physics and electronics. *Phys. Rev. Lett., 58*, 2059.

Yang, H., Liu, H., Kang, H., & Tan, W., (2008). Engineering target-responsive hydrogels based on aptamer-target interactions. *J. Am. Chem. Soc., 130*, 6320–6321.

Yang, Y., Yang, D., Tian, H., & Ji, Y., (2013). Photonic crystal stress sensor with high sensitivity in double directions based on shoulder-coupled aslant nanocavity. *Sens. Actuators A: Phys., 193*, 149–154.

Yao, S., & Zhu, Y., (2014). Wearable multifunctional sensors using printed stretchable conductors made of silver nanowires. *Nanoscale, 6*, 2345.

Yetisen, A. K., Akram, M. S., & Lowe, C. R., (2013). Paper-based microfluidic point-of-care diagnostic devices. *Lab Chip, 13*, 2210–2251.

Yetisen, A. K., Butt, H., & Yun, S. H., (2016). Photonic crystal flakes. *ACS Sens., 1*, 493–497.

Yetisen, A. K., Montelongo, Y., Da Cruz, V. F., Martinez-Hurtado, J. L., Neupane, S., Butt, H., Qasim, M. M., et al., (2014). Reusable, robust, and accurate laser-generated photonic nanosensor. *Nano Lett., 14*, 3587–3593.

Yetisen, K., Martinez-Hurtado, J. L., Da Cruz, V. F., Simsekler, M. C. E., Akram, M. S., & Lowe, C. R., (2014). The regulation of mobile medical applications. *Lab Chip, 14*, 833–840.

Zhang, D., & Liu, Q., (2016). Biosensors and bioelectronics on smartphone for portable biochemical detection. *Biosens. Bioelectron., 75*, 273–284.

Zhang, J., Sun, Z., & Yang, B., (2009). Self-assembly of photonic crystals from polymer colloids. *Curr. Opin. Colloid Interface Sci., 14*, 103–114.

Zhang, Y., Zhao, Y., & Wanga, Q., (2015). Measurement of methane concentration with cryptophane E infiltrated photonic crystal microcavity. *Sens. Actuators B: Chemical, 209*, 431–437.

Zi, J., Yu, X., Li, Y., Hu, X., Xu, C., Wang, X., Liu, X., & Fu, R., (2003). Coloration strategies in peacock feathers. *Proc. Natl. Acad. Sci. U.S.A., 100*, 12576–12578.

Zou, Y., Chakravarty, S., Kwong, D. N., Lai, W. C., Xu, X., Lin, X., Hosseini, A., & Chen, R. T., (2014). Cavity-waveguide coupling engineered high sensitivity silicon photonic crystal microcavity biosensors with high yield. *IEEE J. Sel. Top. Quantum Electron., 20*, 6900710 (1–10).

CHAPTER 4

Metal Oxide Nanostructures for Gas Sensing Applications

MEENAKSHI SRIVASTAVA[1] and NARENDRA SINGH[1,2]

[1]Centre for Advanced Studies, Dr. A. P. J. Abdul Kalam Technical University, Lucknow, Uttar Pradesh, India

[2]Department of Chemical Engineering, Indian Institute of Technology Kanpur, Kanpur–208016, Uttar Pradesh, India, Tel.: +91-9936337743, E-mail: narendra.hbti.be@gmail.com

ABSTRACT

Gas sensing is an important process to monitor the environment, indoor chemical gases, chemical processes, agriculture, and pharmaceutical processes. Various materials have been used for gas sensing, such as metal oxides, carbon-based nanomaterials (e.g., GN, carbon nanotubes (CNTs), etc.), and many more. Metal oxide nanostructures (MON) (e.g., ZnO, SnO_2, WO_3, etc.), have been extensively used for gas sensing application to detect toxic gases over the last few decades. These materials have advantages over other materials owing to their economically viable and easy device fabrication process with high sensitivity. The different processes were used to fabricate such materials will be summarized in this chapter. Different properties such as morphology, crystal structure, etc., of the MON have specific selectivity and hence selectivity toward the specific gases due to varying surface structures, which further dependent on adsorption sites and surface area of the material. Further, other modifications such as heterostructures will also be summarized in terms of selectivity, sensitivity towards the enhancement of the gas sensing effect. This chapter will discuss in detail about the various MON for the gas sensing applications.

4.1 INTRODUCTION

Gas sensors are devices that quantitatively analyze the presence of a gaseous analyte by changing the physical parameters of the sensor and are monitored by an externally connected device (Hulanicki et al., 1991; Barsan et al., 2016). Metal oxides gas sensors are the most prominent solid-state gas sensing devices for households, commercial, and industrial applications, which shows the features like low cost, compact size, etc. In the present scenario, most industries are using the metal oxide-based gas sensors, which are fabricated by screen printing route, and others are based on ceramic substrates. Basically, the gas sensors based on nanomaterials are prominently evolving directions to advances in the sensing characteristics such as low cost, high selectivity, long-term durability, low response time, etc. However, there is a range of several chemical toxins from the industries, automobiles, and households, which releases into the atmosphere, and affecting the global environment which causes, for example, acid rain, greenhouse effect and ozone depletion, etc., (Tamaekong et al., 2010; Koplin et al., 2006; Liu et al., 2012; Fine et al., 2010; Kanan et al., 2009) These are affecting the human, animal, and aquatic life. Lethal and toxic gases from auto and industries may be dissipate into the environment, can cause serious accident like Bhopal gas tragedy (Kanan et al., 2009; Dhara et al., 2002). So it is necessary to sense such threats through a high-quality gas sensor. With the purpose of evaluation and controlling of these gases, an individual needs to identify the quantity and categories of gases present in the local and global surroundings. Therefore, the necessity of observing and handling these gases in time has preceded to investigate and expansion of different types of sensing instrument using a wide range of materials and technologies. To build-up the efficient and capable instruments for the measurement or detection of harmful gases, one need to lower the expense, appearance, dimension, mass, etc., of the gas sensing devices, it is very important to install the sensor devices in the domestic use, industries, etc., so that we can control it within time and reduces or eliminates the risk. Carbon monoxide (CO), Carbon dioxide (CO_2), Chlorine (Cl_2), Ethanol (C_2H_5OH), Ammonia (NH_3), etc., are toxic and polluting gases evolving from the different industries (Fine et al., 2010; Chou et al., 2006; Fraiwan et al., 2011). The discharge of these fumes, when reach to hazardous level closer to 100 ppm, may cause the severe health hazards for all life (animal, human, etc.). Exposure of few such gases up to 150 ppm and above can cause death. Unwanted gases liberated by the industries and vehicles, smoke, and particulate matters are the foremost pollutants in the environment. The gases need to be regulated up to the assured limit otherwise it can cause adverse and disastrous effects on human and environment, are called air pollutants.

Even though, there are previously some publications reported on metal oxide gas sensor, it is still important to methodically encapsulate the properties of metal oxides from the outlook of nanoscience and technology involvement (Yamazoe et al., 2003; Wang et al., 2010; Tricoli et al., 2010; Barsan et al., 2001). Various types of MON have been prepared for enhancement of the gas sensing performance like sensitivity, gas response, recovery time, selectivity, and so on (Sun et al., 2012; Korotcenkov and Cho, 2011; Comini, 2006). We will focus on the basic properties of sensors and include an overview on the metal oxide-based gas sensors in this chapter.

4.2 SENSORS

The sensor can be defined as an apparatus which accepts an indication or a response that acts inform of automated or optical signal. According to the International Electrochemical Committee (IEC), "the sensor is the primary part of a measuring chain which converts the input variable into a signal for measurement" (Terms and definitions in Industrial Process Measurement and Control (ICE draft 65/84) (IEC, 1982). According to Gopel et al., "a sensor is an element with housing and electrical connections included" and "a sensor system is a sensor which incorporates some kind of signal processing (analog or digital)" (Gopel and Zemel, 1989). The sensor is built-in the sensor system and it is the foremost component to record the facts calculated. The illustration of the sensor can be viewed from Figure 4.1.

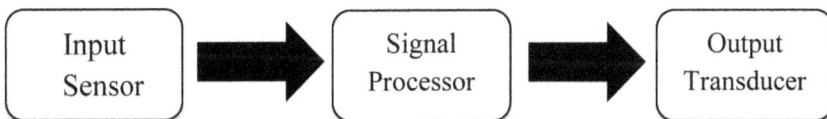

| Input Sensor | ➡ | Signal Processor | ➡ | Output Transducer |

FIGURE 4.1   Block diagram of sensor system.

4.3 NEED OF SENSORS

At the present time, there is an outlook in the technical and engineering community that there is a crucial necessity to develop the inexpensive, reliable, durable, stable, etc., sensors for the mechanism or computing systems, mechanization facilities and for the industrial and scientific machineries. The sensors are essential mainly for the dimensions of physical quantities and also used to control particular process. At present, the environmental waste has become a worldwide matter of subject from different industries for their exhausts/hazard waste discharge. The reducing gases such as CO, H_2, C_2H_5OH, oxygenic gases such as CO_2, NO_X, O_2, CH_3OH, CH_4, odorous gases such as NH_3, H_2S, dangerous gases such as C_2H_2, C_2H_4, C_3H_6, C_3H_8, LPG, toxic gases such CO, H_2S, Cl_2, NO_2, and chemical warfare agents, and their simulants, etc., (Prudenziati and Morten, 1986; Moseley, 1997; Morten et al., 1990; White et al., 1997; Zhang et al., 1997; Setty, 1994; Patil et al., 1998; Kuwabara, 1987; Sorita and Kawano, 1996; Chiu and Chang, 1999; Inaba and Saji, 1999; Kong and Shen, 1996; Ishihara, 1997; Martinelli et al., 1999; Yamaura et al., 1995; Noguchi et al., 1999; Tomchenko et al., 2005; Nimal et al., 2009; Seto et al., 2005; Lavoie et al., 2007; Hill et al., 2002; Cordell et al., 2007). Must be restrained for the healthy existence of all the living beings. Hence, there is accumulative interest in minimizing the emission toxic, reducing, oxygenic, odorous gases and as well to minimize discharge of such unburnt hydrocarbons from industrial exhausts. For detecting, measuring, and controlling these gases, an individual must aware about the type and their concentration level existing in the surroundings. Thus, the necessity of monitoring and controlling the exposure of these gases has led to investigation and growth of various types of sensors by means of diverse resources and equipment.

4.4 CATEGORIZATION OF SENSORS

Sensors are classified in different ways, such as external power requirement, applications, etc. We will discuss about the classification of sensors in this section.

4.4.1 ON THE BASIS OF EXTERNAL POWER REQUIREMENT

The sensors are categorized on the basis of external power requirement:

- Passive sensor; and
- Active sensor.

4.4.1.1 PASSIVE SENSORS

An external control is required to produce an output signal in relation to the input signal, are referred as passive sensors. Passive sensor is also called parametric sensor, because of their change in its own features in response to an input signal (concentration, form of materials, etc.), and its variation in the characteristics which is transformed into output signals (e.g., thick, and thin-film sensors, etc.).

4.4.1.2 ACTIVE SENSORS

Active sensors generate exactly an output signal with none requirement of the external energy source in relation to the input signals (e.g., thermocouple or a pH-meter, etc.).

4.4.2 ON THE BASIS OF APPLICATIONS

On the basis of applications, sensors are grouped into physical sensors and chemical sensors which is classified in Table 4.1.

TABLE 4.1 Classification of Different Types of Sensor with Their Detection Features (Hulanicki et al., 1991)

Sensor Class	Detected Features
Chemical Sensors	
• Gas;	• Organic and inorganic gas;
• Humidity.	• Water molecule.
Physical Sensors	
• Optical;	• Light intensity, wavelength, polarization, etc.
• Mechanical;	• Length, acceleration, flow, force, pressure, etc.
• Magnetic;	• Magnetic flux, density, magnetic moment, etc.
• Thermal;	• Temperature, specific heat, heat flow, etc.
• Electrical.	• Charge, current, voltage, resistance, inductance, etc.

4.4.2.1 CHEMICAL SENSOR

The chemical sensor can be defined as an analyzer that acts in response to a particular analyte in a selective and two-sided means and alters the input chemical quantity, varying from the concentration of a particular sample constituent to a complete mixture study, into a methodically electrical signal.

4.4.2.2   PHYSICAL SENSOR

A physical sensor is a tool which can assesses a physical quantity (like temperature, charge, current, etc.), and transforms it into a signal that can be examined by an equipment or instrument. Physical sensors make use of various physical effects, for example, piezoelectric, magnetostriction, ionization, thermoelectric, photoelectric, magnetoelectric, etc., for sensing.

4.5   CLASSIFICATION OF GAS SENSOR

Currently, solid-state based gas sensors are being progressed. The solid state-based gas sensors are advanced due to their small size, less expensive, and more reliable to industries. The solid-state gas sensors are of three types:

- Solid-electrolyte sensor;
- Catalytic combustion gas sensor; and
- Metal oxide semiconductor (MOS) gas sensor.

4.5.1   SOLID ELECTROLYTE SENSOR

These types of sensors operate on the principle mechanism of electrochemistry or ionic conductivity of the solid electrolyte materials in the existence of gas, which changes the electrochemical or conductivity properties of the sensors. Solid electrolytes are the constituents, which let the conduction of ions across it but it does not allow the conduction of electrons. The necessary function of the solid electrolyte is to partition the two regions of different action of the species to be examined/studied and also accept the excessive mobility of ions of the species between two regions.

4.5.2   CATALYTIC COMBUSTION GAS SENSOR

These types of sensors include catalyst materials along with sensor material. In this type of sensor, combustible gas is subjected to the sensor, which then responds with catalyst causing the burning of fuel gas, which finally boosts the resistance of the sensing materials. The increase in resistance is then measured and further co-related/analyzed with a concentration of the combustible fuel gas.

4.5.3 METAL OXIDE SEMICONDUCTOR (MOS) GAS SENSOR

These sensors are grounded on the semiconductor oxides. The working principle of such sensors is based on adsorption phenomenon. The electrical properties of the surface are altered/modified due to the adsorption of distant kinds (e.g., gases, liquids, etc.), over the surface of the semiconductor material. The solid-state gas sensors are manufactured in the outline of pellets, thin or thick films, etc. Liu et al. has categorized the gas sensors based on their sensing methods and parted them into two units (2012).

- Methods based on variation in electrical properties; and
- Methods based on variation in other properties which can be depicted from Figure 4.2.

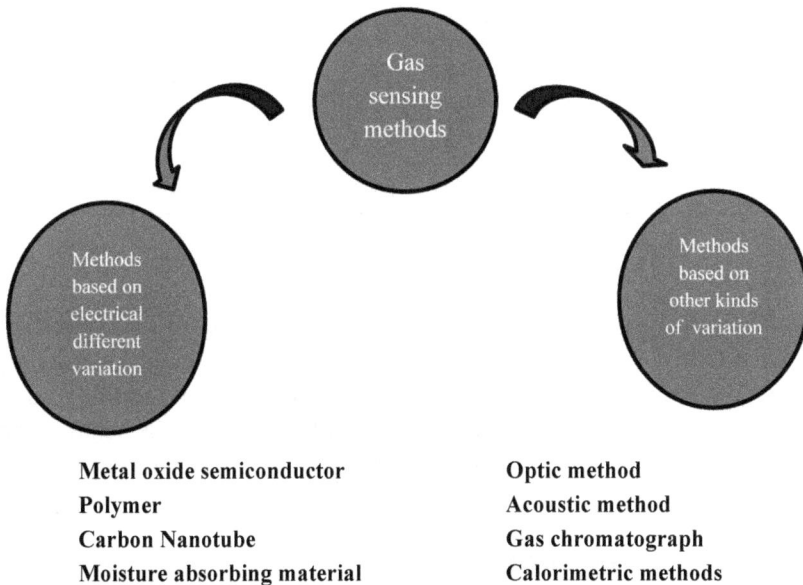

Metal oxide semiconductor	Optic method
Polymer	Acoustic method
Carbon Nanotube	Gas chromatograph
Moisture absorbing material	Calorimetric methods

FIGURE 4.2 Classification of gas sensing method.
Source: Reproduced with permission from: Liu et al. (2012).

Materials like semiconductor metal oxides (SMOs), carbon nanotubes (CNTs), and polymers are able to sense a wide range of gases, owing to variation of its electrical properties. Another deviations in its properties are optic, acoustic, gas chromatographic and calorimetric, which can also generate signals and hence detect the gas. Comini grouped the gas sensors corresponding to the measurement ways such as: (a) DC conductometric gas sensors; (b) field-effect-transistors (FET) based gas sensors; (c) photoluminescence (PL) based gas sensors. The contrast of different types of gas sensors is mentioned in Table 4.2 and has been reviewed by G. Korotcenkov (Comini et al., 2006; Korotcenkov, 2007).

TABLE 4.2   Comparison of Various Types of Gas Sensor

Parameters	Types of Gas Sensors				
	Semi-Conductor	Catalytic Combustion	Electro-chemical	Thermal Conductive	Infrared Absorption
Sensitivity	e	g	g	b	e
Accuracy	g	g	g	g	e
Selectivity	p	b	g	b	e
Response time	e	g	p	g	p
Stability	g	g	b	g	g
Durability	g	g	p	g	e
Maintenance	e	e	g	g	p
Cost	e	e	g	g	p
Suitability to portable instruments	e	g	p	g	b

Note: e: excellent; g: good; p: poor; b: bad.

All the factors are employed to illustrate the features of a specific material or a tool. A standard chemical sensor must acquire the following properties like high sensitivity, dynamic range, selectivity, and stability, lower detection limit, appropriate linear response, lesser hysteresis behavior and response time, and long-life cycle (Korotcenkov, 2007; Dey, 2018).

4.6   ROLE OF METAL OXIDES

Metal oxides materials are the major basis for domestic, commercial, industrial applications. The research on metal oxides revolve around reviewing their properties and methods of increasing the influencing factors such as sensitivity, selectivity, response time, durability, etc., towards specific gases at different operating conditions. Earlier, the metal oxide-based sensors did not show very good results and having problems like humidity sensitivity, high cross-sensitivity, slow response, etc. To increase the sensor functioning, a wide range of several MOSs have been developed over the last 40 years (Mizsei, 2016; Meixner and Lampe, 1996). After the first publication of SnO_2 based sensors, these sensors are the best-known as metal oxide-based gas sensors. The sensor properties of the metal oxide-based gas sensors can be altered by modifying the dopants, fabrication techniques, operating temperature, crystal structures, etc. Metal oxides such as Cr_2O_3, MnO_2, CO_3O_4, NiO, CuO, SrO, WO_3, TiO_2, SnO_2, ZnO, CeO_2, etc., are well known examples that are suitable for sensing response and can be determined by their different properties (e.g., electronic structure) (Korotcenkov, 2007).

4.6.1 NANOSTRUCTURED METAL OXIDES-BASED GAS SENSORS

4.6.1.1 TIN DIOXIDE (SNO₂)

Tin oxide (SnO_2) is mostly utilized materials by the gas sensor industries, as it is n-type having wide bandgap semiconductor. SnO_2 is a transparent conductive oxide with a rutile structure and having interesting thermal and gas sensing properties. Wei et al. has synthesized SnO_2 nanowires (NWs) over the oxidized silicon substrate at 900°C in an Argon flow at atmospheric pressure using Tin grains through thermal evaporation technique (2013). The structural feature of SnO_2 NWs shows the tetragonal arrangement of about 30 to 200 nm in diameter measurement and having a length of few micrometers. The SnO_2 nanowire gas sensor shows the changeable reaction towards H_2 gas at working temperature, which is near about 300°C and the peak sensitivity found to be low at 150°C. The sensor sensitivity increases with increase in H_2 concentration. It has been concluded that the SnO_2 nano-wires are able to utilize for the good gas sensor applications (Wei et al., 2013). Khuspe et al. stated the fabrication of SnO_2 thin film employed by sol-gel combined with spin coating technique, which is the environment friendly and effective process for fabricating it (2013). The gas sensing for SnO_2 film is found to be selective for lower concentrations of NO_2 gas at 200°C. SnO_2 based thin film sensor demonstrates a maximum 19% gas response with 77.90% stability towards NO_2 gas. The fastest response time was found to be 7 s, while recovery time calculated as 1202 s for the NO_2 concentration of 100 ppm. The response time and recovery time was found 32 s and 302 s, respectively, for the 10 ppm NO_2 concentration. This fall in response time may occur because of the high availability of vacant sites as depicted by the FESEM (field emission scanning electron microscope) and TEM microimages (Figures 4.3 and 4.4) on the film for the adsorption of gas (Khuspe et al., 2013).

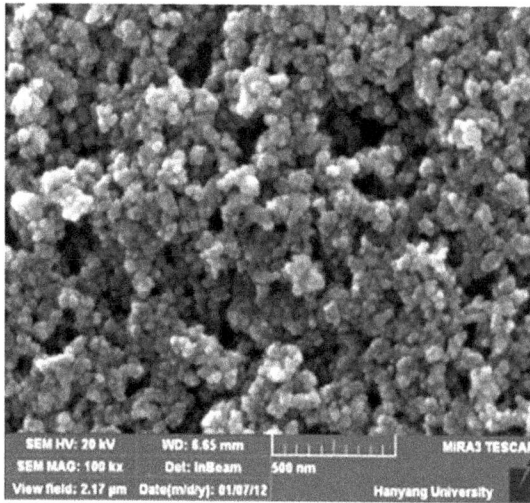

FIGURE 4.3   FESEM of SnO_2 thin films.
Source: Reproduced with permission from: Khuspe et al. (2013). © Elsevier.

The microwave-assisted hydrothermal method under different conditions has been carried out for the synthesis of nanostructured SnO_2. Synthesized SnO_2 nanoparticles (NPs) was found to be platelet-like and hierarchical structure (Man et al., 2013). The surface-controlled sensing mechanism for SnO_2 has been observed here, and it has been investigated that the sensitivity of the sensor was highly dependent on the adsorption and desorption phenomena of the gas molecules. There are three different samples prepared. It can be concluded that all samples exhibit the fast response time as well as fast recovery time. As the alcohol concentration was increased, the gas sensitivity also increases and it revealed the stability of the gas sensor is good. The results showed that samples constituting the hierarchical structure have higher sensitivity in comparison to the other sample (Man et al., 2013). The quasi-molecular imprinting mechanism design have been carried out in the following study for the development of highly sensitive SnO_2 semiconductor for the target gas of carbon monooxide (CO) by varying the gas concentration from 50 ppm to 3000 ppm (Li et al., 2015). SnO_2 NPs have been synthesized through hydrothermal method and different gas sensor film devices were prepared as Sc (after the suspension coating of SnO_2 which was fully dried, was exposed to target gas CO for 12 h) and S_A (after suspension coating of SnO_2 film which is found to be fully dried, was exposed to the air atmosphere) which consist of the SnO_2 NPs. In the different range of CO concentration, the response of Sc is higher. It had been found out that Sc showed the shorter response time and recovery time in comparison with S_A at various CO concentration (Li et al., 2015). The other research showed a thin film micro-electro-mechanical system (MEMS) based gas sensor, which was utilized for acetone gas detection (Sachdeva et al., 2019). As MEMS technique have been recommended in the manufacturing of gas sensor in view of its practical applications. MEMS was commonly prepared through a number of processes, which involves like lithography, oxidation, etching, sputtering, depositions, etc. Acetone gas was detected through the prepared SnO_2 and it showed a very good response towards the target gas. Various concentration levels of acetone gas have been analyzed by varying different level from 1.5 ppm to 20 ppm concentration and

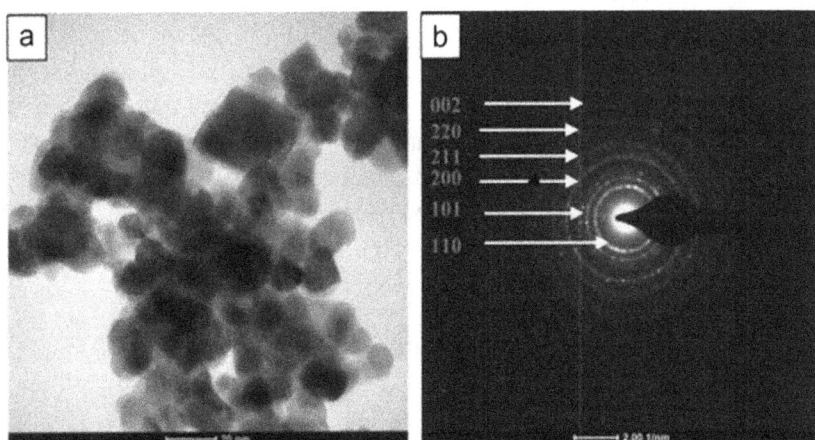

FIGURE 4.4 (a) TEM image of SnO_2; and (b) SAED pattern.

Source: Reproduced with permission from: Khuspe et al. (2013). © Elsevier.

response was achieved around 30% to 45%, respectively. SnO_2 thin films have been annealed at 300°C to achieve an optimum grain size of 86.3 nm as depicted by AFM. The response time in the detection of acetone gas was approximately found to be 3 mins and the recovery time was 4 mins. The following work has investigated the synthesis process using a glancing angle deposition (GLAD) along with an RF sputtering method for the growth and transformation of column-like SnO_2 nanostructure in the detection of CO gas at low temperature (Singh et al., 2018). In the growth of nonporous column-like structure of SnO_2 thin film under the GLAD configuration, the enhanced sensing response operating at lower temperature have been seen, which concluded being in contact of target CO gas molecules with the larger surface area in sensing SnO_2 thin film.

4.6.1.2   ZINC OXIDE (ZnO)

Zinc oxide (ZnO) is an adaptable material amongst the metal oxides and is used for numerous applications such as environmental pollutants degradation, sensing, solar cells, etc. (Schmidt-Mende et al., 2007). ZnO is n-type semiconducting material with chemical stability, tunable transport properties and large exciton binding energy. These properties made ZnO one such promising key material for the purpose of gas sensing (Shankar et al., 2015). For ZnO tetrapod fabrication, the ideal vapor phase growth have been employed so as to carry out huge output, with a good reproducibility and a single morphology (Calestani et al., 2010). The sensing properties for these sensors have been evaluated with high response as $S = 25$ at 1 ppm concentration and $S = 100$ at 5 ppm on comparing with the largest value of undoped ZnO nanorods (NRs) and sensitivity towards H_2S have also been investigated (Calestani et al., 2010). In the following research study, ZnO thin films have been synthesized with the help of sol-gel spin coating technique onto a glass substrate using zinc acetate dehydrate $[Zn(CH_3COO)_2.2H_2O]$ as precursor (Nimbalkar et al., 2017). Microstructural analysis showed the structured morphology of ZnO thin film being inhomogeneous form and having porosity which turned out to be appropriate in gas sensing applications depicting from Figure 4.5. The morphology of the ZnO film having porous structure improves the H_2S gas sensing carried out at 300C. The sensor shows the highest gas response of 3.2 with 59% stability have been revealed by the sensor in exposure to 100 ppm of H_2S gas concentration (Nimbalkar et al., 2017).

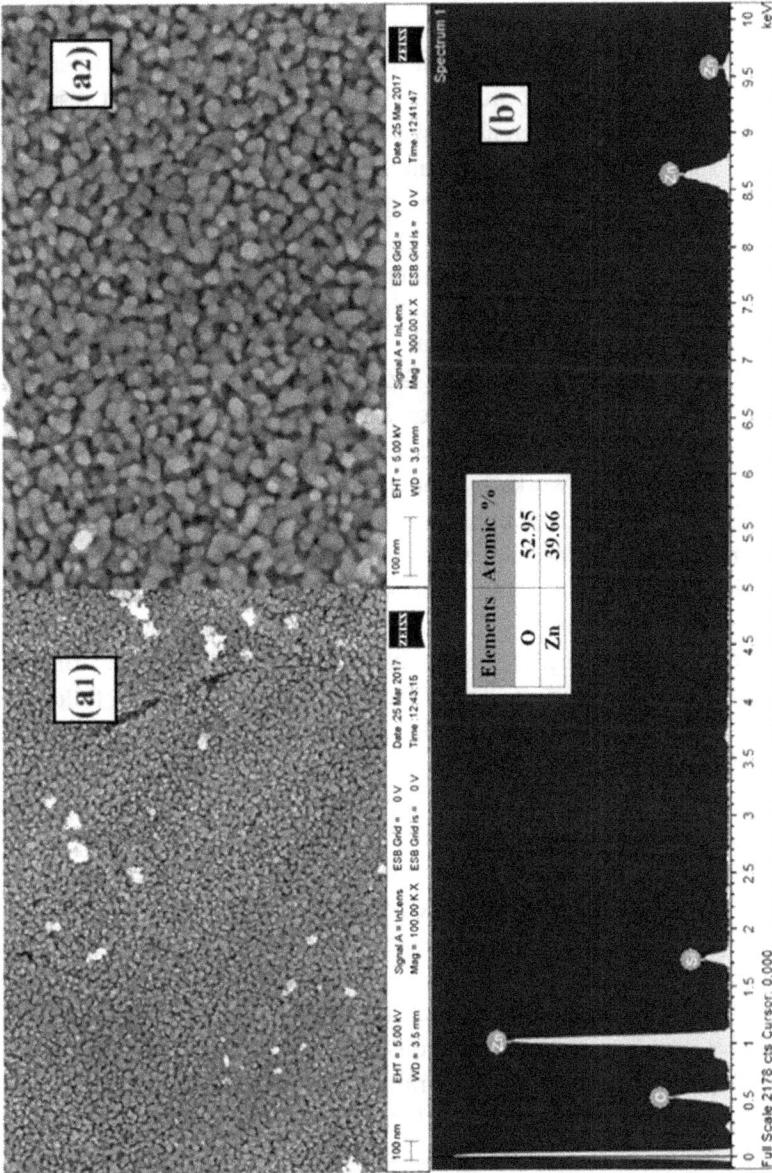

FIGURE 4.5 (a1 and a2) High-magnification FESEM images; and (b) EDX spectrum of ZnO thin film.

Source: Reproduced with permission from: Nimbalkar and Patil (2017). © Elsevier.

In the other paper, the two different synthesis techniques, i.e., simple heat treatment and thermal evaporation-two zone furnaces have been employed for preparing ZnO NPs (Bhatia et al., 2017). For controlling shape configuration and mass of ZnO NPs, the NPs were produced with the help of these two methods for two-zone split furnace by altering zone temperature (Zone 1–800°C and Zone 2–400°C). The high sensitivity, fastest response and recovery time have been also investigated at an operating temperature of 250°C and this confirms that thermal evaporation technique for 50 ppm ethanol found to be an effective method sensing applications in every field of technology (Hatia et al., 2017). For the development in adsorption and desorption of gaseous species, the fabrication of 3-D interconnected networks of ZnO tetrapods have been the most effective step. ZnO-T-Fe_2O_3 and ZnO-T-CuO compound structure showed the higher gas response towards ethanol vapor, while ZnO-T-$ZnAl_2O_4$ hybrid networks exhibited good selectivity towards H_2 gas (for ZnO: Al (20:1)) and towards CH_4 (for ZnO: Al (10:1)). The achieved results have shown the gas sensing response of ZnO-T networks by doping and alloying with Fe, Cu, or Al metals and it has been found that it provides better sensors for industrial and environmental monitoring (Lupan et al., 2017). In current years, wearable electronic devices, such as smartwatches, smart glass, and wearable cameras have been emerged promptly in the application area of health monitoring (Zheng et al., 2015). More studies have directed on emerging of new wearable electronic devices. From the research study of the following chapter, UV-light controlled, flexible, transparent, and working at room-temperature ethanol gas sensor have been fabricated by simply coating ZnO NPs on flexible and transparent PET-ITO substrates. The fabricated sensor showed the fastest photoresponse with the highest sensing response towards ethanol under UV irradiation. Meanwhile, its transmittance exceeds 62% in the visible spectral range, and the sensing performance exhibits the same curve at a curvature angle of 90° (Zheng et al., 2015).

ZnO hierarchical structures, holding the higher surface area and less accumulation which can also be used functioning of gas sensor. The key parameters such as sensitivity response, selectivity, and stability, which affect the performances of ZnO hierarchical structures-based gas sensors have been analyzed. The various performance factors affecting the sensing features such as long-term stability, sensitivity, etc., of ZnO hierarchical structure-based gas sensor is summarized in Table 4.3 (Zhang et al., 2018). An ultraviolet-enhanced (UV-enhanced) nitric oxide (NO) sensor based on silver-doped ZnO nano-flowers has been fabricated with the help of less expensive hydrothermal method (Tsai et al., 2018). The optimized operating temperature has been varied from 200°C to 150°C using UV light illumination, and it was found that the response has been increasing from 73.91% to 89.04%for NO gas sensor under UV illumination at 150°C operable temperature (Tsai et al., 2018). In 2006, Zhong Lin Wang's group has projected a unique model for nano-generators (NGs), including piezoelectric nano-generator and triboelectric nano-generator, as to transform automated spark into an electric output. In the following review chapter, the advancement in the progress for NG-based self-powered gas sensors new concept has been systematically summarized. Being a new field, in coupling piezoelectric or triboelectric with semiconducting gas sensing attributes, the NG-based self-powered gas sensing system has been established with various sensor feature such as flexible, lightweight, high-efficient, cost-effective, and environmental outgoing designs.

TABLE 4.3 A Summary About Factors Affecting Gas Sensing Performances of ZnO Hierarchical Structure-based Gas Sensors and Improvement Approaches

Main Characteristics Indexes which Reflect the Performances	Influencing Factors and Improvement Approaches	References
Sensitivity	Modulation of the dimensional and the exposed crystal facet of their constituting building blocks.	Zhang et al. (2009) Lei et al. (2017); Song et al. (2018) Lin et al. (2015)
	Enhancing the porosity of hierarchical structures.	
	Modification by doping with noble metals and loading of other p-type and n-type MOS materials.	
Selectivity	Control of grain size.	Mirzaei et al. (2018) Li et al. (2015) Chen et al. (2016); Espid et al. (2017)
	Dope with noble metals and p-type metal oxide.	
	Lowering the operating temperature by activating the sensing material under UV illumination.	
Long term stability	Calcination/Annealing as the post-processing treatment.	Gu et al. (2011) Chen et al. (2016) Dey (2018)
	Reduces the working temperature of gas sensing element.	
	Dope noble metal or synthesis of metal oxides.	

4.6.1.3   INDIUM OXIDE (IN₂O₃)

Indium oxide has been an n-type semiconducting material constituting of direct bandgap of 3.6 eV and indirect bandgap of about 2.6 eV. Using the ambient ultrasonic spray pyrolysis technique co-relating with a low decomposition temperature (200–300°C) indium nitrate-based precursor solution, Indium oxide thin-film transistors have been fabricated (Faber et al., 2015). In the characterization study, it was identified that the two primaries aims for the improved transistor performance analysis are the presence of a reduced concentration of In-OH groups along with the development of denser films at 250C. Researcher reported the In_2O_3 films grown at 250°C have been highly continuous, smooth, i.e., (surface roughness found to be rms value < 2 nm), extremely thin near about 6–8 nm and highly crystalline in nature. For the development of low operating voltage of approximately <2 V transistors, the sprayed In_2O_3 layers with solution of processed AlO_x/ZrO_2 high-k dielectrics have been studied (Faber et al., 2015). The following chapter investigated the detection for ppb levels concentration of acetone, a biomarker for diabetes, revealing the higher sensitivity of subspherical sections of In_2O_3-Pt NPs (Karmaoui et al., 2016). The form of monodispersed metal oxide In_2O_3 NPs with diameters of 6 nm to 8 nm, patterned with 2% by mass ratio, Pt-based metal NPs of 2 nm to 3 nm on the surface, have been synthesized via a hydrate sol-gel routing technique. The hybrid In_2O_3-Pt NPs being practical applications, in chemo-resistive devices for monitoring acetone at ppb levels in human breath conditions, which helps in the diagnosis and monitoring of diabetes. The response of the sensor towards 1.56 ppm of acetone, on comparing with the pure In_2O_3, lying in the range from 100°C to 250°C, have investigated in Figure 4.6 (Karmaoui et al., 2016).

A coral-like In_2O_3 was realistically synthesized by a solvothermal method, after 2 hrs of treating the precursor at 550°C which can be seen from Figure 4.7 (Zhang et al., 2017). The gas sensing properties of sensors based on the as-synthesized In_2O_3 towards NO_2 were analyzed. The sensor demonstrates tremendous NO_2 sensing properties at 130°C. The response of the sensor is found to be 2.41 towards 10 ppb concentration of NO_2 at 130°C. The response time was examined about 40s and recovery time were about 22 s (Zhang et al., 2017).

Solvothermal technique fabricated the uniform size HFP-In_2O_3 with L-lysine, ethylene glycol and annealing of the precursors at 400°C for 2 h

(Xu and Sun, 2015). The probable synthetic mechanism can be analyzed from Figure 4.8. The gas sensing features were examined and closely compared and revealed that 500 ppb concentration of NO_2 at 40°C have a response value of about 50.5, which exhibits higher than other gases. The following material have shown higher selectivity response towards NO_2 (Xu and Sun, 2015).

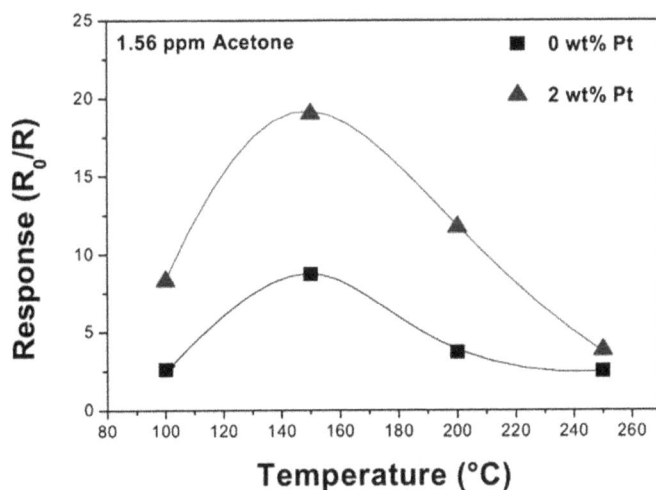

FIGURE 4.6 Comparison of tested sensor responses as a function of temperature.
Source: Reproduced with permission from: Karmaoui et al. (2016). © Elsevier.

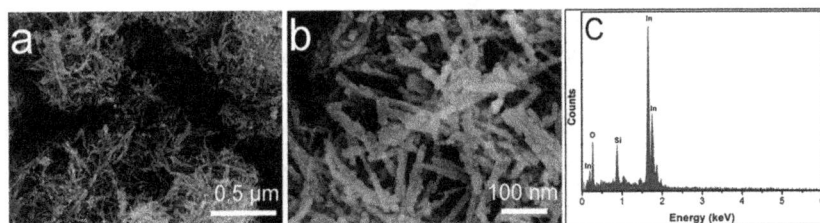

FIGURE 4.7 FESEM images of a and b of the as-synthesized In_2O_3. The EDX pattern of the coral-like In_2O_3.
Source: Reproduced with permission from: Zhang et al. (2017). © The Royal Society of Chemistry 2017. Open access.

In_2O_3/Au NRs along with pure In_2O_3 have been fabricated by using a simplistic co-precipitation procedure (Xing et al., 2015). It is found that

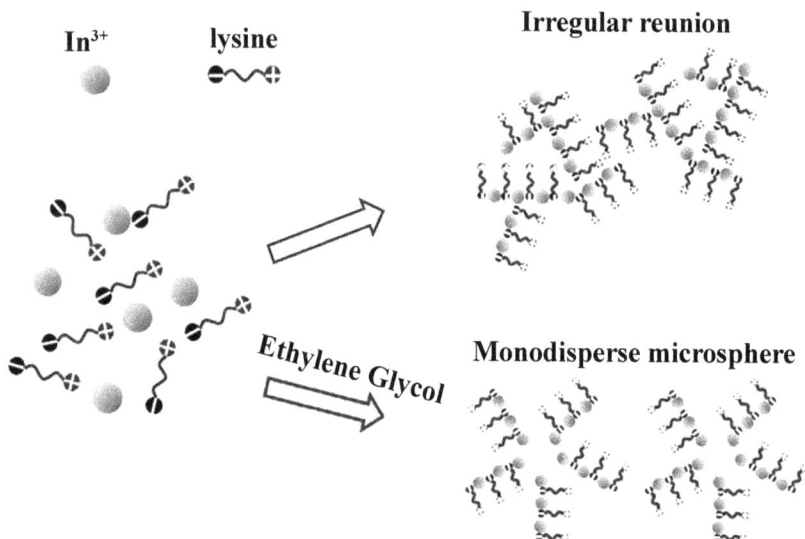

FIGURE 4.8   Synthetic mechanism of the material.
Source: Reproduced with permission from: Xu, Li, and Sun (2015). © Royal Society of Chemistry.

the initial $In(NO_3)_3$ amount and reaction time will have a little effect in the structure of In_2O_3/Au NR. The GNPs were uniformly dispersed in In_2O_3/Au NRs for very low concentration of acetone and ethanol. The results demonstrated that the optimal In_2O_3/Au NRs sensor detected the acetone at 250°C and ethanol at 400°C, which showed the gas response from 1 ppm to 2.8 ppm acetone, and 5 ppm to 9.8 ppm ethanol. It is also found that it can detect with very low concentration limit of 0.1 ppm of acetone and 0.05 ppm of ethanol (Xing et al., 2015). Bulk In_2O_3 was synthesized by calcination (573K, 3h, static air) of $In(OH)_3$, which had been precipitated by adding the excess of NH_4OH to $In(NO_3)_3 \cdot xH_2O$ dissolved in a 1:3 mixture of deionized water and ethanol (Martin et al., 2016). In the reaction, it is found that the In_2O_3 catalysts have been stimulated in Ar at 573 K and at 0.5 MPa for 1 h, while the Cu-ZnO-Al_2O_3 catalyst have been pre-processed in 5 vol% H_2/Ar under the same operating conditions. In_2O_3 revealed the 100% selectivity towards methanol by varying the testing temperature, whereas the ternary catalyst found to be maximum of 47% only at 200°C to that of RWGS reaction (Martin et al., 2016). In the following chapter, mesoporous In_2O_3 nanostructures have been fabricated by an In^{3+} ions catalytic FAR-template route (Zhang et al., 2016). Here, a facile, high-yield method is used to manufacture mesoporous In_2O_3 nano-structures with significant amount. The sensors were designed by coating the acquired In_2O_3 sample on a ceramic tube which consists of Pt lead wires, two Au electrodes and heating wire. The author reported the vertically aligned Si-NWs as an operational assistance for In_2O_3-x(OH)y-based gas-phase photo-catalysts in the reduction of CO_2 to CO via RWGS reaction (Hoch et al., 2016). The higher magnification of $In_2O_{3-x}(OH)_y$/SiNW bilayer films indicates that it have porosity and particle size are uniform (Figure 4.9).

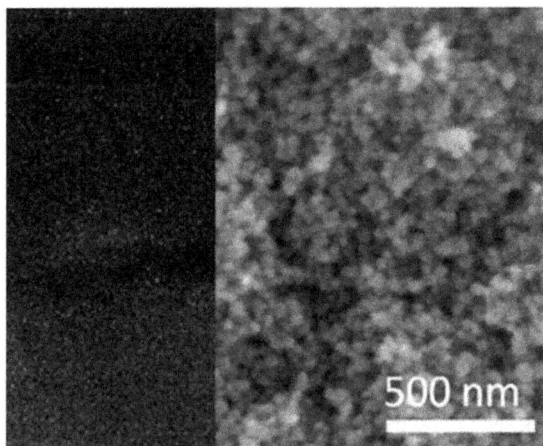

FIGURE 4.9 $In_2O_{3-x}(OH)_y$/SiNW bilayer films.
Source: Reproduced with permission from: Hoch et al. (2016). © American Chemical Society.

4.6.1.4 TUNGSTEN TRIOXIDE (WO₃)

WO_3, n-type semiconducting material consisting of a bandgap of 2.7 eV, have attracted the scholars to investigate its sensing properties. "W" sites with different oxidation states of the non-stoichiometric WO_3 stimulated the author to examine the chemistry of the surface reactions. In the following work, thermal oxidation method have been employed for the synthesis process of WO_3 NRs and investigated for gas sensing application (Hoch et al., 2016). For the following fabrication procedure, on oxidized Si substrate tungsten film has been deposited through sputtering method and therefore followed by thermal oxidation process at 500°C in an ambient conditions.

The WO_3 NRs based sensor revealed the sensitivity and selectivity much higher towards NO_2 gas in comparison to other analytes. At an optimum working temperature, the sensor detected a small amount of concentration of NO_2 gas (2 ppm). It was identified that the WO_3 NRs were highly sensitive towards NO_2 gas, and lower sensitive response towards NH_3, H_2S, ethanol, methanol, and acetone have been examined (Behera and Chandra, 2018). In another study, Cu-doped WO_3 hollow fibers have been prepared by electrospinning technique along with sol-gel and sintering process (Bai et al., 2014). The sensing characteristics of the sensor built on 3 mol% of Cu doped triclinic WO_3 hollow fibers revealed the high gas response, good selectivity and fastest response time of 5s and recovery time around 20s towards 20 ppm concentration of acetone (Figure 4.10) (Bai et al., 2014).

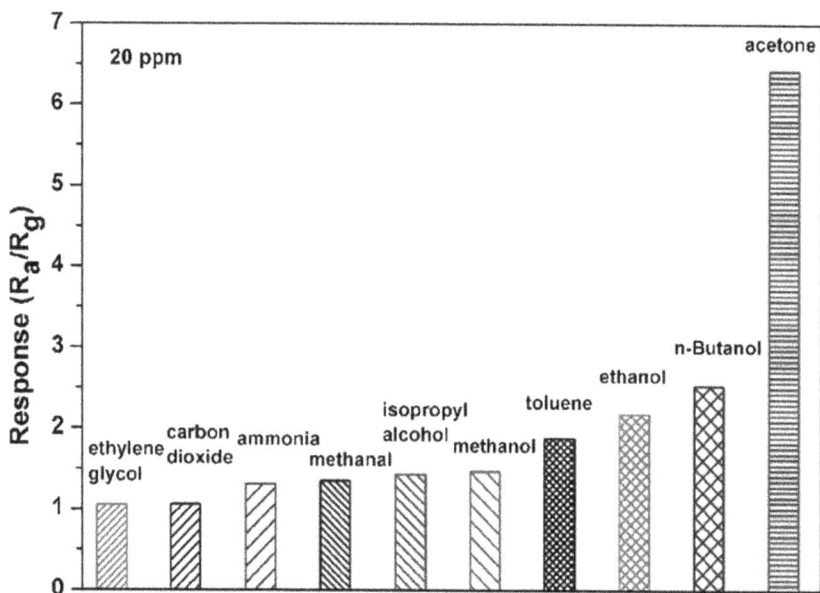

FIGURE 4.10   Response values of 3 mol% Cu-doped WO_3 sensor to 20 ppm of different gases.

Source: Reproduced with permission from: Bai, Ji, Gao, Zhang, and Sun (2014). © Elsevier.

Hexagonal tungsten oxide NWs patterned with PdO or PtO_x NPs turn out to be the best choice in the detection of H_2 gas and a high sensitivity and good selectivity was also examined in comparison to the NO, CO, and CH_4 analytes. Both NPs pattern lead to similar sensor performance. Since the sensor response towards H_2 shown a large effect, even at 150°C, the author also conducted the measurements at 30°C, 70°C and 130°C moreover, to identify whether the devices could handle the further experiment without external heating (Kukkola et al., 2013). The author reported the synthesis of single-crystalline ultrathin $W_{18}O_{49}$ NWs by an aliphatic amine using benzyl alcohol routing having high proportionality factor. The sensor, comprising of 10 layers of aligned NWs, revealed the sensitivity towards H_2 at ambient temperature in humid air (Cheng et al., 2015). Deng et al. reported the sensing of formaldehyde (HCHO) using mesoporous silica WO_3, which were examined via activation of illumination at room temperature (2012). It is investigated that the response of the WO_3 gas sensors reached to 1.3×10^{-7} $\Omega^{-1}s^{-1}$ for HCHO (100 ppm) under white light (100 Wm^{-2}) while response was found to be $9.5 \times 10^{-8} \Omega^{-1}s^{-1}$ under blue light (100 Wm^{-2}), which was found to be 4 and 9 times in comparison to the commercial WO_3. This was related with the presence of the mesopores and higher surface area. Moreover, the responses towards acetone, ethanol, and toluene at 100 ppm concentrations each, for mesoporous and commercial WO_3 sensors were also evaluated. Figure 4.11 shows a graph of response time of mesoporous and commercial WO_3 against HCHO, acetone, and toluene.

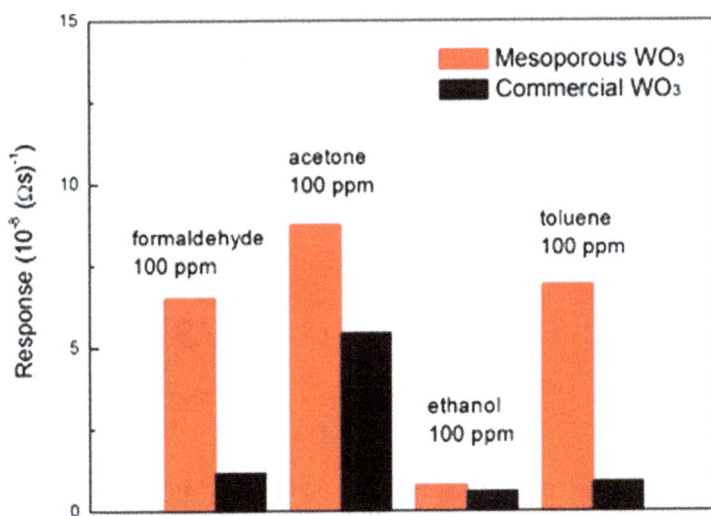

FIGURE 4.11 Responses of the mesoporous and commercial WO_3 to formaldehyde (100 ppm), acetone (100 ppm), ethanol (100 ppm) and toluene (100 ppm) activated by blue light (40 W/m^2).

Source: Reproduced with permission from: Deng et al. (2012). © Elsevier.

For the synthesis of hierarchical self-assembled hollow spheres (HS) of tungsten oxide nano-sheets, the hydrothermal procedure has been employed (Li et al., 2015). The gas sensing properties of the self-assembled hierarchical WO_3 HS (by calcined prototypes at 500°C) were also examined. The response performance of WO_3 HS was experienced at 140°C, in which response time was calculated 90s and recovery time was 400s for 100 ppb NO_2 concentration. To control the morphology of the hydrothermal procedure outcome, the oxalic coordination composite which controls the hydrothermal rate of nucleation has been observed and finally forms the self-assembled hollow sphere structure (Li et al., 2015). Zhong et al. reported that the WO_3 and Ag-WO_3 (mixed solid solutions Ag with WO_3) NPs are suitably fabricated by sol-gel method (2018). The XRD of pure WO_3 and Ag-WO_3 NPs is presented in Figure 4.12. The XRD pattern reveals that in the temperature range from 300°C to 500°C, the phase transition of hexagonal to monoclinic has been identified. The crystallinity magnitude for WO_3 NPs found to be increased by increasing calcination temperature and decreased a little by stirring Ag with it (Lu et al., 201).

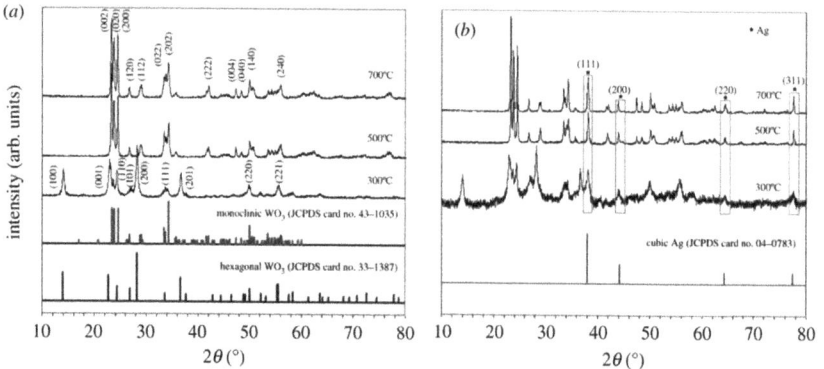

FIGURE 4.12   XRD diffraction patterns of (a) pure WO_3 and (b) Ag-WO_3 nanoparticles at different calcination temperatures.

Source: Reproduced with permission from: Lu, Zhong, Shang, Wang, and Tang (2018). © 2018 The Authors. https://creativecommons.org/licenses/by/4.0/

The thin films of tungsten oxide (WO_3) having structure like 2D nanoplates were fabricated via hydrothermal technique with sodium tungstate dihydrate ($Na_2WO_4.2H_2O$) has been taken as a precursor on soda-lime glass substrate at the reaction temperature of 1000°C and the reaction time varied from 3 h to 7 h have been seen (Shendage et al., 2017). The excellent NO_2 sensing properties at a low operating temperature of 100°C for WO_3 thin-film sensor have been evaluated during synthesis. The sensor response calculated to be 10 for 5 ppm NO_2 concentration and when reached to 100 ppm concentration of NO_2, the response was 131.75 at the working temperature of 100°C. In the following work, B. Urasinska-Wojick et al. reported the response of a tungsten oxide-based MEMS gas sensor towards ppb level concentration of nitrogen dioxide (NO_2) operated at different environment conditions (2017). The response was estimated at ca. 500% to a 100-ppb pulse of NO_2 in air at 350C operating temperature. It was investigated that under various working temperatures, ranging from 250°C and 450°C, the author revealed the gas sensor response at low oxygen levels, i.e., below 1%. It was seen that there was a small change in sensitivity feature to changes in humidity (ca. 0.2%/%RH) but there is cross-sensitivity found to be negligible towards CO, H_2, CH_4 and acetone at much higher ppm levels. The chapter presented the diameter-controlled synthesis of hierarchical and plenty amount of nanoporous tungsten oxide nanorod bundles for the applications of NO_2 gas sensor (Van Tong et al., 2013). It has been examined that by changing the amount of P123 surfactant used throughout the hydrothermal procedure, the morphologies for the synthesized NRs have been controlled. The gas sensor device manufactured with the help of nanoporous tungsten oxide nanorod bundles revealed the sensing features such as high sensitivity, selectivity, and stability in the detection of NO_2 gas at low concentrations. The response of the sensor at 1 ppm was 4, 24, at 2.5 ppm was 42.08 and at 5 ppm concentration was 111.34, respectively towards NO_2 gas at 250°C.

4.6.1.5   COPPER OXIDE (CuO)

Copper oxide (CuO), a p-type material exists as cupric (CuO) and cuprous (Cu_2O) oxide form with narrow bandgap of 1.2 eV to 1.5 eV and 2.12 eV, correspondingly. The exchange of oxygen from atmosphere and lattice oxygen vacancy in the course of the sensing process, switches cupric to cuprous oxide material. Nemade et al. synthesized the NPs of CuO were effectively synthesized via a spray pyrolysis method (2014). An average elemental size of the following NPs found to be approximately 6 nm. As prepared CuO sensor film exhibited a good sensing response towards the CO_2 gas. The sensing response showed the highest value of 3.5 at 1000 ppm level of CO_2 gas. Likewise, the optimum operable temperature for the sensor attained at 423 K for 500 ppm concentration. The response time witnessed for this sensor was about 16s, whereas, recovery time was about 20s shown by the sensor (Nemade et al., 2014). In another work, the less expensive sol-gel spin coating technique followed by annealing has been used in the synthesis of thin films of nanocrystalline CuO at various temperatures ranging between 300°C and 700°C. From Figure 4.13, the electrical gas response of CuO was analyzed in response to 20, 40, 60, 80 and 100 ppm of H_2S and found that CuO film was more sensitive and also responsive to H_2S gas in the environment. The maximum response for H_2S was near about 25.2% at 100 ppm gas concentration and also faster in comparison to other gases (Patil et al., 2011).

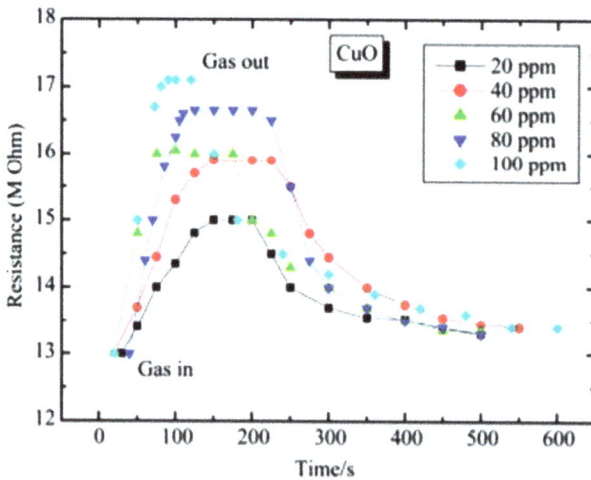

FIGURE 4.13   Gas responses of CuO sensor film to 20–100 ppm of H_2S.

Zeggar et al. reported the CuO thin film fabrication for the ethanol (C_2H_5OH) vapor detection (2016). This film was deposited on heated glass substrate via spray ultrasonic pyrolysis technique at optimum temperature. The microstructural analysis has been characterized by X-ray diffraction (XRD) and atomic force microscopy (AFM), which shows the presence of intense peaks in the XRD patterns, which showed that film is polycrystalline in nature. Vapor-sensing test was carried out using static vapor-sensing system, at different temperatures in the range of 100°C to 175°C at 300 ppm concentration of ethanol vapor. The optimal gas response was found to be with a value of 45% at 150°C (Zeggar et al., 2016). In another work, Zhang et al. investigated the flower-like CuO constituted of many nano-flakes with average thickness of 40 nm was synthesized via a hydrothermal process (Zhang et al., 2011). In comparison with other electrodes, it was found that CuO/GCE showed the analogous or less detection limit along with linear range to be wider, which is summarized in Table 4.4.

TABLE 4.4 Comparison of Sensing Performances of Different Electrochemical Sensors for Nitrites

Electrode	Linear Range (µM)	Detection Limit (µM)	References
Nano-Au/Ch/GC	0.4–750	0.1	Wang et al. (2009)
Nano-Au/P3MT/GC	5–500	2.3	Huang et al. (2008)
Pt-disk electrode	10–10,000	4.8	Abbaspour et al. (2005)
Cu-TI composite film-GCE	1000–10,000	250	Casella et al. (2004)
CuO-graphite composite CE	100–1250	0.6	Sljukic et al. (2007)
MnO$_2$-graphite composite CE	–	1.2	Langley et al. (2007)
CuO-GCE	1.0–91.5	0.36	Zhang et al. (2011)

Reprinted with permission from Zhang et al., 2011. © Springer Nature.

In the following work, the CuO microspheres covered with Cu$_2$O/CuO nanocrystals and CuO NWs networks have been successfully synthesized the simple thermal oxidation process has been employed for synthesizing the CuO microspheres covering withCu$_2$O/CuO nanocrystals and CuO NWs shaping network on pre-patterned glass substrates with Au/Cr pads. The optimal working temperature for the development of the thread like and intense nanowire arrays was found to be 425°C in air at an oxidation time of 5 h (Oleg et al., 2015). In this chapter, the author has gone through the summarized research on the fabrication process with the effect of different factors or the properties, and few favorable applications of CuO nanostructures (Tran et al., 2014). For the nanostructure synthesis, the microwave method in which copper hydroxide nanostructures have been fabricated following the precursor solution and changes has been observed by microwave into CuO which has been considered as a favorable method to investigate additionally (Tran et al., 2014).

4.6.2 NANOCOMPOSITES MATERIALS

Nanocomposites are the multiphase solid materials that combines dimension of less than 100 nanometers particles into the molds of material in a traditional way. The outcome of the nanoparticle supplements is an extreme development in the possessions which holds mechanical strength, toughness, and electrical or thermal conductivity. The efficiency of the nanoscale particles can be determined by the addition of the quantity of material which is normally found within 0.5 and 5% range on mass scale. NPs have an enormously high surface to volume ratio, which considerably altered the several characteristics, on differentiating with the same large sized particles. It also transforms the approach in which the NPs are co-related with almost all big size materials. Therefore, the composites can be intensified in comparison to parts of the element.

In this chapter, Gu et al. reported the appropriately-structured the fabrication of indium oxide-reduced GN oxide (In_2O_3-rGO) nanocomposites through hydrothermal technique (2015). The fundamental, configurational analysis, chemical composition study revealed that In_2O_3-rGO nanocomposites-based gas sensor has revealed the sensing features in the detection of NO_2 at ambient temperature such as excellent selectivity, high response, relatively short response and recovery time. The gas response was found to be 8.25 with 30 ppm of NO_2 gas at the room temperature condition and the response and recovery time found to be 4 min and 24 min, respectively (Gu et al., 2015). The following research article investigated the layer-by-layer spin-coating deposition technique which has been used for the fabrication of SnO_2 quantum wire fixed on reduced graphene (rGO) nanosheets in the H_2S gas detection at responsive room temperature (Song et al., 2016). It was also investigated that observed morphology-related quantum confinement evolution of crystallized SnO_2, which could be well controlled by tuning the reaction time with the aid of the steric hindrance of rGO in the one-step synthesis. The sensing characteristics like dynamic response and recovery time at room temperature were also observed in the following study research, and the response time was found to be 2s to 13s on the basis of H_2S gas concentration. The sensor response dependency on the H_2S gas concentration lies in the range of 20 ppm to 100 ppm, which was found to be almost linear, the slope and correlation coefficient (R^2) of the linear fit was analyzed to be 0.69 ppm^{-1} and 0.959. The sensor response towards 50 ppm of NH_3, SO_2, NO_2 and ethanol vapor were determined as 1.27, 1.47, 0.65, and 0.94, respectively at ambient temperature, which revealed that the H_2S-sensing selectivity is ideal as compared to the other gases such as NH_3, SO_2, NO_2 and ethanol vapor at ambient temperature (Song et al., 2016). Y. Zhou et al. reported the rGO/MoS_2 composite film was prepared as a sensing layer for detecting NO_2 (2017). The experiment study investigated that rGO/MoS_2 composite film was engaged by a large contact area, having more sorption site and mass of p-n heterojunction, and hence in the sensing response of 59.8% towards 2 ppm NO_2 at 60°C (optimal operating temperature), was found to be 200% better in relating with simpler GO sample. Therefore, the exploration of NO_2 detection (at ppb level), the detection level was examined near about 5.7 ppb which is nearly low (Zhou et al., 2017). The following chapter investigated the undoped and In-doped ZnO including NPs and NRs, which were synthesized by means of sol-gel process (Shokry et al., 2014). For the highest sensitivity of gas, the effect of doping ratios of 1%, 5% and 10% for indium as a dopant element has been improved. The gas sensitivity for O_2, CO_2, and H_2 gases were measured for the fabrication of gas sensor devices as a function of temperature for In-doped ZnO nano-powders, the gas sensitivity for O_2, CO_2, H_2 gases has been identified and further they have been compared with un-doped ZnO films. The sensitivity evaluated for Zn:In is 95.5 by weight which is found to be maximum, and, 93 in percentage at 190°C (Shokry et al., 2014). The high-class graphene nanoplatelet (GNP) from exfoliation of flake graphite and GNP/SnO_2 nanocomposites have been fabricated with the help of superficial solid-state method (Zhang et al., 2018). It has been observed that 2D GNP has no change in basic structure during exfoliating process from flake graphite, and on the surface of GNP the SnO_2 NPs were dispersed fully. The GNP/SNO_2 core sensor has shown the tremendous sensing performance towards ethanol and the gas sensing properties has been improved due to definite surface area. For GNP/SnO_2 based sensors, the response time and recovery time has been evaluated as 26 s and 64 s, respectively (Zhang et al., 2018).

The different microporous substrates are used in the fabrication of rGO/SnO_2 nanocomposites thin films for investigating the sensing performance in the detection of NO_2 (Zhu et al., 2017). The selectivity of rGO/SnO_2 sensor towards NO_2 with 1 ppm concentration at 60°C among various gases such as H_2O, CO, NH_3, H_2S, HCHO was found to be excellent in comparison to other gases which can be depicted from Figure 4.14. The detection limit was also calculated as 15.7 ppb depending on the prepared sensor (Zhu et al., 2017). Hu et al. reported the synthesis process of hybrid Pd^{+2}/SnO_2/CNT using a sol-gel technique comprising of different Pd-loaded levels and CNT doped levels, investigating the CO sensors (2014). It is found that the hybrid $Pd^{+2}/SnO_2/CNT$ sensors revealed the higher sensitivity, selectivity, repeatability, a lower detection (at 5 ppm, Ra/Rg= 1.95), and a fast response-recovery which is less than or near about 2s towards CO at 100°C. The material sensitivity found to be higher, i.e., 80 times in comparison to pure tin oxide for 500 ppm of CO concentration. The characterization analysis showed that the SnO_2 particles was prevented by CNTs from establishing agglomerations because during CNT surface functionalization, it was found that SnO_2 particles has been likely to be attached with hydroxyl and carboxylic groups which can be depicted from Figure 4.15.

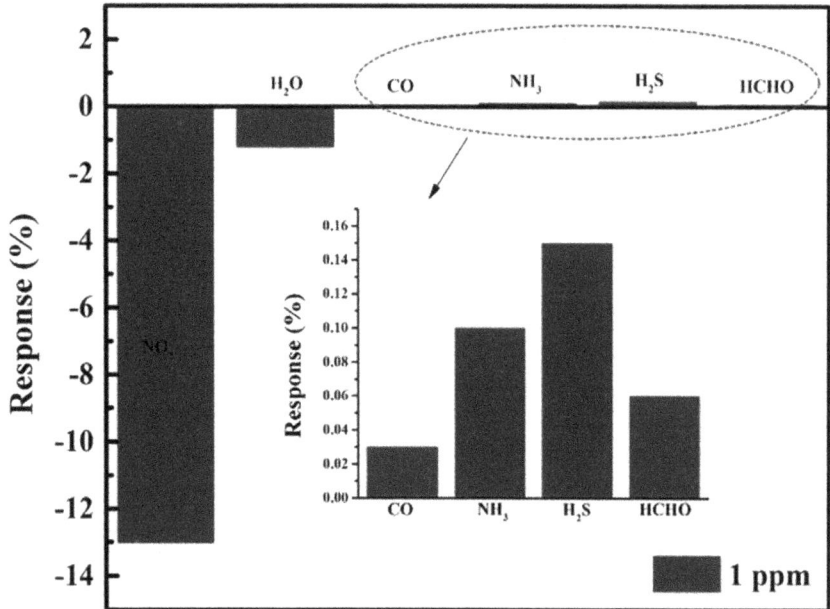

FIGURE 4.14   Selectivity investigation of rGO/SnO_2 composite film towards 1 ppm NO_2 gas.

Source: Reproduced with permission from: Zhu, Guo, Ren, Gao, and Zhou (2017). © Elseiver.

Graphene/ZnO nanocomposite was prepared by *in situ* reduction of zinc acetate (($CH_3COO)_2Zn \cdot 2H_2O$) and graphene oxide (GO) during refluxing (Anand et al., 2014). The morphological, compositional, and elemental analysis have been analyzed and the synthesized samples were illustrated by XRD, FESEM, and EDX spectroscopy depicting from Figure 4.16. The detecting results investigated that sensor based on 1.2% by weight, graphene/ZnO composite have shown the best response towards 200 ppm of hydrogen gas at an operating temperature of 150°C and compared with the prepared samples by varying their concentrations (Anand et al., 2014). In their study, it was reported that the synthesis of Fe-doped ZnO/reduced graphene oxide (rGO) nanocomposites with shared and improved sensing performance in the detection of HCHO via one-pot hydrothermal process has been carried out. The sensor created on 5 atomic% of Fe in Fe-ZnO/ rGO unveils the response of gas, i.e., 12.7 ppm to 5 ppm HCHO at 120°C, and the response time and recovery time found to be 34s and 37 s which is less, and the stability and selectivity showed the good behavior in sensing performance, but the sensor also deteriorated the gas sensing performance above 40% RH (Guo et al., 2019).

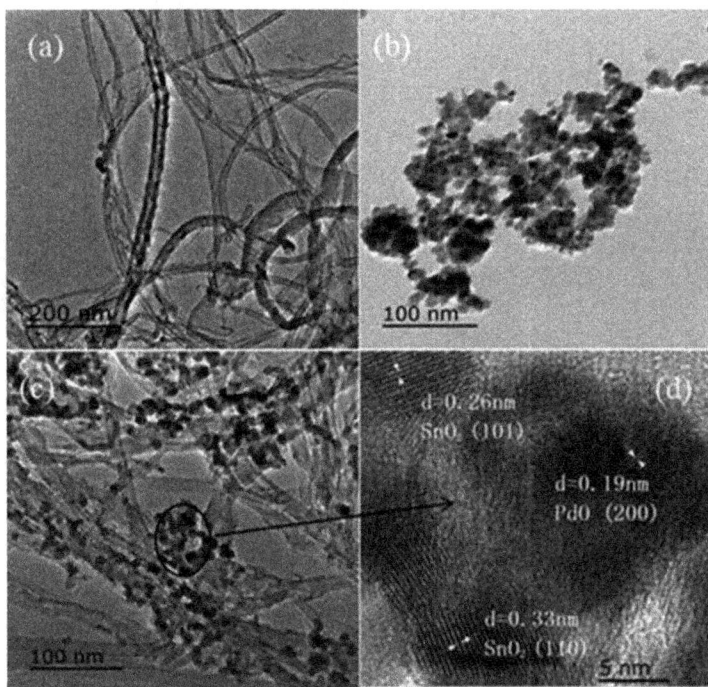

FIGURE 4.15 TEM images of (a) CNTs; (b) 1.0 mol% Pd^{+2}/SnO_2; (c) 1.0 mol% $Pd^{+2}/$ SnO_2/CNT (CNT/Sn = 0.12); and (d) HR-TEM of the $Pd^{+2}/SnO_2/CNT$ nanocomposites. *Source*: Reproduced with permission from: Hu, Liu, and Lian (2014). © John Wiley.

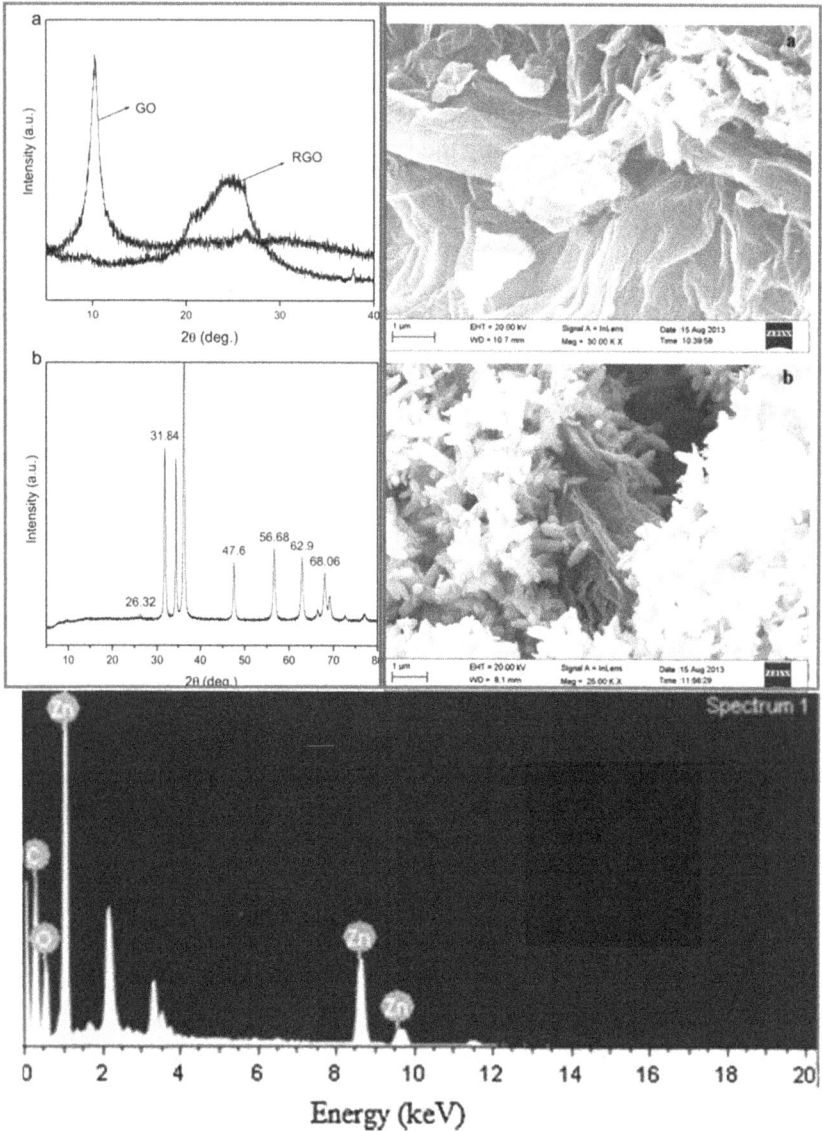

FIGURE 4.16 XRD patterns of (a) GO and rGO (b) RGO/ZnO composite. FESEM image of (a) RGO sheets; and (b) RGO/ZnO composite powder and EDX spectra of RGO/ZnO composite.

Source: Reproduced with permission from: Anand et al. (2014). © Elsevier.

4.7 CONCLUSIONS

The metal oxide-based gas sensors are very important designed for sensing a wide range of gases, which depends on their physical and chemical properties. The materials morphology, crystal structure affect the detecting features, for example, selectivity, sensitivity, reliability, durability, etc. We discussed the different metal oxides such as SnO_2, ZnO, In_2O_3, WO_3, CuO, Cu_2O, and nanocomposites materials for the different gas detection. It has been found that these metal oxide-based materials have advantages such as low cost, high sensitivity, and selectivity, low response time, etc.

KEYWORDS

- **carbon monoxide**
- **field-effect-transistors**
- **gas sensors**
- **metal oxide nanostructures**
- **photoluminescence**
- **sensitive gas sensors**

REFERENCES

Abbaspour, A., & Mehrgardi, M. A., (2005). Electrocatalytic activity of Ce(III)–EDTA complex toward the oxidation of nitrite ion. *Talanta, 67*, 579–584.

Anand, K., Singh, O., Singh, M. P., Kaur, J., & Singh, R. C., (2014). Hydrogen sensor based on graphene/ZnO nanocomposite. *Sensors and Actuators B: Chemical, 195*, 409–415.

Bai, X., Ji, H., Gao, P., Zhang, Y., & Sun, X., (2014). Morphology, phase structure and acetone sensitive properties of copper-doped tungsten oxide sensors. *Sensors and Actuators B: Chemical, 193*, 100–106.

Barsan, N., & Weimar, U., (2001). Conduction model of metal oxide gas sensors. *Journal of Electroceramics, 7*, 143–167.

Barsan, N., Gauglitz, G., Oprea, A., Ostertag, E., Proll, G., Rebner, K., Schierbaum, K., Schleifenbaum, F., & Weimar, U., (2016). Chemical and biochemical sensors, fundamentals. In: *Ullmann's Encyclopedia of Industrial Chemistry* (pp. 1–81).

Behera, B., & Chandra, S., (2018). Synthesis of WO_3 nanorods by thermal oxidation technique for NO_2 gas sensing application. *Materials Science in Semiconductor Processing, 86*, 79–84.

Bhatia, S., Verma, N., & Bedi, R. K., (2017). Ethanol gas sensor based upon ZnO nanoparticles prepared by different techniques. *Results in Physics, 7*, 801–806.

Calestani, D., Zha, M., Mosca, R., Zappettini, A., Carotta, M. C., Di Natale, V., & Zanotti, L., (2010). Growth of ZnO tetrapods for nanostructure-based gas sensors. *Sensors and Actuators B: Chemical, 144*, 472–478.

Casella, I. G., & Gatta, M., (2004). Electrochemical reduction of NO_3^- and NO_2^- on a composite copper thallium electrode in alkaline solutions. *Journal of Electroanalytical Chemistry, 568*, 183–188.

Chen, Y., Li, X., Li, X., Wang, J., & Tang, Z., (2016). UV activated hollow ZnO microspheres for selective ethanol sensors at low temperatures. *Sensors and Actuators B: Chemical, 232*, 158–164.

Cheng, W., Ju, Y., Payamyar, P., Primc, D., Rao, J., Willa, C., Koziej, D., & Niederberger, M., (2015). Large-area alignment of tungsten oxide nanowires over flat and patterned substrates for room-temperature gas sensing. *Angewandte Chemie International Edition, 54*, 340–344.

Chiu, C. M., & Chang, Y. H., (1999). The structure, electrical and sensing properties for CO of the $La_{0.8}Sr_{0.2}Co_{1-x}Ni_xO_{3-\delta}$ system. *Materials Science and Engineering: A, 266*, 93–98.

Chou, S. M., Teoh, L. G., Lai, W. H., Su, Y. H., & Hon, M. H., (2006). ZnO: Al thin film gas sensor for detection of ethanol vapor. *Sensors, 6*, 1420–1427.

Comini, E., (2006). Metal oxide nanocrystals for gas sensing. *Analytica Chimica Acta, 568*, 28–40.

Cordell, R. L., Willis, K. A., Wyche, K. P., Blake, R. S., Ellis, A. M., & Monks, P. S., (2007). Detection of chemical weapon agents and simulants using chemical ionization reaction time-of-flight mass spectrometry. *Analytical Chemistry, 79*, 8359–8366.

Deng, L., Ding, X., Zeng, D., Tian, S., Li, H., & Xie, C., (2012). Visible-light activate mesoporous WO_3 sensors with enhanced formaldehyde-sensing property at room temperature. *Sensors and Actuators B: Chemical, 163*, 260–266.

Dey, A., (2018). Semiconductor metal oxide gas sensors: A review. *Materials Science and Engineering: B, 229*, 206–217.

Dhara, V. R., & Dhara, R., (2002). The union carbide disaster in Bhopal: A review of health effects. *Archives of Environmental Health: An International Journal, 57*, 391–404.

Espid, E., & Taghipour, F., (2017). Development of highly sensitive ZnO/In_2O_3 composite gas sensor activated by UV-LED. *Sensors and Actuators B: Chemical, 241*, 828–839.

Faber, H., Lin, Y. H., Thomas, S. R., Zhao, K., Pliatsikas, N., McLachlan, M. A., Amassian, A., et al., (2015). Indium oxide thin-film transistors processed at low temperature via ultrasonic spray pyrolysis. *ACS Applied Materials and Interfaces, 7*, 782–790.

Fine, G. F., Cavanagh, L. M., Afonja, A., & Binions, R., (2010). Metal oxide semiconductor gas sensors in environmental monitoring. *Sensors, 10*, 5469–5502.

Fraiwan, L., Lweesy, K., Bani-Salma, A., & Mani, N., (2011). In A wireless home safety gas leakage detection system. *2011 1st Middle East Conference on Biomedical Engineering*, 11–14.

Gopel, J. H., & Zemel, J. N., (1989). Sensors, A comprehensive survey. *Fundamental and General Aspects., 1*, 3–4.

Gu, C., Huang, J., Wu, Y., Zhai, M., Sun, Y., & Liu, J., (2011). Preparation of porous flower-like ZnO nanostructures and their gas-sensing property. *Journal of Alloys and Compounds, 509*, 4499–4504.

Gu, F., Nie, R., Han, D., & Wang, Z., (2015). In$_2$O$_3$-graphene nanocomposite-based gas sensor for selective detection of NO$_2$ at room temperature. *Sensors and Actuators B: Chemical, 219*, 94–99.

Guo, W., Zhao, B., Zhou, Q., He, Y., Wang, Z., & Radacsi, N., (2019). Fe-Doped ZnO/ reduced graphene oxide nanocomposite with synergic enhanced gas-sensing performance for the effective detection of formaldehyde. *ACS Omega, 4*, 10252–10262.

Hill, H. H., & Martin, S. J., (2002). Conventional analytical methods for chemical warfare agents. *Pure and Applied Chemistry, 74*, 2281–2291.

Hoch, L. B., O'Brien, P. G., Jelle, A., Sandhel, A., Perovic, D. D., Mims, C. A., & Ozin, G. A., (2016). Nanostructured indium oxide-coated silicon nanowire arrays: A hybrid photothermal/photochemical approach to solar fuels. *ACS Nano, 10*, 9017–9025.

Hu, Q., Liu, S., & Lian, Y., (2014). Sensors for carbon monoxide based on Pd/SnO$_2$/CNT nanocomposites. *Physica Status Solidi (a), 211*, 2729–2734.

Huang, X., Li, Y., Chen, Y., & Wang, L., (2008). Electrochemical determination of nitrite and iodate by use of gold nanoparticles/poly(3-methyl thiophene) composites coated glassy carbon electrode. *Sensors and Actuators B: Chemical, 134*, 780–786.

Hulanicki, A., Glab, S., & Ingman, F., (1991). Chemical sensors: Definitions and classification. *Pure and Applied Chemistry, 63*, 1247–1250.

Inaba, T., Saji, K., & Takahashi, H., (1999). Limiting current-type gas sensor using a high temperature-type proton conductor thin film. *Electrochemistry-Tokyo, 67*, 458–462.

International Electrochemical Committee, (1982). *Terms and Definitions in Industrial Process Measurement and Control (ICE draft 65/84).*

Ishihara, N., Nishiguchi, H., & Takita, Y., (1997). Detection mechanism of CuO-BaTiO$_3$ capacitive type gas sensor. *Proceedings of Ceramic Sensors III* (pp. 6–11). San Antonio, TX, USA.

Kanan, S. M., El-Kadri, O. M., Abu-Yousef, I. A., & Kanan, M. C., (2009). Semiconducting metal oxide-based sensors for selective gas pollutant detection. *Sensors, 9*, 8158–8196.

Karmaoui, M., Leonardi, S. G., Latino, M., Tobaldi, D. M., Donato, N., Pullar, R. C., Seabra, M. P., et al., (2016). Pt-decorated In$_2$O$_3$ nanoparticles and their ability as a highly sensitive (<10 ppb) acetone sensor for biomedical applications. *Sensors and Actuators B: Chemical, 230*, 697–705.

Khuspe, G. D., Sakhare, R. D., Navale, S. T., Chougule, M. A., Kolekar, Y. D., Mulik, R. N., Pawar, R. C., et al., (2013). Nanostructured SnO$_2$ thin films for NO$_2$ gas sensing applications. *Ceramics International, 39*, 8673–8679.

Kong, L. B., & Shen, Y., (1996). Gas-sensing property and mechanism of Ca$_x$La$_{1-x}$FeO$_3$ ceramics. *Sensors and Actuators B: Chemical, 30*, 217–221.

Koplin, T. J., Siemons, M., Océn-Valéntin, C., Sanders, D., & Simon, U., (2006). Workflow for high throughput screening of gas sensing materials. *Sensors, 6*, 298–307.

Korotcenkov, G., & Cho, B. K., (2011). Instability of metal oxide-based conductometric gas sensors and approaches to stability improvement (short survey). *Sensors and Actuators B: Chemical, 156*, 527–538.

Korotcenkov, G., (2007). Metal oxides for solid-state gas sensors: What determines our choice? *Materials Science and Engineering: B, 139*, 1–23.

Kukkola, J., Mohl, M., Rautio, A. R., Mäklin, J., Halonen, N., Shchukarev, A., Kónya, Z., Jantunen, H., & Kordás, K., (2013). Room temperature hydrogen sensors based on metal decorated WO$_3$ nanowires. *Sensors and Actuators B: Chemical, 186*, 90–95.

Kuwabara, M., (1987). CO gas sensitivity in porous semiconducting barium titanate. *Am. Ceram. Soc. Bull., 65*, 1401–1405.

Langley, C. E., Scaron, Ljukic, B., Banks, C. E., & Compton, R. G., (2007). Manganese dioxide graphite composite electrodes: Application to the electroanalysis of hydrogen peroxide, ascorbic acid and nitrite. *Analytical Sciences, 23*, 165–170.

Lavoie, H., Thériault, J. M., & Dubé, D., (2007). *Measurement of Toxic Industrial Chemicals, Chemical Warfare Agents and Their Simulants*, 2006–2634.

Lei, C., Pi, M., Jiang, C., Cheng, B., & Yu, J., (2017). Synthesis of hierarchical porous zinc oxide (ZnO) microspheres with highly efficient adsorption of congo red. *Journal of Colloid and Interface Science, 490*, 242–251.

Li, C., Lv, M., Zuo, J., & Huang, X., (2015). SnO_2 highly sensitive CO gas sensor based on quasi-molecular-imprinting mechanism design. *Sensors (Basel), 15*, 3789–3800.

Li, J., Liu, X., Cui, J., & Sun, J., (2015). Hydrothermal synthesis of self-assembled hierarchical tungsten oxides hollow spheres and their gas sensing properties. *ACS Applied Materials and Interfaces, 7*, 10108–10114.

Li, T., Zeng, W., & Wang, Z., (2015). Quasi-one-dimensional metal-oxide-based heterostructural gas-sensing materials: A review. *Sensors and Actuators B: Chemical, 221*, 1570–1585.

Lin, Y., Wei, W., Wang, Y., Zhou, J., Sun, D., Zhang, X., & Ruan, S., (2015). Highly stabilized and rapid sensing acetone sensor based on Au nanoparticle-decorated flower-like ZnO microstructures. *Journal of Alloys and Compounds, 650*, 37–44.

Liu, X., Cheng, S., Liu, H., Hu, S., Zhang, D., & Ning, H., (2012). A survey on gas sensing technology. *Sensors, 12*, 9635–9665.

Lu, R., Zhong, X., Shang, S., Wang, S., & Tang, M., (2018). Effects of sintering temperature on sensing properties of WO_3 and $Ag-WO_3$ electrode for NO_2 sensor. *Royal Society Open Science, 5*, 171691.

Lupan, O., Postica, V., Gröttrup, J., Mishra, A. K., De Leeuw, N. H., Carreira, J. F. C., Rodrigues, J., et al., (2017). Hybridization of zinc oxide tetrapods for selective gas sensing applications. *ACS Applied Materials and Interfaces, 9*, 4084–4099.

Man, L., Zhang, J., Wang, J., Xu, H., & Cao, B., (2013). Microwave-assisted hydrothermal synthesis and gas sensitivity of nanostructured SnO_2. *Particuology, 11*, 242–248.

Martin, O., Martín, A. J., Mondelli, C., Mitchell, S., Segawa, T. F., Hauert, R., Drouilly, C., et al., (2016). Indium oxide as a superior catalyst for methanol synthesis by CO_2 hydrogenation. *Angewandte Chemie International Edition, 55*, 6261–6265.

Martinelli, G., Carotta, M. C., Ferroni, M., Sadaoka, Y., & Traversa, E., (1999). Screen-printed perovskite-type thick films as gas sensors for environmental monitoring. *Sensors and Actuators B: Chemical, 55*, 99–110.

Meixner, H., & Lampe, U., (1996). Metal oxide sensors. *Sensors and Actuators B: Chemical, 33*, 198–202.

Mirzaei, A., Kim, J. H., Kim, H. W., & Kim, S. S., (2018). How shell thickness can affect the gas sensing properties of nanostructured materials: Survey of literature. *Sensors and Actuators B: Chemical, 258*, 270–294.

Mizsei, J., (2016). Forty years of adventure with semiconductor gas sensors. *Procedia Engineering, 168*, 221–226.

Morten, B., Prudenziati, M., Sirotti, F., De Cicco, G., Alberigi-Quaranta, A., & Olumekor, L., (1990). Magneto resistive properties of Ni-based thick films. *Journal of Materials Science: Materials in Electronics, 1*, 118–122.

Moseley, P. T., (1997). Solid-state gas sensors. *Measurement Science and Technology, 8,* 223–237.

Nemade, K., & Waghuley, D. S., (2014). Optical and gas sensing properties of CuO nanoparticles grown by spray pyrolysis of cupric nitrate solution. *International Journal of Materials Science and Engineering, 2.*

Nimal, A. T., Mittal, U., Singh, M., Khaneja, M., Kannan, G. K., Kapoor, J. C., Dubey, V., et al., (2009). Development of handheld SAW vapor sensors for explosives and CW agents. *Sensors and Actuators B: Chemical, 135,* 399–410.

Nimbalkar, A. R., & Patil, M. G., (2017). Synthesis of ZnO thin film by sol-gel spin coating technique for H_2S gas sensing application. *Physica B: Condensed Matter, 527,* 7–15.

Noguchi, Y., Kuroiwa, H., & Takata, M., (1999). Sensing properties of oxygen sensor using hot spot on $La_{0.2}Sr_{0.8}Co_{0.8}Fe_{0.2}O_{3-\delta}$ ceramic rod. *Key Engineering Materials, 169–170,* 79–82.

Oleg, L., Postica, V., Cretu, V., Wolff, N., Duppel, V., Kienle, L., & Adelung, R., (2015). Single and networked CuO nanowires for highly sensitive p-type semiconductor gas sensor applications. *Physica Status Solidi (RRL)-Rapid Research Letters, 10,* 260–266.

Patil, L. A., Wani, P. A., Sainkar, S. R., Mitra, A., Phatak, G. J., & Amalnerkar, D. P., (1998). Studies on 'fritted' thick films of photo conducting CdS. *Materials Chemistry and Physics, 55,* 79–83.

Patil, V., Jundale, D., Pawar, S., Chougule, M., Godse, P., Patil, S., Raut, B., & Sen, S., (2011). Nanocrystalline CuO Thin Films for H_2S monitoring: Microstructural and optoelectronic characterization. *Journal of Sensor Technology, 1,* 11.

Prudenziati, M., & Morten, B., (1986). Thick-film sensors: An overview. *Sensors and Actuators, 10,* 65–82.

Ran, T. H., & Nguyen, V. T., (2014). Copper oxide nanomaterials prepared by solution methods, some properties, and potential applications: A brief review. *International Scholarly Research Notices, 2014,* 14.

Sachdeva, S., Agarwal, R., & Agarwal, A., (2019). MEMS based tin oxide thin film gas sensor for diabetes mellitus applications. *Microsystem Technologies, 25,* 2571–2586.

Schmidt-Mende, L., & MacManus-Driscoll, J. L., (2007). ZnO-nanostructures, defects, and devices. *Materials Today, 10,* 40–48.

Seto, Y., Kanamori-Kataoka, M., Tsuge, K., Ohsawa, I., Matsushita, K., Sekiguchi, H., Itoi, T., et al., (2005). Sensing technology for chemical-warfare agents and its evaluation using authentic agents. *Sensors and Actuators B: Chemical, 108,* 193–197.

Setty, D. P. A., (1994). *Thick Film Sensors, 3.* Elsevier.

Shankar, P., & Rayappan, J. B. B., (2015). Gas sensing mechanism of metal oxides: The role of ambient atmosphere, type of semiconductor and gases: A review. *Science Letters, 4,* 126.

Shendage, S. S., Patil, V. L., Vanalakar, S. A., Patil, S. P., Harale, N. S., Bhosale, J. L., Kim, J. H., & Patil, P. S., (2017). Sensitive and selective NO_2 gas sensor based on WO_3 nanoplates. *Sensors and Actuators B: Chemical, 240,* 426–433.

Shokry Hassan, H., et al., (2014). Synthesis, characterization and fabrication of gas sensor devices using ZnO and ZnO:In nanomaterials. Beni-Suef University. *Journal of Basic and Applied Sciences, 3*(3), p. 216–221.

Singh, A., Sharma, A., Tomar, M., & Gupta, V., (2018). Tunable nanostructured columnar growth of SnO_2 for efficient detection of CO gas. *Nanotechnology, 29,* 065502.

Šljukić, B., Banks, C. E., Crossley, A., & Compton, R. G., (2007). Copper oxide-graphite composite electrodes: Application to nitrite sensing. *Electroanalysis, 19,* 79–84.

Song, L., Yue, H., Li, H., Liu, L., Li, Y., Du, L., Duan, H., & Klyui, N. I., (2018). Hierarchical porous ZnO micro flowers with ultra-high ethanol gas-sensing at low concentration. *Chemical Physics Letters, 699*, 1–7.

Song, Z., Wei, Z., Wang, B., Luo, Z., Xu, S., Zhang, W., Yu, H., et al., (2016). Sensitive room-temperature H_2S gas sensors employing SnO_2 quantum wire/reduced graphene oxide nanocomposites. *Chemistry of Materials, 28*, 1205–1212.

Sorita, R., & Kawano, T., (1996). A highly selective CO sensor: Screening of electrode materials. *Sensors and Actuators B: Chemical, 36*, 274–277.

Sun, Y. F., Liu, S. B., Meng, F. L., Liu, J. Y., Jin, Z., Kong, L. T., & Liu, J. H., (2012). Metal oxide nanostructures and their gas sensing properties: A review. *Sensors, 12*, 2610–2631.

Tamaekong, N., Liewhiran, C., Wisitsoraat, A., & Phanichphant, S., (2010). Flame-spray-made undoped zinc oxide films for gas sensing applications. *Sensors, 10*, 7863–7873.

Tomchenko, A. A., Harmer, G. P., & Marquis, B. T., (2005). Detection of chemical warfare agents using nanostructured metal oxide sensors. *Sensors and Actuators B: Chemical, 108*, 41–55.

Tricoli, A., Righettoni, M., & Teleki, A., (2010). Semiconductor gas sensors: Dry synthesis and application. *Angewandte Chemie International Edition, 49*, 7632–7659.

Tsai, Y. T., Chang, S. J., Ji, L. W., Hsiao, Y. J., Tang, I. T., Lu, H. Y., & Chu, Y. L., (2018). High sensitivity of NO gas sensors based on novel Ag-doped ZnO nanoflowers enhanced with a UV light-emitting diode. *ACS Omega, 3*, 13798–13807.

Urasinska-Wojcik, B., Vincent, T. A., Chowdhury, M. F., & Gardner, J. W., (2017). Ultrasensitive WO_3 gas sensors for NO_2 detection in air and low oxygen environment. *Sensors and Actuators B: Chemical, 239*, 1051–1059.

Van, T. P., Hoa, N. D., Van, Q. V., Van, D. N., & Van, H. N., (2013). Diameter controlled synthesis of tungsten oxide nanorod bundles for highly sensitive NO_2 gas sensors. *Sensors and Actuators B: Chemical, 183*, 372–380.

Wang, C., Yin, L., Zhang, L., Xiang, D., & Gao, R., (2010). Metal oxide gas sensors: Sensitivity and influencing factors. *Sensors, 10*, 2088–2106.

Wang, P., Mai, Z., Dai, Z., Li, Y., & Zou, X., (2009). Construction of Au nanoparticles on choline chloride modified glassy carbon electrode for sensitive detection of nitrite. *Biosensors and Bioelectronics, 24*, 3242–3247.

Wei, D., Shen, Y., Li, M., Liu, W., Gao, S., Jia, L., Han, C., & Cui, B., (2013). Synthesis and characterization of single-crystalline SnO_2 nanowires. *Journal of Nanomaterials, 2013*, 6.

Wen, Z., Shen, Q., & Sun, X., (2017). Nanogenerators for self-powered gas sensing. *Nano-Micro Letters, 9*, 45.

White, N. M., & Turner, J. D., (1997). Thick-film sensors: Past, present and future. *Measurement Science and Technology, 8*, 1–20.

Xing, R., Xu, L., Song, J., Zhou, C., Li, Q., Liu, D., & Wei, S. H., (2015). Preparation and gas sensing properties of In_2O_3/Au nanorods for detection of volatile organic compounds in exhaled breath. *Scientific Reports, 5*, 10717–10717.

Xu, W., Li, J., & Sun, J., (2015). Fabrication of monodispersed hollow flower-like porous In_2O_3 nanostructures and their application as gas sensors. *RSC Advances, 5*, 81407–81414.

Yamaura, H., Tamaki, J., Miura, N., & Yamazoe, N., (1995). *NO_x Sensing Properties of Metal Titanate-Based Semiconductor Sensor at Elevated Temperature* (pp. 341–346). Engineering Science Reports, Kyushu University, Japan.

Yamazoe, N., Sakai, G., & Shimanoe, K., (2003). Oxide semiconductor gas sensors. *Catalysis Surveys from Asia, 7*, 63–75.

Zeggar, M. L., Bourfaa, F., Adjimi, A., Aida, M. S., & Attaf, N., (2016). Copper oxide thin films for ethanol sensing. *IOP Conference Series: Materials Science and Engineering, 108*, 012004.

Zhang, H., Chen, W. G., Li, Y. Q., & Song, Z. H., (2018). Gas sensing performances of ZnO hierarchical structures for detecting dissolved gases in transformer oil: A mini-review. *Front Chem., 6*, 508–508.

Zhang, H., Xu, X., Zhu, Y., Bao, K., Lu, Z., Sun, P., Sun, Y., & Lu, G., (2017). Synthesis and NO_2 gas-sensing properties of coral-like indium oxide via a facile solvothermal method. *RSC Advances, 7*, 49273–49278.

Zhang, L., Yuan, F., Zhang, X., & Yang, L., (2011). Facile synthesis of flower like copper oxide and their application to hydrogen peroxide and nitrite sensing. *Chemistry Central Journal, 5*, 75.

Zhang, R., Jia, J. B., Cao, J. L., & Wang, Y., (2018). SnO_2/graphene nanoplatelet nanocomposites: Solid-state method synthesis with high ethanol gas-sensing performance. *Front Chem., 6*.

Zhang, S., Song, P., Yan, H., Yang, Z., & Wang, Q., (2016). A simple large-scale synthesis of mesoporous In_2O_3 for gas sensing applications. *Applied Surface Science, 378*.

Zhang, Y. C., Tagawa, H., Asakura, S., Mizusaki, J., & Narita, H., (1997). Solid-state electrochemical CO_2 sensor by coupling lithium-ion conductor (Li_2CO_3-Li_3PO_4-Asl_2O_3) with oxide ion-electron mixed conductor ($La_{0.9}Sr_{0.1}MnO_3$). *Solid State Ionics, 100*, 275–281.

Zhang, Y., Xu, J., Xiang, Q., Li, H., Pan, Q., & Xu, P., (2009). Brush-like hierarchical ZnO nanostructures: Synthesis, photoluminescence and gas sensor properties. *The Journal of Physical Chemistry C, 113*, 3430–3435.

Zheng, Z. Q., Yao, J. D., Wang, B., & Yang, G. W., (2015). Light-controlling, flexible and transparent ethanol gas sensor based on ZnO nanoparticles for wearable devices. *Scientific Reports, 5*, 11070.

Zhou, Y., Liu, G., Zhu, X., & Guo, Y., (2017). Ultrasensitive NO_2 gas sensing based on rGO/MoS_2 nanocomposite film at low temperature. *Sensors and Actuators B: Chemical, 251*.

Zhu, X., Guo, Y., Ren, H., Gao, C., & Zhou, Y., (2017). Enhancing the NO_2 gas sensing properties of rGO/SnO_2 nanocomposite films by using microporous substrates. *Sensors and Actuators B: Chemical, 248*.

CHAPTER 5

Optical Biosensors for Diagnostic Applications

SUDHA KUMARI and SAPAN MOHAN SAINI

Department of Physics, National Institute of Technology, Raipur, Chhattisgarh–492010, India, E-mail: kumari.sudha93@gmail.com (S. Kumari)

ABSTRACT

Optical biosensors based on plasmonics are employed for sensing using optical properties of metallic thin films or nanostructures. Surface plasmon resonance (SPR) sensing techniques are generally used for the detection of target chemical and biological molecules at the surface of metal thin film interfaced with dielectric medium. Due to its highly sensitive nature, SPR sensors have emanated as an influential sensing method in the biological sensor applications resulting in a very cost-effective way. Plasmonics materials such as silver (Ag), gold (Au), and aluminum (Al), etc., consisting of thin films and nanostructures supports SPR at metal-dielectric interface. The properties of surface plasmon are very sensitive to the surrounding dielectric medium which is in contact with the metallic surface. In addition, the metal nanostructures help to confine the light which significantly increases the electric field, thereby enhancing the sensitivity of the sensing device. This makes SPR based plasmonic devices, a promising candidate for developing a label free optical biosensor. Additionally, the development of cost-effective, label free and highly sensitive optical biosensor is highly demanding for routine clinical diagnosis for fast and real-time identification of biomarkers specific to certain diseases, e.g., cancer, Alzheimer, and Tuberculosis (TB), etc.

5.1   INTRODUCTION

Biosensors are the investigative devices having immobilized biological material (such as enzyme, nucleic acid, antibody, hormone, or bio-cell) which can precisely interact with an analyte and yield electrical, physical, or chemical signals that can be measured. The analyte may be the compound (such as pesticide, drug, glucose, urea, or drug) whose concentration has to be measured. Basically, the biosensors comprise the quantitative examination of some substances by altering their biological activities into the measurable signals. The performance of a biosensor is typically dependent on the sensitivity and specificity of the biological reaction. Based on the mechanism of transduction, there are several sorts of biosensors, including resonant biosensors, thermal detection biosensors, electrochemical biosensors, ion-sensitive biosensors, and optical biosensors. The optical biosensors exploit the principle of optical measurements (fluorescence, absorbance, chemiluminescence, etc.). They employ the use of optical waveguide and optoelectronic transducers. This chapter is devoted to the plasmonic-based optical biosensors.

5.2   SURFACE PLASMON RESONANCE (SPR)

Plasmonic is a subfield of nanophotonics that exploits the unique optical properties of metallic nanostructures to manipulate light at nanometer length scales. This field of the science and technology is emerging rapidly for the challenging biosensing applications. The term plasmonic refers to the resonant interaction (under certain conditions) between an electromagnetic (EM) radiation (e.g., light) and the free electrons at the interface between a metal and a dielectric. When the metal is segregated into fine discrete particles that have dimensions close to the wavelength of light, there will be a marked change in the mirror-like smooth morphology of the metal (Jeffrey et al., 2008). There has been a growing interest towards the surface plasmon resonance (SPR) phenomenon in the visible and/or near-infrared wavelength range. This is due to the fact that favorable optical confinement takes place at these wavelengths. All conductive materials, such as metals (i.e., copper, silver, gold, and aluminum), support Plasmon because their plasmon resonance lies closer to the visible region of the spectrum (Lal et al., 2007). The plasmonic materials often refer to gold and silver, but copper and platinum, palladium, and aluminum are sometimes used (Debruijn et al., 1992; Saambles et al., 1991). Silver has higher properties in near-infrared region and has sharper resonance peak but generally gold is preferred due its chemical stability resistance to oxidation. SPR based sensing is a real time and label-free detection technique to measure bio-molecular interactions on the gold surface. Label-free detection techniques monitor biomolecular interactions by eliminating the need for secondary reactants. Moreover, they provide quantitative information for the binding kinetics (Helmerhorst et al., 2012; Lee et al., 2012). Surface plasmon polarities (SPP) are traveling charge density waves at the surface of conducting materials present at the interface of two media (metal-dielectric) with permittivities of opposite sign (Abbs et al., 2011).

At low-frequency region, metals act like perfect or good conductors. When low-frequency EM waves hit onto metals, they reflect back with little amounts of penetration depths and negligible minor loss of energy. In the visible part of the spectrum, penetration increases, this leads to more loss. Whereas in the UV part of the spectrum, metals converge to dielectrics and turn out to be transparent at a certain frequency threshold. This extremely dispersive behavior leads to generate a dispersion model for metal which needs the formulation of frequency, ω. This frequency is known as a plasma frequency as shown in the Eqn. (1). Below the plasma frequency, ωp, the dielectric function is negative and the field cannot enter the metal and is totally reflected. However, above the plasma frequency, ωp, the light waves can enter the solid and transmittance occurs according to the Eqn. (2).

$$\omega_p^2 = \frac{ne^2}{m\varepsilon_o} \tag{1}$$

$$\varepsilon(\omega) = 1 - \frac{\omega_p^2}{\omega^2} \tag{2}$$

When the EM field is illuminated on the metal surface, the free electrons exist on the metal surface starts to move back and forth 180° out of phase, and photons of incident EM wave is coupled with plasmons. The plasmons can be defined as the quasi-particles that represent the quantum of a typical plasma oscillation, which consists of a large number of interacting mobile charged particles. The collective oscillation eigenmodes generated by the free electron gas inside a metal can be interpreted in terms of material excitations as quasiparticles, called plasmons. Electron oscillations in metals lead to three types of plasmons: (i) volume plasmons, (ii) surface plasmons (SPs), and (iii) localized plasmons which are discussed in subsections.

5.2.1   VOLUME PLASMONS

The volume plasmon is the collective longitudinal oscillation of the conduction electron gas that propagates in the volume of a solid against the rigid positive ion cores in plasma slab and can be excited at plasma frequency. Figure 5.1 shows the collective displacement of electron clouds by a distance 'u' that creates a surface charge density of $\sigma = \pm neu$ at the slab boundaries and produced a uniform electric field E inside the slab. Consequently, the displaced electrons experienced a restoring force which leads to the oscillation of free conductions in a metal solid. The quantum of this charge oscillation is known as volume plasmon (Jackson, 1962; Maier, 2005).

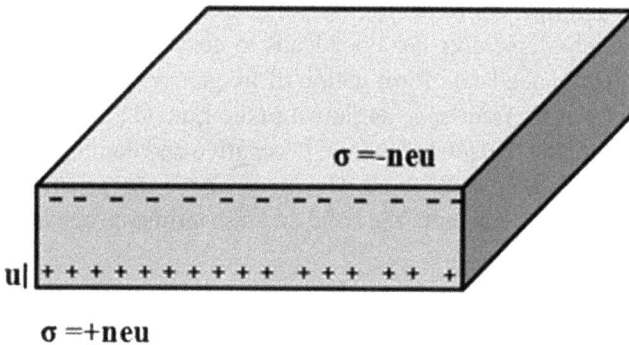

FIGURE 5.1   Schematic diagram showing longitudinal oscillation of conduction electrons in a metal solid.

5.2.2   SURFACE PLASMONS (SPS)

The surface plasmons (SPs)are excited EM waves that propagate along the interface of the metal and dielectric materials, which arise due to the coherent oscillations of the free conduction electrons at the metal (or highly doped semiconductor) surface. It is excited due to the coupling of EM fields with free conduction electrons on the metal surface. Since it is confined close to the metal surface and propagates along the metal-dielectric interface, it is also referred to as surface plasmon polaritons (SPPs).

5.2.3 LOCALIZED PLASMONS

The SP in nanometer-sized metallic structures, such as metallic nanoparticles (NPs), is called localized SP which is the consequence of SP confinement in a nanoparticle having equal or lesser than the wavelength of incident light. The two most distinguishing characteristics of the localized surface plasmon are; (i) there is an increase in the strength of the electric fields near the particle's surface, and (ii) optical absorption of the particle reaches a maximum value at the plasmon resonant frequency. This enhancement in the optical fields rapidly decays with distance away from the surface of the metal NPs. To study the physical properties of SPPs excited on metal-dielectric interface, we have to solve Maxwell's equation on the plane boundary between a conductor and a dielectric (Figure 5.2) (Zayatsa et al., 2005). The description of the interaction between light and matter can be summarized by Maxwell's equations which can be expressed in the differential form, as follows:

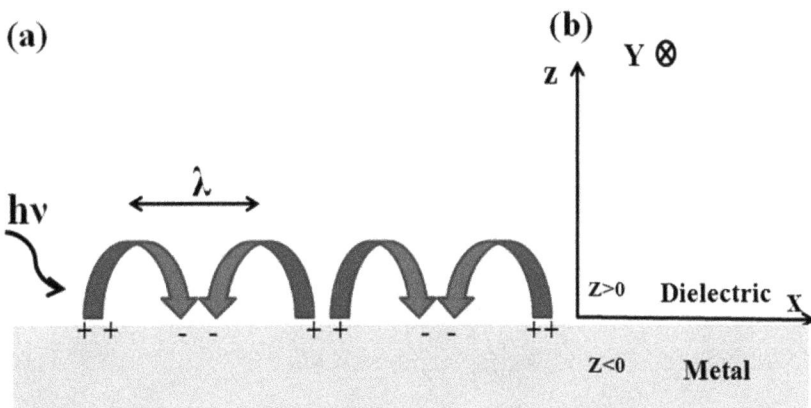

FIGURE 5.2 (a) Charge density oscillations at the metal/dielectric surface; and *(b)* shows the wave propagation at both the interfaces.

$$\nabla.D = \rho \tag{3}$$

$$\nabla.B = 0 \tag{4}$$

$$\nabla \times E = -\frac{\partial B}{\partial t} \tag{5}$$

$$\nabla \times H = J + \frac{\partial D}{dt} \tag{6}$$

Here these equations have the four macroscopic quantities including D, E, H, and B.D is the dielectric displacement, E is the electric field, H is the magnetic field and B is the magnetic induction or magnetic flux density. While the other quantities, ρ and J, are the external charge and current densities, respectively. In the absence of ρ and J, Maxwell equation reduces to:

$$\nabla.(\varepsilon_0 \varepsilon E) = 0 \tag{7}$$

$$\nabla.(\mu H) = 0 \tag{8}$$

$$\nabla \times E = -\mu \frac{\partial H}{\partial t} \tag{9}$$

$$\nabla \times H = \varepsilon_0 \varepsilon \frac{\partial E}{dt} \tag{10}$$

where; ε_0 and μ_0 are the electric permittivity and magnetic permeability of vacuum, respectively. Considering the magnetic permeability μ is equivalent to the free space permeability μ_o for the non-magnetic materials If we suppose harmonic time dependence of the field vectors in the form of $e^{-i\omega t}$, where ω is the frequency, then we can write the following couple equations using curl equation from Eqns. (9) and (10):

$$\frac{\partial E_z}{\partial y} - \frac{\partial E_y}{\partial z} = i\omega\mu_o H_x \tag{11a}$$

$$\frac{\partial E_X}{\partial Z} - \frac{\partial E_Z}{\partial X} = i\omega\mu_o H_y \tag{11b}$$

$$\frac{\partial E_Y}{\partial x} - \frac{\partial E_x}{\partial y} = i\omega\mu_o H_z \tag{11c}$$

$$\frac{\partial H_z}{\partial Y} - \frac{\partial H_Y}{\partial Z} = -i\omega\varepsilon_o \varepsilon E_x \tag{11d}$$

$$\frac{\partial H_x}{\partial z} - \frac{\partial H_z}{\partial x} = -i\omega\varepsilon_o \varepsilon E_y \tag{11e}$$

$$\frac{\partial H_y}{\partial x} - \frac{\partial H_x}{\partial y} = -i\omega\varepsilon_o \varepsilon E_z \tag{11f}$$

If we consider the wave propagation along the x-direction with propagation constant, i.e., the component of the wave vector in the direction of propagation ($\frac{\partial}{\partial x} = i\beta$) and homogeneity in the Y-direction ($\frac{\partial}{\partial y} = 0$), then the above equation simplifies to:

$$\frac{\partial E_y}{\partial z} = -i\omega\mu_o H_x \tag{12a}$$

$$\frac{\partial E_x}{\partial z} - i\beta E_z = i\omega\mu_o H_y \tag{12b}$$

$$-i\beta E_y = i\omega\mu_o H_z \tag{12c}$$

$$\frac{\partial H_y}{\partial z} = i\omega\varepsilon_o\varepsilon E_x \tag{12d}$$

$$\frac{\partial H_x}{\partial z} - i\beta H_z = -i\omega\varepsilon_o\varepsilon E_y \tag{12e}$$

$$i\beta H_y = -i\omega\varepsilon_o\varepsilon E_z \tag{12f}$$

The above equation was two sets of self-consistent solutions. For transverse magnetic (TM) mode or P-polarization, the field components, E_x, E_z, H_y, are non-zero and the system of governing equation reduces to:

$$\frac{\partial H_y}{\partial z} = -i\omega\varepsilon_o\varepsilon E_x \Rightarrow E_x = -\frac{i}{\omega\varepsilon_o\varepsilon}\frac{\partial H_y}{\partial z} \tag{13}$$

$$i\beta H_y = -i\omega\varepsilon_o\varepsilon E \Rightarrow E_z = -\frac{\beta}{\omega\varepsilon_o\varepsilon}H_y \tag{14}$$

$$\frac{\partial E_x}{\partial z} - i\beta E_z = i\omega\mu_o H_y \Rightarrow \frac{\partial^2 H_y}{\partial z^2} + (k_o^2\varepsilon - \beta)^2 H_y = 0 \tag{15}$$

$k_O^2 = \frac{\omega^2}{c^2}$ and $c = \frac{1}{\sqrt{\mu_o\varepsilon_o}}$ and c is the speed of light in free space.

For transverse electric (TE) mode or S-polarization, field components of H_x, H_z and E_y are non-zero and gives an additional set of the equation:

$$H_x = -\frac{i}{\omega\mu_o}\frac{\partial E_y}{\partial z} \tag{16}$$

$$H_z = -\frac{\beta}{\omega\mu_o}E_y \tag{17}$$

$$\Rightarrow \frac{\partial^2 E_y}{\partial z^2} + (k^2{}_o \varepsilon - \beta)^2 E_y \tag{18}$$

Consider a wave propagating along the X-direction and no spatial variation along Y-direction on the flat interface between a dielectric, non-absorbing half-space (z > 0) with ε_d an adjacent conducting half-space (z <0) with ε_m to describe the metallic character below the bulk plasmon frequency ω_p. For TM mode, solutions in both the half-spaces yield.

for z > 0,

$$H_y(z) = A_d e^{i\beta x - k_d z} \tag{19}$$

$$E_x(z) = iA_d \frac{i}{\omega \varepsilon_o \varepsilon_d} k_d e^{i\beta x - k_d z} \tag{20}$$

$$E_z(z) = -A_d \frac{\beta}{\omega \varepsilon_o \varepsilon_d} e^{i\beta x - k_d z} \tag{21}$$

where;
    A_d= Amplitudes of the propagating waves in the dielectric medium.
    k_d = Propagating wave vector in the dielectric medium.

for z < 0,

$$H_y(z) = A_m e^{i\beta x + k_m z} \tag{22}$$

$$E_x(z) = -iA_m \frac{i}{\omega \varepsilon_o \varepsilon_m} k_m e^{i\beta x + k_m z} \tag{23}$$

$$E_z(z) = -A_m \frac{\beta}{\omega \varepsilon_o \varepsilon_m} e^{i\beta x + k_m z} \tag{24}$$

where;
    A_m = Amplitudes of the propagating wave in the metallic region.
    k_m = Propagating wave vector perpendicular to the metal-dielectric surface.

Applying continuity of H_y and E_x at the interface, z = 0 and $A_d = A_m$.

$$\frac{k_d}{k_m} = -\frac{\varepsilon_m}{\varepsilon_d} \tag{25}$$

The expression of the H_y needs to fulfill the wave Eqn. (25)

$$k_m^2 = \beta^2 - k_O^2 \varepsilon_m \tag{26a}$$

$$k_d^2 = \beta^2 - k_O^2 \varepsilon_d \tag{26b}$$

Combining Eqns. (2.25) and (2.26)

$$\varepsilon_d^2 \beta^2 - k_0^2 \varepsilon_d^2 \varepsilon_m = \varepsilon_m^2 \beta^2 - k_0^2 \varepsilon_m^2 \varepsilon_d$$

$$\beta^2 = k_0^2 \varepsilon_d \varepsilon_m \frac{\varepsilon_d - \varepsilon_m}{\varepsilon_d^2 - \varepsilon_m^2}$$

$$k_{sp} = \beta = k_0 \sqrt{\frac{\varepsilon_d \varepsilon_m}{\varepsilon_d + \varepsilon_m}} = \frac{\omega}{c} \sqrt{\frac{\varepsilon_d \varepsilon_m}{\varepsilon_d + \varepsilon_m}} \quad (27)$$

This gives the dispersion relation of the SPPs propagating at the metal-dielectric interfaces and applicable for both real and complex ε_m, i.e., for without and with attenuation. Hence, Maxwell's assumption shows that electron charges on the interface of metal-dielectric can carry out coherent oscillation (Abbs et al., 2011; Jackson, 1962). This oscillation frequency ω is related to its wave vector k by a dispersion relation. The convention of the signs used for this equation is obligatory and sufficient that Re $[k_m]$ < 0 if $\varepsilon_2 > 0$ for the existence of SPPs. This indicates that the surface wave exists only at the interfaces between two materials with reverse signs of the real part of their dielectric contrast or permittivity, such as a conductor and an insulator. Eqn. (27) can be defined as the surface frequency $\omega = \omega_{sp}$, when $\varepsilon_m = -\varepsilon_d$.

In the case of low-frequency region, i.e., low ω, then Eqn. (27) can be written as:

$$k_{sp} = = \frac{\omega}{c} \lim \varepsilon_{m \to -\infty} \sqrt{\frac{\varepsilon_d \varepsilon_m}{\varepsilon_d + \varepsilon_m}} = \frac{\omega}{c} \sqrt{\varepsilon_d} \quad (28)$$

Hence, the plasmonic dispersion curve exists on the right side of the light line of the dielectric part of the interface (see Figure 5.3). Hence, beam directly incident on the metal-dielectric interface cannot excite SP directly, because they do not match with the energy and momentum conservation.

$$k_x = \frac{\omega}{c} \sqrt{\varepsilon_d} \quad (29)$$

Since the momentum of SP, $k_{sp} > k_x$, therefore, it is not possible to excite surface plasmon by directly shining the beam on metal film. To excite the SP, two optical coupling techniques such as prism coupling and gratings coupling are in general adopted which are explained in subsections.

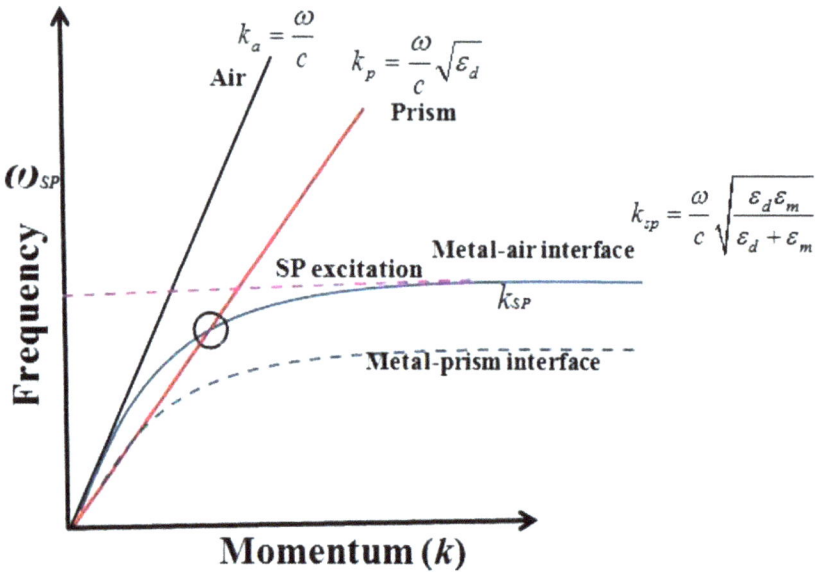

FIGURE 5.3 Excitation of surface plasmons by light. Prism and grating coupling can efficiently excite surface plasmons after increasing the wave vector of the surface plasmon k_{sp}.

5.3 EXCITATION OF SURFACE PLASMONS (SPS)

To excite the SP, criteria of both energy and momentum conservation must be fulfilled. The wave vector, k_{sp}, of the SP is larger than the wave vector, k, of incoming light in free space as seen from Eqn. (27).

$$k_{sp} = \frac{\omega}{c}\sqrt{\frac{\varepsilon_d \varepsilon_m}{\varepsilon_d + \varepsilon_m}} \geq k_p = \frac{\omega}{c}\sqrt{\varepsilon_d} \tag{30}$$

This can be understood by analyzing the dispersion relation of the SPPs as shown in Figure 5.3. In the small energy limit, light line is asymptotically approached the SP dispersion given. The excitation of SP is feasible if the wave vector of the incident light matches to the wave vector of the SP. This state is called phase matching coupling condition. This can be accomplished by using optical techniques like prism coupling and grating coupling scheme. The electric field (E-field) of SP wave excited on a thin metallic layer is analytically described by an exponential function which is mathematically expressed as (Homola, 2006; Jatschka et al., 2016).

$$E = E_{max}\, exp\left(-\frac{h}{z}\right) \tag{31}$$

where; E_{max} is the maximum E-field at the metal surface, z is the penetration depth, h, depicts the thickness of the layer within which refractive index change occurs on the metal surface. The above equation evidently indicates that the E-field of the SP wave has maximum value at the interface (i.e., $z = 0$) and it decays exponentially into the dielectric medium. The E-field decay outline is defined by the penetration depth z, which depends on optical properties of both metal and dielectric media at a given wavelength. In other words, the E-field of the SP wave is squeezed to a volume much smaller below the diffraction limit by $(\lambda_0/2n)^3$, where n $= \sqrt{\varepsilon}$ is the refractive index (RI) of the surrounding medium. This strong confinement of E-field at the metal-dielectric interface enables a variety of applications in optical sensing. Similarly, the localized SP wave excited in metal nanoparticle also has the strongest E-field at the metal NPs surface and exponentially decays into the dielectric medium. In the electrostatic approximation, the E-field profile of the localized SP wave excited on metal nanoparticle can be described by a simple analytical expression (Homola, 2006; Jatschka et al., 2016):

$$E = E_{max}\, exp\left(1+\frac{h}{r}\right)^{-(p+2)} \tag{32}$$

where; r is the radius of the nanoparticle and p represent the order of the plasmon mode. From this equation, it is observed that the E-field decay in metal nanoparticle depends on the order of the plasmon mode (p) and the radius of the nanoparticle (r). Thus, the localized SP wave can be spatially confined much stronger than the propagating plasmons SP waves and the strength of the E-field confinement is determined by the nanoparticle size.

5.3.1 PRISM COUPLING

There are two types of the prism coupling schemes; (i) Otto configuration and (ii) Kretschmann configuration. In the Otto setup, a spacer layer with RI n is employed between a metal and a prism (Figure 5.4(a)) (Otto, 1968). Prism has higher RI than spacer layer (rarer medium) and hence the component of momentum along the interface between the media can be increased. When light is shine at an angle of incidence, θ, which is greater than the critical angle, such that only an evanescent field penetrates into the spacer layer, and this evanescent field will be able to couple to the SPP at the metal interface. The coupling strength depends on the width of the air gap. When the gap width between two interfaces is larger, the evanescent field provides the weak response. By adjusting an angle of incidence of the reflected light within the prism, the resonance criteria for excitation of SP can be fulfilled. When the space between the metal and prism is too small, the resonance gets broadened due to radiation damping of the SPPs. The evanescent wave changes into a propagating wave and quickly decays in a radiative manner due to the existence of the half-space between the interfaces. Moreover, when the gap space between the interfaces is too large, the SP can no longer be able to excite and resonance disappears. So, due to the difficulties in precise controlling of the small gap between the two surfaces, Otto configuration is considered to be practically inconvenient.

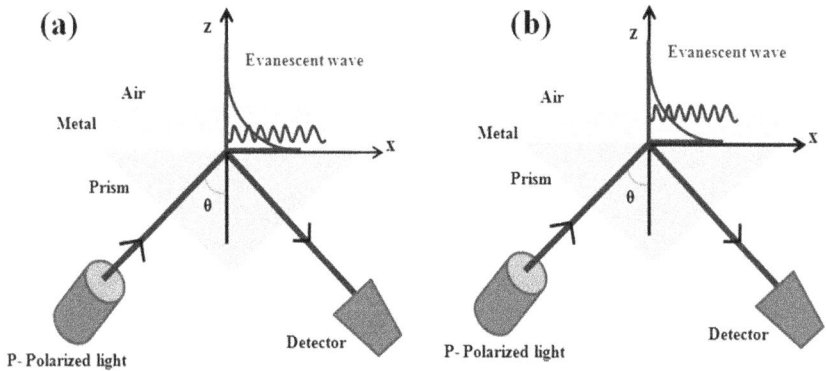

FIGURE 5.4 Prism coupling techniques: (a) Otto configuration; and (b) Kretschmann configuration.

The Kretschmann configuration is generally used in which a metal thin layer is coated on the base surface of the prism, and the light is shine at an angle greater than the critical angle (Dondapati et al., 2010). This resulted in the total internal reflection (TIR) of incident light at the interface of prism-metal and the evanescent fields arise along the longitudinal direction that penetrates through the metal film and able to excite propagating SP on the bottom surface of the metal as shown in Figure 5.4(b). The thickness of metal layer must be lesser than the skin depth of the evanescent field. When a light intensity is incident reflected at the interface of metal-dielectric through a prism having an in-plane momentum of the light, $k_x = k\sqrt{\varepsilon} \sin(\theta)$ is sufficient enough to satisfy phase-matching condition via $k_{sp} = k\sqrt{\varepsilon} \sin\theta$ for excitation of SPPs on the surface of the metal. A minimum drop of the reflected beam intensity is the SPPs excitation. The least energy of the reflected light is owing to destructive interference between the leakage waves in the prism and the reflected excitation light. For an optimal metal film thickness, there will be zero intensity in the reflected beam that can be possible with the ideal destructive interference in which the leakage energy is not detectable. Therefore, there will be an absolute transfer of the energy from the incoming light via tunneling of the excitation fields into a SP excited in metal-dielectric surface, and this state is commonly defined as the SPR.

5.3.2 GRATING COUPLING

There is another method of optical excitation of SP from the grating (Hibbins, 1999). Light incident at an angle θ normal of the plane of the grating surface, diffracted from the grating with various components of its wave vector by integer multiples of the grating wave vector k. The diffracted wave produces the various diffraction orders. The order of diffraction having wave vector larger than that of the incident light in the same dielectric medium, will not propagate and transform into an evanescent field. These evanescent fields with the increased momentum may couple to the SPPs of the grating surface. The difference in the wave vector between the in-plane momentum $k_x = k \sin(\theta)$ of the incident photons and propagation constant k_{sp} of the SP can be overcome by using the metal surface with the grating. When a light of wave vector k is incident on the metallic grating having periodicity Λ with an angle of incidence θ, there are various diffracted orders as shown in Figure 5.5.

The wavevector of the diffracted light of mth order is:

$$k_g = k_x + m\,G \tag{33}$$

where; represents an integer of the diffraction order for $m = 0, \pm1, \pm2 \ldots$ and G indicates the grating vector. The grating vector remains in the x-y line and is perpendicular to the grating. The magnitude of the grating vector for geometry can be expressed as:

$$\vec{G} = \frac{2\pi}{\Lambda}\vec{x} \text{ and } \left|\vec{G}\right| = \frac{2\pi}{\Lambda} \tag{34}$$

where; x is the unit vector along the x-direction. Using Eqn. (33), the wave vector of the diffracted light along the grating k_g can be written as:

$$k_g = k_x + m\frac{2\pi}{\Lambda} \tag{35}$$

$$k_g = \frac{\omega}{c}\sqrt{\varepsilon_d}\sin\theta + m\frac{2\pi}{\Lambda} \tag{36}$$

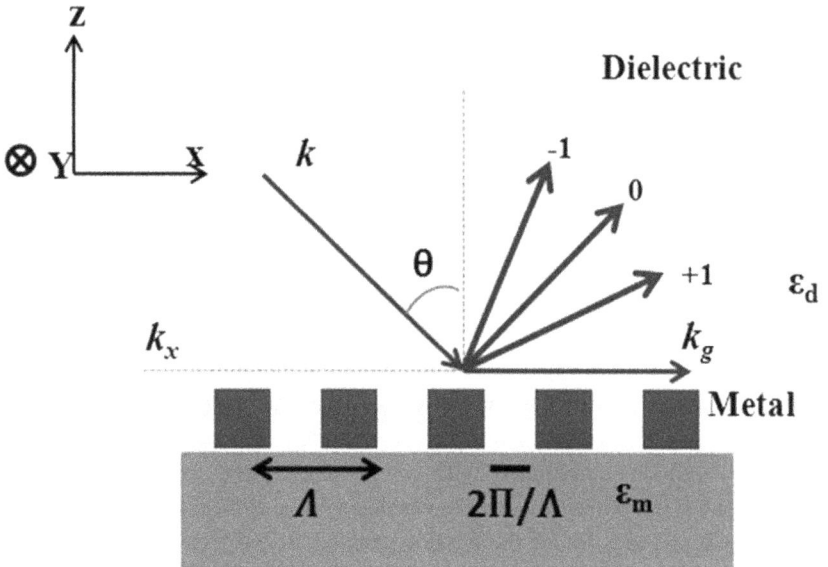

FIGURE 5.5   Grating coupling technique.

Hence, when the propagation constant k_g of the diffracted wave traveling in the plane of the grating can be is equivalent to that of the SPs k_{sp}, hence, we can write:

$$\frac{2\pi}{\lambda}n_d\sin\theta + m\frac{2\pi}{\Lambda} = k_{sp} = \frac{\omega}{c}Re\left(\sqrt{\frac{\varepsilon_d\varepsilon_m}{\varepsilon_d + \varepsilon_m}}\right) \tag{37}$$

Similar to prism coupling, the excitation of SPPs in grating coupling scheme also observed as the minimum in the reflected light during the measurement.

5.4   LOCALIZED SURFACE PLASMONS (SPS)

SPR in nanometer-scaled structures is called localized surface plasmon resonances (LSPR). Localized surface plasmon is excited when an incident light interacts with surface electrons in the conduction band of metallic NPs or nanostructures that is they show strong dipolar excitations (Kelly et al., 2003; Liz-Marzan et al., 2006; El-Sayed et al., 2004; Jain et al., 2010). This phenomenon is possible only when the size of metal NPs is smaller or equal to the wavelength of incident light. Hence, upon incidence of the light, the EM field penetrates into the nanoparticle and displaces the bound electrons relative to the metal ion lattice. The produced opposite charges of the NPs (see Figure 5.6) generate a restoring local field inside the nanoparticle, which increases with more displacement of the bound electrons relative to the metal ion lattice. The coherently displaced electrons along with the produced restoring field represent an oscillator. Thus, when the frequency of incident light matches the natural frequency of electrons oscillations against the restoring force, a resonance condition can be attained. Due to this resonance, there is an amplification of EM fields both inside and in the near field zone outside the nanoparticle which is generally called LSPR. The resonance frequency of the oscillation can be tuned by varying the dielectric properties of the metal, surrounding medium and by size and shape of the particle (Hu et al., 2006). For gold and silver NPs, the resonance occurs in the visible range of the EM spectrum, therefore, the bright colors are manifested by NPs under both transmitted (scattering) and reflected (absorption) light. Due to its distinctive characteristic, it has been used in diverse applications in the past hundreds of years, including colorful windows or ornamental cups.

5.5   BIOSENSORS

The term biosensor, can be defined as a detection technique in which a specific set of materials are put as receptacles that are designed to bind to a target species of interest through a physical transduction process. This process of biochemical interaction is then subsequently translated into a quantifiable signal (Chakraborty et al., 2017). SPR-based biosensor are currently in demand due to their unique features and advantages over other sensing techniques. Because the measurements are based on the RI changes so the analyte does not require any special characteristics and labels; hence it can be detected directly without the need of any multistep detection protocols. It also gives the real time or kinetic measurement. The measurement can be performed in real-time, allowing the user to collect data as well as thermodynamic data. The optical setup for biosensing experiment is shown in Figure 5.7, in which microfluidic chip is used for checking reflectance or transmittance measurement. Through this optical set up bulk refractive index sensitivity (RIS) can be recorded.

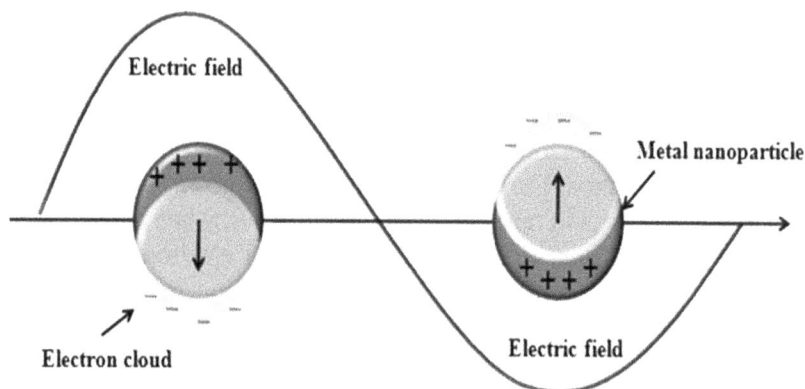

FIGURE 5.6 Illustration of a dipole oscillation in the nanoparticle under the influence of incident light, showing the movement of the conduction electron cloud relative to the nuclei.

There are several factors that need to be taken care of while developing a biosensing device. These factors include the generation and optimiza-tion of the conversion signal (increase of signal, decrease of noise, etc.), fluidics design (i.e., sample injection and drainage, optimized sample consumption, facilitation of analyte transportation, fast detection, etc.), surface immobilization chemistry (effective analyte capture, suppression of non-specific binding, etc.), detection format (direct binding, sandwich-type binding, competitive binding, etc.), and data analysis. Biorecognition molecules, such as antibodies (primary antibodies), are immobilized on the sensor surface. First of all, the sensor surface is filled with a buffer solution. When the receptors are exposed to the concerned analytes, the analyte molecules bind to the receptor molecules, where they replace the molecules inside the buffer solution from a few nanometers to a few thousands of nanometers from the surface. The target analyte (Secondary antibodies) have a different RI than that of the buffer solution resulting in a RI change near the sensor surface because changed medium will change the optical properties of the sensor layer, which can be detected optically as the sensing transduction signal (Peltomaa et al., 2018).

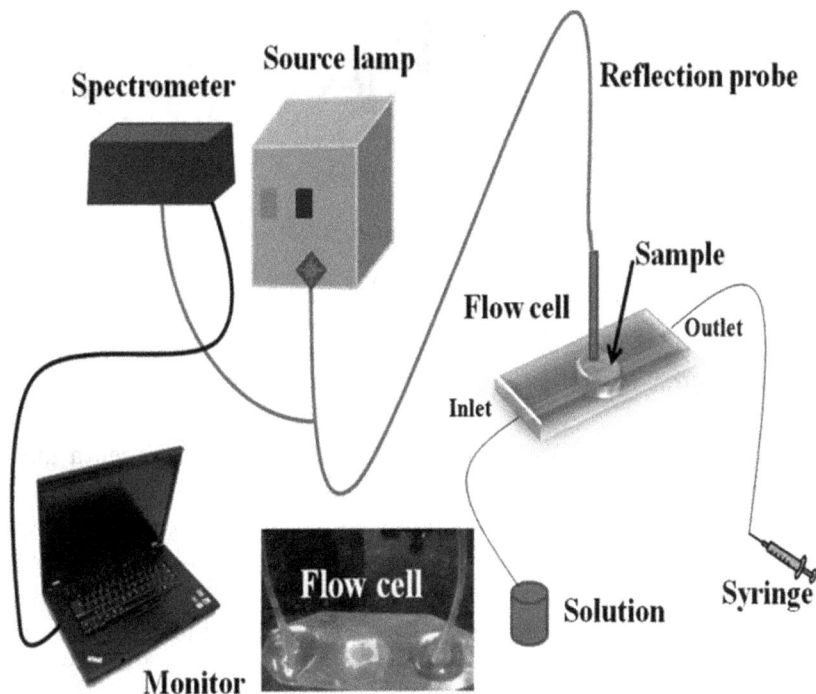

FIGURE 5.7 Optical setup for biosensing.

Source: Reprinted with permission from Mohapatra et al., 2017. © IOP Publishing.

The binding constant between the surface trapped ligand and the solvent dispersed target molecule determines the detection limit. Detection and monitoring of biomolecules are shown in Figure 5.8. Since most of the biomolecules possess a RI that is higher than the buffer solution, there will be a noticeable increment in the local RI value when the biomolecules bind to NPs. This triggers a redshift in both the extinction and the scattering spectrum. The real time and precise monitoring of binding at the molecular level can be done by implementing simple and affordable transmission spectrometry, which measures extinction, the sum of absorption and scattering. Hence, the plasmonic NPs behave like a transducer that converts a small change in the surface properties into spectral shifts as well as change in the intensity of light reflected from the nanostructures (Kvítek et al., 2013; Mongra, 2012; Jana et al., 2016).

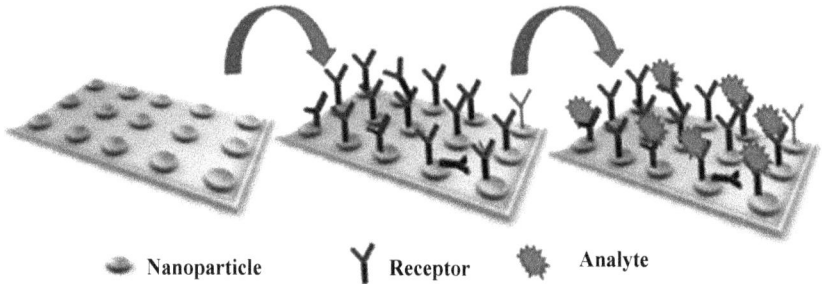

Nanoparticle   **Y** **Receptor**   **Analyte**

FIGURE 5.8   The detection of receptor and analyte.

5.5.1   *DESIGN PRINCIPLE FOR SENSING PERFORMANCE*

In SPR sensors, the SP wave excited at the interface between a metal film and a dielectric medium is very sensitive to changes in bulk or local RI of the dielectric surrounding medium interfaced with the metal film. Assuming that there is a local change in RI of Δn upon binding of chemical or biological molecules in the surrounding dielectric medium (with bulk RI n). Then, a change in the RI $n + \Delta n$ in the local surrounding medium produces a change in the propagation constant $\beta + \Delta\beta$ of SP wave at metal(gold)-dielectric (liquid media) interface. Subsequently, this leads to the change in the phase-matching condition require exciting SPR at different resonance wavelength or angle, which results in red-shifting of SPR reflection dip. Based on the characteristics of the light interacting with SP wave, SPR sensor can be classified with different schemes such as angular, wavelength, intensity, phase, or polarization modulation. In angular interrogation-based SPR sensor, a monochromatic light wave is used to excite SP wave at metal-dielectric interface. The strength of coupling between the incident light and SP wave is recorded with respect to multiple angle of incidence of light. The SPR resonance angle is appeared as a dip in the reflectance intensity in the angular spectra. By recording the shift in the angle or reflection intensity as sensor signal, we can monitor the binding of chemical or biological molecules on the sensor surface. Similarly, wavelength interrogation-based SPR sensor, SP wave is excited via a collimated broadband light source at constant incident angle of the light. The strength of coupling between the incident wave and SP wave is recorded with respect to multiple wavelengths. The shifting wavelength that corresponds to the SPR peak is employed as a sensor signal to monitor various chemical or biological process occurred on the sensor surface. SPR sensors based on intensity modulation measures the coupling strength between the incident light and a SP wave at a fixed angle of incidence and wavelength. The change in the intensity of light at SPR condition is employed a sensor signal with respect to the biological or chemical molecules attachment on the sensor surface. In phase modulation based SPR, the shift in phase or change in the polarization of lightwave interacting with the SP is measured at both constant wavelength and incident angle with respect to bulk RI change or attachment of biological/ chemical molecules on the sensor surface (Homo, 2003).

The SPs confined to the EM field carry the corresponding energy and are rapidly converted into high-energy EM waves, leading to an enormous localized EM enhancement. The sensitivity and resolution are determined by the properties of the SPR sensor and can be used further for the real-time measurement. Although there are improvements in the present technology and instrumentation of SPR biosensor still needs significant advances in miniaturization of SPR biosensing platforms, biomolecular recognition elements with high specificity and assimilation of SPR sensor set up with microfluidic devices. Furthermore, the bulky size and high cost of the instruments restrict their usage for portable, affordable, and low-cost applications. In biosensing, biomolecular binding events can be monitored in terms of spectral or intensity changes, as shown in Figure 5.9. When a biological molecule or analyte is immobilized on the surface of the metal nanoparticle or nanostructure, local surrounding dielectric constants are changed in the proximity of metal NPs or nanostructures surface. Since LSPR peak wavelength (λ_{max}) is very sensitive to the changes in the local surrounding dielectric constant described, the successive binding of biological molecules on the sensor surface will cause shifting in the LSPR peak position. The shift in LSPR peak upon target binding can be understood by the following relation (Unser et al., 2015).

$$\Delta\lambda = S(\Delta n)\left[1 - exp(\frac{-2d}{\delta_d})\right] \quad (38)$$

where; S is the RIS (RIU), Δn is the change in RI due to the biomolecular binding, d is the biomolecular film thickness and δ_d represent the EM field decay length. The quantity S generally can be obtained from the slope ($\Delta\lambda/\Delta n$), which can be determined by linearly fitting of data points of LSPR wavelength shift versus the RI change. When the size of NPs is approximately comparable to the size of biomolecules, δ_d provides the good sensitivity to sense the attached biomolecules to the surface. If the decay length is small or large in comparison to the metal film thickness, there will be rapid exponential decay that leads to small sensing volume or weak response. Thus, for the best outcome, an appropriate transducer (metal NPs) has to be chosen so that the collective RIS and decay length offer superior LSPR response. Though, SPR sensor provides higher sensitivity to changes in the bulk RI in comparison to the LSPR sensor. The sensing capability of both techniques becomes comparable but for the biomolecular detection. LSPR sensitivity can be improved to cut the need for low cost and reasonable sensor device. Hence, the objective of the thesis will be to design and execute SPR and LSPR biosensor using the simpler approach of nanofabrication techniques. In sensing sensitivity, figure of merit (FOM) and resolution can be termed as design principle for sensing performance.

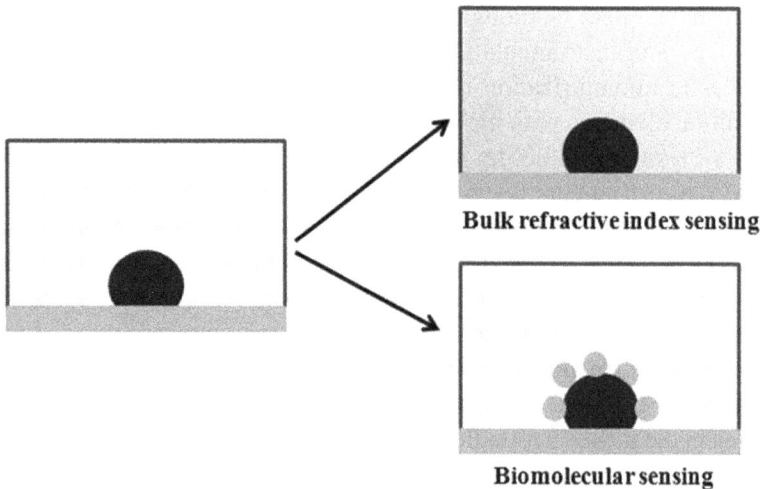

Bulk refractive index sensing

Biomolecular sensing

FIGURE 5.9   Bulk refractive index sensing and biomolecular sensing.

5.5.2   SENSITIVITY

The important characteristics pertaining to SPR biosensors include sensitivity, accuracy, precision, repeatability, resolution, signal to noise ratio (SNR) and the lowest detection limit. Sensor sensitivity, S, is the ratio of the change in the sensor output (e.g., angle of incidence, wavelength, intensity, intensity, phase, and polarization of light waves interacting with an SPW.) to the change in measurand (e.g., analyte concentration) (Prabowo et al., 2018). The sensor has a high sensitivity at larger resonant incident angle if negative diffraction order of metallic grating is used to excite the surface plasmon. The sensitivity of the negative diffraction order (m < 0) is tens of times higher than that of positive diffraction order (m > 0) at larger resonant angle, which is also much higher than that of conventional prism-based SPR sensor. The sensitivity of a sensor is defined as the smallest change in sensor input which produces significant changes in the sensor output. Therefore, in basic terms, the sensitivity is merely the minimum fractional change in a device that can be measured. Mathematically, it can be written as:

$$S = \frac{\Delta Y}{\Delta X} \tag{39}$$

where; ΔY is the sensor output and ΔX is the sensor input. In SPR sensors, the RIS is the major key factor to decide the performance of the sensor. For wavelength interrogation based on SPR sensor, the sensitivity of the sensor can be defined as:

$$S = \frac{\Delta \lambda}{\Delta n} \tag{40}$$

i.e., $\Delta \lambda$ is the change in wavelength to change in RI Δn in the surrounding medium of the sensor surface.

5.5.3 LIMIT OF DETECTION (LOD)

The LOD is defined as the least concentration level of the analyte that can be detected with reliable certainty.

5.5.4 FIGURE OF MERIT (FOM)

To achieve high coupling efficiency, the sensor should have a narrow resonant dip with a full width at half maximum (FWHM). FOM is generally defined as the ratio of the sensitivity (S) over the resonance line width ($\delta \lambda$):

$$FOM = \frac{S}{\delta \lambda} \tag{41}$$

FOM of metallic nanostructures in wavelength units is defined as ($\Delta\lambda$ SPR/Δn)/$\Delta\lambda$, where $\Delta\lambda$ is the FWHM bandwidth. The FWHM is related to the loss of SPR. The intensity sensitivity is defined as ($\Delta I/I_0$)/Δn, where $\Delta I/I_0$ is the normalized intensity change. It is determined by both the wavelength sensitivity and resonant bandwidth.

5.5.5 RESOLUTION

The term, resolution, can be defined as the limit of detection (LOD), which can be enhanced through the tuning of the shape and size of the concerned nanostructures. Therefore, sensor resolution can be explained in terms of the ability to determine the minimum change in the parameter that can be resolved by a sensing device. Here, some sensitivity based on RI is listed from different chapters:

Nanostructures Sensitivity (nm per RIU) References

Hollow gold nanoshell 408 (Sun et al., 2002)
Gold nanorings 880 (Larsson et al., 2007)
Gold nanoring trimers 345 (Lin et al., 2010)
Gold nanodisk trimers 170 and 373.9 (Tripathy et al., 2010)
Arrays of gold nanodisk 167 and 327 (Lee et al., 2011)
Nanocubes 165 (Galush et al., 2009)
Nanostars 218 (Dondapati et al., 2010)
Nanocrescents 879 (Bukasov et al., 2010)
Double Nanopillars with nanogaps 652 and 1056 (Kubo and Fujikawa, 2011)
Arrays of Plasmonic nanotubes 250 (McPhillips et al., 2010)
Nanopillars arrays 675 (Cetin et al., 2011)
Plasmonic nanorods metamaterial 30000 (Kabashin et al., 2009)
EOT gold nanoholes arrays 1580 (Chen et al., 2019)
Triple narrow band plasmonic perfect absorber 1194 (Cheng et al., 2019)
Gold grating on nitride substrate 1140 nm/RIU (Sharma et al., 2019)
Rectangular plasmonic interferometer 4923 nm/RIU (Khajemiri et al., 2019)

5.5.6 SENSING OF BIOMARKERS

The hormones and neurotransmitters are produced by the glands in the endocrine and the nervous system, respectively. These hormones and neurotransmitters control many functions of the body. The concentrations of the hormones and neurotransmitters in the body indicate the state of the body, henceforth the use of the term 'biomarker.' The excess concentrations of the biomarkers (such as cortisol, epinephrine, serotonin, and dopamine (DA)) released by the body in response to the variety of conditions including euphoria, stress, and other dangerous diseases. A biomarker is an indicator of a biological state of disease. A biomarker can be a protein, a fragment of a protein, DNA, or RNA-based. It is characteristic of a specific state and therefore can be used as a marker for a target disease. Traditionally used immunoassay techniques such as ELISA and fluorescence immunoassay help in the precise biomedical diagnosis; however, the growing demand for early, affordable, and accurate screening methods of molecular biomarkers is compelling the development of ultrasensitive sensors through signal amplification or exploitation of novel detection techniques. One of the disadvantages of these traditional immunoassay methods is label-based technique that can be overcome by using SPR methods. To investigate the effectiveness of LSPR sensor towards the detection of molecular biomarker, a common model system comprising biotin-streptavidin is used mostly. The interaction mechanism between the biotin-streptavidin complex and the subsequent resultant effect is of great significance for LSPR sensors, because of the small dimension of biotin, which can be conjugated to the nanoparticle surface. However, streptavidin is a comparatively larger molecule than biotin and can be detected easily by measuring the changes in its RI. But the harnessing of LSPR sensors has been done in the form of generally antigen and antibody. Antigen-antibody has the advantage of kinetic measurements giving real-time analysis, whereas Biotin-streptavidin has some diffusion limitations and has weak binding affinity in comparison of antigen-antibody interactions. Based on these techniques, LSPR sensing technology has been applied to diagnosis the specific diseases (Unser et al., 2015).

For the study and diagnosis of the cancer, tissue biopsy is a very excellent technique. However, the removal of patient tissue offers significant limitations in terms of the sample acquisition and information obtained. For example, the main challenges in the tissue biopsy is cancer heterogeneity, which can be present within the same tumor and between metastases in the same patient. Consequently, the extraction of tissue from a specific lonely tumor may not offer the complete information of the condition of the patient. Nevertheless, multiple tissue abstractions are not suggested to overcome cancer heterogeneity because every abstraction enhances the risk of spreading the disease to the other parts of the body. The alternative to tissue or solid biopsy, the liquid biopsy is lower invasive and extra robust in contradiction of the cancer heterogeneity. The investigation and quantification of the cancer-related biomarkers from several body fluids such as blood, saliva, urine, and cerebrospinal fluid provide substantial advantages. The body fluids are a fresh foundation of the biomarkers. The liquid sample can be obtained at any point throughout the course of the therapy, which provides a dynamic information related to the evolution of the tumor. However, all the above-mentioned benefits are vulnerable by the deficiency of specificity or sensitivity of most of the protein cancer biomarkers including prostate specific antigen or carcinoembryonic antigen. In this way, liquid biopsies for these proteins are only used as accompanying diagnostic tools. Additionally, the investigation of the cancer biomarkers has been generally focused on the disease diagnosis, rather than prognosis, which could have the prospective to improve the treatment and disease management. During the current decade, an ample amount of research articles has been published related to the new sorts of circulating biomarkers, including cell-free and circulating tumor DNA, microRNA (miRNA), exosomes, and circulating tumor cells (CTCs).

In recent years, wearable sensing devices for human health and routine monitoring have grown significant attention. The key things that have aided the advance of such platforms are (i) ubiquitous wireless data transmission; (ii) information processing infrastructure, and (iii) healthcare and monitoring models that care the growth of in-home patient treatment. In order to spread the application zones for wearable sensing devices, developing technologies must pursue non-invasive methods to evaluate health and the physical conditions of the patients. In this perspective, sweat sensing offers a ridiculous source of the biomarkers that are effortlessly available exterior to the body, and consequently may avoid the typical regulatory sanction process. Earlier reports of the technologies that permit observing of the human health and the physical situations from sweat are (i) electrochemical glucose sensor "tattoos," and (ii) hybrid integrated hydration sensors, using ion-selective electrodes (ISEs). Whereas these above-mentioned example of the sensors have established the recognition of targeted analytes in the sweat, most of the applications need to concurrently measure a range of biological signatures essential to make exact evaluations of the health or the physical conditions, or necessitate monitoring of a target biomarker for much longer time periods. With the intention of achieving these goals, the sensing platforms are required to have a higher level of the system integration leading to a collective manufacturing platform to initiative low-cost and keeping better performance. Such an inconspicuous sensing platform is best for the consumer applications, including point-of-care diagnostics, personal health, and the fitness surveillance.

Steckl et al. reviewed the basic characteristics of 12 primary stress-induced biomarkers including (i) origin in the body (hormones, neurotransmitters, or both), (ii) chemical composition, (iii) molecular weight (small/medium size molecules and polymers), and (iv) hydro-or lipophilic nature (2018). When the body is in the effect of the stress, it releases certain molecules which play an important role in mediating the effect of stress. This comprises hormones released by the glandular (endocrine system), and neurotransmitters released by the nervous system. The endocrine system possesses manifold glands which control, trigger, or regulate many functions in the body. The endocrine and the nervous system cooperate in order to uphold a steady equilibrium condition in the body. The thyroid gland controls the metabolism while adrenal glands trigger the 'fight-or-flight' retort to the stressful state. Such control function is capable of the generation of the hormones (molecules) that communicate the signal from the gland to the target cell in selected tissues and organs. The hormones are usually released into the blood circulation, where they travel until they touch their target. Some hormones are hydrophilic and can be move voluntarily in the bold vessels. The hydrophilic hormones communicate their signal, when they reach the cell target, by attaching with the cell surface receptors. The hydrophobic hormones move in the bloodstream with the assistance of the carrier proteins and are inserted into the cell nucleus, where they attach to nuclear receptors. For the detection and measurement of biomarkers, the customary analytical techniques are X-ray diffraction (XRD), nuclear magnetic resonance, mass spectrometry, and liquid or gas chromatography. The above-mentioned analytical techniques can deliver lots of information about the analytes (such as structure, concentration, molecular weight, etc.), which is present in a sample under test.

Nonetheless, the equipment related to these approaches represents a substantial investment, needs operation by trained personnel, and recurrently necessitates particular laboratory space. Furthermore, other than the high-cost feature there is the need of long time for the full analysis. So as to bring the biomarker measurement procedure closer to the specific and to decrease the cost, therefore, there has been significant development for the investigation of the point of care diagnostic platform for the stress and the human routine observation. The point of care diagnostics plays a vital character in supervisory the timely patient care in the crucial care settings. The point of care devices for the biosensing applications designed to identify and quantify the target molecules such as proteins, disease specific antigens, and nucleic acids are the main tools of the wide attention in the medical diagnostics. The substantial advancement has been done in the design and development of the sensitive and definite point of care detection systems, with careful and selective focus on the detection of the biomarkers in the biological fluids where recognition specificity is a crucial factor. To identify and quantified the concentration of various biomarkers, sensing system requires the transducers for converting energy from one form to another. Sensing systems are usually made-up by immobilizing the biological receptor on the surface of the appropriate transducer that can convert a generated biochemical signal into the measurable electronic signals. Traditionally, transducers provide the conversion between the mechanical signal and the electrical signal. As shown in Figure 5.10, the presence of the biomarkers in biological fluids can be detected by using the various kind of transduction methods.

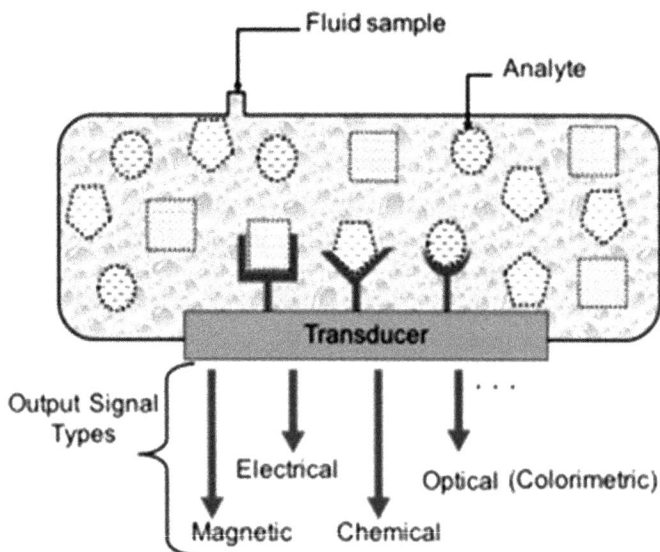

FIGURE 5.10   Biomarker sensing methods.
Source: Reproduced with permission from: Steckl and Ray (2018). © American Chemical Society.

It is to be noted that the different kinds of biomarkers can have very different concentrations in any one fluid (by as much as 5 orders of the magnitude), and the concentration of the certain biomarker is probable to change meaningfully from fluid to fluid. It has been found that the serotonin is existing with relatively high concentrations (approx. 100 ng/ mL) in blood, tissue interstitial fluid, and urine, while it is effectively absent in the sweat and saliva. Stimulatingly, cortisol is also found in crudely the similar concentration in the sweat sample, but the serotonin is absent. It is very clear that the high sensitivity is required for the accurate detection of biomarker. It is also possible that no one single concept of the sensor will work for the recognition of all the biomarkers. Nevertheless, it may be conceivable to define the subsets that can be assisted by one key biomarker type (such as small molecules vs. hormones or polymers vs. enzymes). In most of the fluids, the concentration of various biomarkers lies in the range of 5–6 orders of magnitude, from hundreds of nanograms per milliliter (~1 μM) down to a few picograms per milliliter (sub-1 pM) (Steckl et al., 2018).

Nowadays, in order to constantly watch the state of patients and treat them well, the healthcare industry is in necessity of technologies for the real-time sensing. The biomarker monitoring can be performed by various ways. One ways of biomarker monitoring is based on the sensing of particle mobility (Visser et al., 2018). This kind of sensing approach for continuous monitoring is based on the resolution of single-molecule. This approach is stable and self-contained because it does not consume or yield any reactants. It is based on affinity interactions, therefore, suitable for a variety of biomarkers. Over the past years, lots of biosensors for sensing the action of muscles, heartbeat, electrocardiography (ECG), blood pressure, body temperature, and respiratory rate have become commercially available. The above-mentioned measure the physical properties rather than indispensable biochemical processes. One of the next important steps is to cultivate biosensors for the uninterrupted *in situ* monitoring of the biochemical markers. Therefore, various research groups in the world are actively working on the sensing of the biomarkers. Visser et al. demonstrated continuous monitoring of the biomarker (DNA and protein), with high sensitivity and accuracy, based on the sensing of particle mobility (2018). This technique is based on single-molecule resolution, self-contained, and affinity interactions. The principle of the sensing of a biomarker is direct and self-contained, without consuming or producing any reactants which has benefits for long-term stability and biocompatibility. One of the important property in this technique is the use of affinity interactions. The benefit of using affinity binders (such as aptamers, antibodies, and recombinant antibody fragments) is that a broad variety of biomarkers can be addressed and that the sensitivity range and response time can be tuned. The design of the biomarker depends on the measurement of particle mobility modulated by the single-molecule interactions.

Another technique is based on the nanopore sensing. This is a very sensitive single-molecule method of sensing that provides the ability to rapidly generate electric read outs for analytes in the solution, in the label-free fashion. When a biomolecule arrives in the space of the nanopore, it may disturb the ionic flow in the pore, subsequent in an ionic current signature. There has been exhaustive research concerning the nanopore-based detection of proteins, nucleic acids, NPs, and DNA-protein complexes. Nevertheless, in most of the cases, the studies of nanopore have been made under the ideal situations that practice only the pure analytes. In fact, using the nanopore techniques, the direct recognition of the analytes in the clinical samples with a complex analyte matrix relics perplexing. Lin et al. in the year of 2017, designed a nanopore system for label-free detection of cancer biomarkers, based on a high selectivity DNA prove and nanoporous membrane, in-clinic samples (Lin et al., 2017). In the study, they showed a solid-state nanopore sensor for direct sensing and quantification of the prostate specific antigen as a cancer biomarker in serum. This technique is based on a high selectivity DNA probe and nanoporous membrane offering a suitable, cost-effective, and fast quantification of cancer biomarkers. It has been expected that the nanopore sensors will open new opportunities for the point-of-care testing of many types of cancer biomarkers for the early diagnosis of cancers. Pallares et al. reviewed the current progress on the metal nanoparticle-based analytical methods for the sensing of circulating cancer biomarkers (including cell-free DNA, circulating tumor DNA, micro RNAs, and exosomes) (2019). The analysis of circulating cancer biomarkers holds the ability in streamlining cancer diagnosis and prognosis using liquid biopsy (body fluid). New analytical apparatuses for proficiently detecting the biomarkers with very low concentrations in the complex sample matrixes are required to enable the clinical application of these biomarkers. Metal NPs have appeared as an extraordinary analytical platform due to their distinctive optical and electronic characteristics and ease of functionalization when perturbed by an external electromagnetic

(EM) radiation. Therefore, several analytical techniques based on metal NPs and their plasmonic properties have been reported in the literature. In contrast to the transition metals whose plasmonic bands lie in the ultraviolet (UV) region, there are several attractive metal NPs (such as gold, silver, and copper NPs), for the application of optical technologies, because of their LSPR bands lie in the visible range of EM spectrum.

The thin and soft wearable sensors that can be closely integrate with the human body provide exceptional abilities. The latest advances in the science of materials engineering, electronics, and the mechanics establish the basics for the stretchable and bendable sensors that can imitate to the complex, textured surface of the skin. For visual information, the wearable sweat sensors rely on the electronics for electrochemical detection or on the calorimetry. Conventional technologies for the analysis of sweat encompass collection using gauze pads to the skin, after that the determination of chemical composition employing benchtop instruments. Even though this is useful in the laboratory and the clinical situations, these tactics cannot afford real-time information. Additionally, their accuracy is limited by loss, degradation, contamination of the samples in the several processes of the analysis, collection, transport, and storage. On the other hand, alternate techniques exploit body-worn sensors for the real-time and on-skin analysis by electrochemical potentiometric techniques. However, these techniques contain the complex collections of hardware, including Bluetooth radios for the data transmission, potentiostats for the signal generation, and rechargeable batteries for the power supply. Since the above-mentioned subsystems are very difficult to shrink, they govern the overall form factor in the way that leads to non-ideal size and the weight for mounting on the skin. Furthermore, potentiometric electrolytic sensors need preconditioning in the typical solutions and standardization before their use, normally with challenges in uncontrolled drifts in the signal. Therefore, potentiometric sensors that use battery-free, and wireless electronics are encouraging as options. However, such sensors can only be able to sense electrolyte levels and fail to sense other physiologically related species such as proteins, drugs, and metabolites. Additionally, the accuracy in capturing the dynamic changes in sweat caused by the lack of controlled routing of newly excreted sweat to the sensor surface is also limited. In this situation, the colorimetric sensors installed in the soft and thin microfluidic networks are required that guide and route sweat into the classified micro-chambers optimally constructed for readout and the measurement. Recently, a battery-free and wireless electronic sensing platform motivated by biofuel cells has been introduced (Bandodkar et al., 2019). Such sensing devices integrate chronometric microfluidic platforms with an embedded colorimetric assays, and combine advantages of microfluidic functionality and electronic in a platform that is meaningfully cheaper, lighter, and smaller than the alternatives.

5.5.6.1   ROLE OF GOLD NANOPARTICLE (AUNP) IN SENSING BIOMARKERS

In nanotechnology, shrinking of the bulk materials to the nanoscale (size of 1–100 nm) offers unique characteristics such as better relative surface area and quantum confinement. Amongst many nanomaterials, the noble metal NPs such as gold nanoparticles are them well-suited for the use of medical diagnostics. Since gold nanoparticles offer remarkable plasmonic properties and large surface to volume ratio; they have been broadly examined for their prospective applications in the detection of biomarker. The optical properties of gold nanoparticles are related to the phenomenon known as LSPR. The most interesting features of AuNP include the large surface area, LSPR, controllable morphology, biological compatibility, high stability, easy functionalization. The above-mentioned properties of gold nanoparticles are strongly dependent on their size, spacing, physical dimensions, and their neighboring environment. The gold nanoparticles provide an exceptional transduction platform for the biosensing. The application of the nanomaterials in the immunoassays and sensors delivers a very large surface area for attachment of antibodies and thus facilitating enhanced access of the analytes to these antibodies. Moreover, nanomaterials also provide better signal amplification and label-free real time protein detection, which leads to the design and development of ultrasensitive sensing of the ultralow levels of the cancer biomarkers. Encouraging ongoing struggles towards microfluidics and the single-molecule biosensing can meaningfully improve the detection of biomarkers to ultra-low levels. The proficient role of the gold nanoparticles (AuNPs) as the nano-carriers of Raman tags, signal amplification in chemiluminescent system components, and the light scattering enhancer by aggregation, have significantly aided in increment the sensitivity of cancer biomarker detection sensors. Regardless of the type of the sensor, the choice of the shape and size of the NPs, composition of the nanocomposites, bioconjugation efficiency, functionalization of NPs, specificity of antibodies or aptamers, have straightforward impact in attaining a sensor with a very high sensitivity and the reliability. The aggregation characteristic of the gold nanoparticles can be exploited in bimolecular sensors as a sensitive and easy to envisage process. When the layer of protein aggregates is bound precisely to the surface of the gold nanoparticle, the hydrodynamic diameter of the nanoparticle-protein complex will be increased, and this variation in the size of the gold nanoparticle probes can be willingly sensed by the dynamic light scattering (DLS). The AuNPs coupled with the DLS measurements aid in the development of a homogeneous immunoassay or sensor to sense free PSA in the range of 0.1 to 10 ng/ml (Devi et al., 2015). There has been a great level of interest, in the field of bio-imaging, growing around the use of AuNPs, because of the excellent optical properties shown by the same. Several key characteristics such as enhanced absorption and scattering processes, controlled through surface-plasmon phenomenon, have provided significant push to these NPs to be used as excellent tools for the fabrication of strong imaging labels and contrast agents. Interestingly, AuNPs possess much better absorption and scattering bands (the band cross-section are found to be at least four to five orders higher in this case) as compared to the commonly implemented organic dyes. AuNPs have been found to be effective in targeting both in-vitro and in-vivo tumor growths when encoded with Raman reporters and subsequent conjugation with ScFv antibodies. This process is carried out in the presence of the epidermal growth factor receptor (EGFR), which is a popular biomarker used to target cancerous cells (Kierny et al., 2012; Qian et al., 2008). In this context, the plasmon resonance coupling, which is usually observed in the case of two closely spaced metal NPs, is used for the in-vitro analytical assays. However, a recent study has reported that the aforementioned plasmon resonance coupling can also prove to be an effective tool for in-vivo molecular imaging of carcinogenesis (Aaron et al., 2007).

Nevertheless, another technique, i.e., DLS analysis, is also effective for biomarker sensing. A one-step immunoassay (homogenous) has been reported for the detection of cancer biomarker, which takes advantage of an effective combination of AuNPs and gold nanorods conjugated with anti-Prostate Specific Antigen (PSA) antibody. The quantitative analysis of the relative ratio between the aggregated and non-aggregated NPs can be easily done with the aid of DLS technique. It is expected that the said ratio between the aggregated and non-aggregated NPs would increase corresponding to the increase in the antigen content in the sample solution, and this relative ratio forms the basis for the homogeneous immunoassay process. This report is based on a study that has been explicitly carried out in a solution phase, contrary to the traditional plate-based immunoassay. Thus, one can afford much better mixing between antigen and antibody. This method is of great significance, since it allows for the biomarker detection at very low concentrations (Choi et al., 2010).

Furthermore, targeted drug delivery and the detection/treatment of a typical cancerous growth can be achieved through the conjugation between quantum dots (QDs) and multifunctional nanoparticle with biomolecules. The excellent optical properties possessed by the QDs have drawn significant attention from the field of bio-imaging and cancer diagnosis. Furthermore, NPs with multifunctional aspects can be synthesized so as to facilitate the precise detection of cancer biomarkers and simultaneous delivery of specific drugs at the targeted cancerous sites (Peng et al., 2010). Koska et al. showed that a sandwich bioassay labeled with AuNPs can be used to detect the cancer biomarkers in serum at ultralow concentrations (2014). The cancer biomarker was firstly recognized by a surface-anchored antibody and then by an antibody in solution that identified a free region of the captured biomarker. This second antibody was tethered to a AuNP that acts as a mass and plasmonic label. The two signatures of biomarker were detected by employing a silicon cantilever. The detection mechanism involves the measurement of the weight of the NPs that have been captured with the help of the aforementioned silicon cantilever, which plays the role of a mechanical resonator in this case. The detection process is also carried out through the use of an optical cavity, which significantly enhances the plasmonic signal generated from the AuNPs (2014). As shown in Figure 5.11, the functionalization of the cantilever is carried out by trapping the antibodies against the concerned protein biomarker through the method of silanization. Additional processes involve the binding of the antibodies on the top surface of the cantilever, and using polyethylene glycol as a blocking agent could minimize non-specific interactions on the bottom surface of the cantilever and voids between the antibodies. Subsequently, the silicon cantilever was then treated with the serum sample to facilitate an immunoreaction process that takes place between the protein biomarker and the captured antibodies. The effectiveness of the immunoreaction process is then tested by exposing the modified silicon cantilever to the detection antibodies against the biomarker that are tethered to AuNPs having an average dimension of 100 nm. The detecting antibodies then help us recognize those specific regions on the captured biomarker (2014).

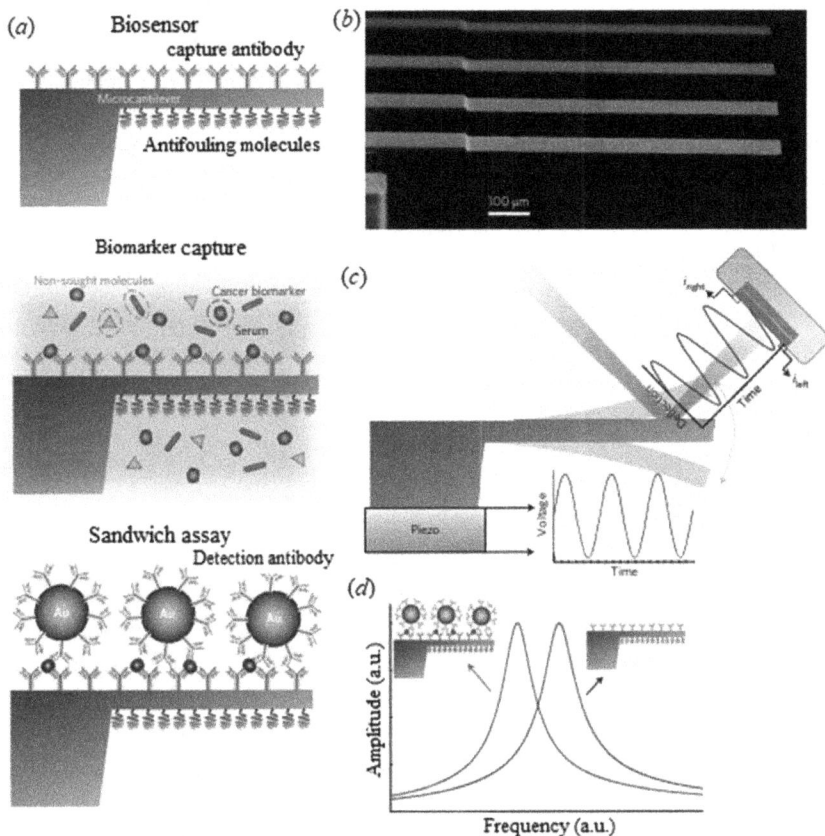

FIGURE 5.11 Schematic representation of the sandwich assay on the cantilevers and the effect of the sandwich assay on the resonance frequency of the cantilever. (a) The cantilever is functionalized with capture antibodies against the sought protein biomarker. (b) SEM image of the silicon cantilevers. (c) The optical beam caused by the cantilever vibration measured by a linear position-sensitive photodetector. (d) The schematics of the effect of the nanoparticle mass loading on the resonance frequency of the cantilever.

Source: Reproduced with permission from: Kosaka et al. (2014). © Springer Nature.

The dimension of the silicon cantilever is typically ~500 μm long, 100 μm wide and 1 μm thick. A laser beam is focused on the free-end region of the cantilever. The deflection of the reflected beam due to the cantilever vibration is then measured by a linear position-sensitive photodetector. The array of the cantilever is driven by a piezoelectric actuator located beneath the base. To derive the resonance frequency and quality factor of the cantilever, the amplitude of the vibrations vs. frequency was close-fitted to the harmonic oscillator model. It has been found that the resulting downshift of the resonance frequency was proportional to the added mass. In this way, by employing the commercially available cantilevers and simple instrumentation, this technique permits ultralow concentrations of the cancer biomarkers to be detected in blood sample. The usage of two different mechanisms of transduction at a single platform sanctions us to determine the existence of the protein with enormously high statistical significance. These characteristics suggest that the hybrid opto-plasmonic and mechanical device could be very suitable in the development of future technologies capable of early detection of cancer through routine blood tests.

5.5.6.2 COMMERCIALLY AVAILABLE BIOSENSOR

Nowadays, the number and diversity of SPR biosensor applications continue to increase. On the basis of the SPR excitation technique, commercial Biacore instruments enable real-time and label-free measurements of biomolecular binding affinity. There are more than 500 companies worldwide presently working in the area of biosensors and bioelectronics. A review suggests that Biacore instruments are the most sensitive in this field. The companies such as 'Affymetrix' and 'Agilent' have developed various commercial micro-array optical detectors and scanners for genomic and proteomic analysis. Some of the companies currently manufacture a variety of biosensor hard-ware (Narsaiah et al., 2012; Mahato et al., 2018) are listed in the following Table 5.1.

5.6 OUTLOOK

In the research field of plasmonic waveguides and devices, there has been a lot of research going on for the betterment of society, especially it is very useful for the spectroscopy, chemical, and biosensing applications.

The sensing behavior of plasmonic-based devices can be used in different areas, including medical, chemical, and environmental sciences. Up to now, many commercialized biosensors have been launched. Plasmonic biosensor or other plasmonic-based sensors are emerging as they offer very fascinating and useful applications in different areas. Based on its sensing mechanism, various biomedical problems can be solved. Through the studies of protein biomolecules on biological samples, disease diagnosis can be done at earlier stages. But there are many challenges to design a sensor-based devices. One of the most significant challenges is nanofabrication, especially the low-cost and high-throughput production of metal nanostructures with tailorable plasmonic properties. At lower concentration detection, ultrasensitive, and cost-effective chip can be designed. In addition to many metal NPs, AuNP is emerging as a very powerful detection agent. Hence based on SPR or localized surface plasmon resonance, metal nanostructures can be used for sensing applications. We hope that this review on the biosensors will be helpful in understanding the basics and working principle of plasmonic sensing devices and provides a valuable perspective.

TABLE 5.1 Commercial Biosensors

Manufacturer Company	Website
Biacore AB	http://www.biacore.com
Bio-Rad	http://www.bio-rad.com
Affinity Sensors	http://www.affinity-sensors.com
Windsor Scientific Limited	http://www.windsor-ltd.co.uk
BioTul AG	http://www.biotul.com
Nippon Laser and Electronics Lab	http://www.rikei.com
Texas Instruments	http://www.ti.com/spr
Agilent	http://www.agilent.com
i-STAT	http://www.abbottpointofcare.com
DiagnoSwiss	http://www.diagnoSwiss.com
GE Life sciences	http://www.gelifesciences.com
Sensor Tech Ltd.	http://www.sensortech.ie
BioNavis	http://www.bionavis.com
GlucoDr	https://www.lelong.com
AimStrip	https://www.leascade.com

KEYWORDS

- gold nanoparticles
- nanoparticles
- protein biomolecules
- surface plasmon polaritons
- surface plasmon resonance
- surface plasmons

REFERENCES

Aaron, J., Nitin, N., Travis, K., Kumar, S., Collier, T., Park, S. Y., Yacaman, M. J., et al., (2007). Plasmon resonance coupling of metal nanoparticles for molecular imaging of carcinogenesis *in vivo*. *J. Biomed Opt., 12*, 034007.

Abbs, A., Lin, M. J., & Quan, (2011). New trends in instrumental design for surface plasmon resonance-based biosensors. *Biosensors and Bioelectronics., 26*, 1815–1824.

Bandodkar, A. J., Gutruf, P., Choi, J., Lee, K., Sekine, Y., Reeder, J. T., Jeang, W. J., et al., (2019). Battery-free, skin-interfaced microfluidic/electronic systems for simultaneous electrochemical, colorimetric, and volumetric analysis of sweat. *Science Advances, 5*, 3294.

Bukasov, R., Ali, T. A., Nordlander, P., & Shumaker-Parry, J. S., (2010). Probing the plasmonic near-field of gold nano crescent antennas. *ACS Nano, 4*, 6639–6650.

Cetin, A. E., Yanik, A. A., Yilmaz, C., Somu, S., Busnaina, A., & Altug, H., (2011). Monopole antenna arrays for optical trapping, spectroscopy and sensing. *Appl. Phys. Lett., 98*, 111110.

Chakraborty, M., Saleem, M., & Hashmi, J., (2017). An overview of biosensors and devices. *Reference Module in Materials Science and Materials Engineering*.

Chen, Z., Zhang, S., Chen, Y., Liu, P., & Duan, H., (2019). Enhanced extraordinary optical transmission and refractive-index sensing sensitivity in tapered plasmonic nanohole arrays. *Nanotechnology, 30*, 33.

Cheng, Y., Chen, H. F., & Gong, R., (2019). Triple narrow-band plasmonic perfect absorber for refractive index sensing applications of optical frequency. *OSA Continuum, 2*, 2114.

Choi, Y. E., Kwak, J. W., & Park, J. W., (2010). Nanotechnology for early cancer detection. *Sensors (Basel), 10*, 428–455.

Debruijn, H. E., Kooyman, R. P. H., & Greve, J., (1992). Choice of metal and wavelength for Surface-plasmon resonance sensors: Some considerations. *Applied Optics, 32*, 440–442.

Devi, R. V., Doble, M., & Verma, R. S., (2015). Nanomaterials for early detection of cancer biomarker with special emphasis on gold nanoparticles in immunoassays/sensors. *Biosensors and Bioelectronics, 68*, 688–698.

Dondapati, S. K., Sau, T. K., Hrelescu, C., Klar, T. A., & Stefani, F. D., (2010). Label-free biosensing based on single gold nanostars as plasmonic transducers. *ACS Nano, 4,* 6318–6322.

El-Sayed, M. A., (2004). Small is different: Shape, size and composition-dependent properties of some colloidal semiconductor nanocrystals. *Acc. Chem. Res., 37,* 326.

Galush, W. J., Shelby, S. A., Mulvihill, M. J., Tao, A., Yang, P., & Groves, J. T., (2009). A nanocube Plasmonic sensor for molecular binding on membrane surfaces. *Nano Letter, 9,* 2077–2082.

Helmerhorst, E., Chandler, D. J., Nussio, M., & Mamotte, C. D., (2012). Real-time and label-free bio-sensing of molecular interactions by surface plasmon resonance: A laboratory medicine perspective. *Clinical Biochemists Review, 33,* 161.

Hibbins, A. P., (1999). *Grating Coupling of Surface Plasmon Polaritons at Visible and Microwave Frequencies.* University of Exeter.

Homo, J., (2003). Present and future of surface plasmon resonance biosensor. *Anal. Bio. Anal. Chem., 377,* 528.

Homola, J., (2006). *Surface Plasmon Resonance Based Sensors* (1st edn., p. 4). Springer: Berlin, Heidelberg, Germany.

Hu, M., Chen, J., Li, Z. Y., Au, L., Hartland, G. V., Li, X., Marqueze, M., & Xia, Y., (2006). Gold nanostructures: engineering their plasmonic properties for biomedical applications. *Chem. Soc. Rev., 35,* 1084–1094.

Jackson, J. D., (1962). *Classical Electrodynamics.* Wiley.

Jain, P. K., & El-Sayed, M. A., (2010). Plasmonic coupling in noble metal nanostructures. *Chemical Physics Letters, 487,* 153–164.

Jana, J., Ganguly, M., & Pal, T., (2016). *Enlightening Surface Plasmon Resonance Effect of Metal Nanoparticles for Practical Spectroscopic Application,* 89.

Jatschka, J., Dathe, A., Csaki, A., Fritzsche, W., & Stranik, O., (2016). Propagating and localized surface plasmon resonance sensing-A critical comparison based on measurements and theory. *Sensing and Bio-Sensing Research, 7,* 62–70.

Jeffrey, N. A., Olga, L., Nilam, C. S., Jing, Z., Van, P., & Richard, D., (2008). Biosensing with plasmonic nanosensors. *Nature Materials, 7,* 442–453.

Kabashin, A. V., Evans, P., Pastkovsky, S., Hendren, W., Wurtz, G. A., Atkinson, R., Pollard, R., et al., (2009). Plasmonic nanorod metamaterial for biosensing. *Nat. Mater., 8,* 867–871.

Kelly, K. L., Coronado, E., Zhao, L., & Schatz, G. C., (2003). The optical properties of metal nanoparticles: the influence of size, shape, and dielectric environment. *J. Phys. Chem B, 107,* 668–677.

Khajemiri, Z., Lee, D., Hamidi, S. M., & Kim, D. S., (2019). Rectangular plasmonic interferometer for highly sensitive glycerol sensor. *Scientific Reports, 9,* 13789.

Kierny, M. R., Cunningham, T. D., & Kay, B. K., (2012). Detection of biomarkers using recombinant antibodies coupled to nanostructured platforms. *Nano Rev., 3,* 3402.

Kosaka, P. M., Pini, V., Ruz, J. J., Da Silva, R. A., González, M. U., Ramos, D., Calleja, M., & Tamayo, J., (2014). Detection of cancer biomarkers in serum using a hybrid mechanical and optoplasmonic nano sensor. *Nature Nanotechnol., 9,* 1047–1053.

Kubo, W., & Fujikawa, S., (2011). Au double nanopillars with nanogap for plasmonic sensor. *Nano Lett., 11,* 8–15.

Kvítek, O., Siegel, J., Hnatowicz, V., & Václav, S., (2013). Noble metal nanostructures influence of structure and environment on their optical properties. *Journal of Nanomaterials,* 743684.

Lal, S., Link, S., & Halas, N. J., (2007). *Nano-optics from sensing to waveguiding. Nature Photonics, 1*, 641–648.

Larsson, E. M., Alegret, J., Kall, M., & Sutherland, D. S., (2007). Sensing characteristics of NIR localized surface plasmon resonances in gold nanorings for application as ultrasensitive biosensors. *Nano Letter, 5*, 1256–1263.

Lee, K. L., Ming, Chih, M. J., Shi, X., Ueno, K., Misawa, L. H., & Wei, P. K., (2012). Improving surface plasmon detection in gold nanostructures using a multi-polarization spectral integration method. *Advanced Materials, 24*, OP253–OP259.

Lee, S. W., Lee, K. S., Ahn, J., Lee, J. J., Kim, M. G., & Shin, Y. B., (2011). Highly sensitive biosensing using arrays of plasmonic Au nanodisks realized by nanoimprint lithography. *ACS Nano, 5*, 897–904.

Lin, V. K., Teo, S. L., Marty, R., Arbouet, A., Girard, C., Alarcon-Llado, E., Liu, S. H., et al., (2010). Gold nanoring trimers: A versatile structure for infrared sensing. *Optics. Express., 18*, 22271–22282.

Lin, Y., Ying, Y. L., Shi, X., Liu, S. C., & Long, Y. T., (2017). Direct sensing of cancer biomarkers in clinical samples with a designed nanopore. *Chem. Commun., 53*, 11564.

Liz-Marzan, L. M., (2006). Tailoring surface plasmons through the morphology and assembly of metal nanoparticles. *Langmuir, 22*, 32–41.

Mahato, K., Maurya, P. K., & Chandra, P., (2018). Fundamentals and commercial aspects of nanobiosensors in point-of-care clinical diagnostics. *3 Biotech, 8*, 149.

Maier, S. A., (2007). *Plasmonics: Fundamentals and Applications*. Springer.

McPhillips, J., Murphy, A., Jonsson, M. P., Hendren, W. R., Fredrik, H. R. A., Zayats, A. V., & Pollard, R. J., (2010). High-performance biosensing using arrays of plasmonic nanotubes. *ACS Nano, 4*, 2210–2216.

Mohapatra, S., & Moirangthem, R. S., (2017). Development of flexible plasmonic plastic sensor using nanograting textured laminating film. *Mazter. Res. Express., 4*, 025008–025014.

Mongra, A. C., (2012). Commercial biosensors: An outlook. *J. Acad. Indus. Res., 1*.

Narsaiah, K., Jha, S. N., Bhardwaj, R., Sharma, R., & Kumar, R., (2012). Optical biosensors for food quality and safety assurance: A review. *J. Food Sci. Technol.*, 383–406.

Otto, A., (1968). Excitation of nonradiative surface plasma waves in silver by the method of frustrated total reflection. *Z. Physik., 216*, 398–410.

Pallares, R. M., Thanh, N. T. K., & Su, X., (2019). Sensing of circulating cancer biomarkers with metal nanoparticles. *Nanoscale, 11*, 22152–22171.

Peltomaa, R., Glahn-Martínez, B., Benito-Peña, E., & Moreno-Bondi, M. C., (2018). Optical biosensors for label-free detection of small molecules. *Sensors., 18*, 4126.

Peng, C. W., & Li, Y., (2010). Application of quantum dots-based biotechnology in cancer diagnosis: Current status and future perspectives. *Journal of Nanomaterials, 1*, 676839.

Prabowo, A., Purwidyantri, A., & Liu, K. C., (2018). Surface plasmon resonance optical sensor: A review on light source technology. *Biosensors, 8*, 80.

Qian, X., Peng, X. H., Ansari, D. O., Goen, Q. Y., Chen, G. Z., Shin, D. M., Yang, L., et al., (2008). In vivo tumor targeting and spectroscopic detection with surface-enhanced Raman nanoparticle tags. *Nature Biotechnology, 26*, 83–90.

Sambles, J. R., Bradbery, G. W., & Yang, F. Z., (1991). Optical excitation of surface plasmons: An introduction. *Contemporary Phys., 32*, 173–183.

Sharma, A. K., & Pandey, A. K., (2019). Design and analysis of plasmonic sensor in communication band with gold grating on nitride substrate. *Superlattices and Microstructures, 130*, 369–376.

Steckl, A. J., & Ray, P., (2018). Stress biomarkers in biological fluids and their point-of-use detection. *ACS Sens., 3*, 2025–2044.

Sun, Y., & Xia, Y., (2002). Increased sensitivity of surface plasmon resonance of gold nanoshells compared to that of gold solid colloids in response to environmental changes. *Anal. Chem., 74*, 5297–5305.

Tripathy, S., & Mlayah, A., (2010). Dual-wavelength sensing based on interacting gold nanodisk trimers. *Nanotechnology, 21*, 305501.

Unser, S., Bruzas, I., He, J., & Sagle, L., (2015). Localized surface plasmon resonance biosensing: Current challenges and approaches. *Sensors, 15*, 15684–15716.

Visser, W. A., Yan, V., Van, I. L. J., & Prins, M. W. J., (2018). Continuous biomarker monitoring by particle mobility sensing with single-molecule resolution. *Nat. Commun., 9*, 2541.

Zayatsa, A. V., Smolyaninovb, I. I., & Maradudinc, A. A., (2005). Nano-optics of surface plasmon polaritons. *Physics Reports, 408*, 131–314.

CHAPTER 6

Metal-Free Electrode Materials for Electrochemical Biosensors

SURJIT SAHOO and SATYAJIT RATHA

School of Basic Sciences, Indian Institute of Technology Bhubaneswar, Argul, Khordha–752050, Odisha, India, E-mail: surjit488@gmail.com (S. Sahoo)

ABSTRACT

An electrochemical biosensor is a potential and innovative analytical device, which has drawn great interest in the field of bio-molecular sensing since the last few decades, due to their high sensitivity and selectivity to diagnose biomarkers and determine biological species. Generally, metal-free electrochemical biosensors, utilizing electrode materials such as carbonaceous nanomaterials (e.g., graphene (GN), CNT, carbon quantum dot (QD), carbon nano-fiber, etc.), and conducting polymers (CPs) are of particular importance in bio-sensing, because of their interesting physical and electrochemical properties. In this chapter, we will study different perspectives of various types of metal-free electrode materials for electrochemical biosensors.

6.1 INTRODUCTION

The evolution of biological or biochemical processes has attracted great interest in medical and biotechnological applications during the last few decades. However, converting a biological response into an electronic signal is not straightforward and can be challenging, due to the difficulty of integrating an electronic device directly with a biological environment. Electrochemical biosensors are a sub-class of chemical sensors that have captivated a great deal of attention due to their high sensitivity and selectivity (Grieshaber et al., 2008; Pingarrón et al., 2008). Electrochemical biosensors transform the biochemical information into electrical signals such as current or voltage, by detecting various biomolecules such as glucose, cholesterol, uric acid (UA), DNA, hemoglobin, blood ketones, and others, in the human body (Pohanka and Skládal, 2008; Yamanaka et al., 2016). Nowadays, electrochemical biosensors are utilized in various fields such as analytical chemistry, industrial process monitoring and control, clinical diagnostics, environmental monitoring and security, and food safety. According to the nature of the biological recognition process, electrochemical biosensors can be divided into two major categories; (i) bio-catalytic sensors, and (ii) affinity sensors. Bio-catalytic sensors incorporate various types of enzymes as the recognition element. Generally, bio-catalytic sensors are simple in design, do not need any expensive instrumentation for their sensing purpose and are easy to use (Ronkainen et al., 2010; Yoon et al., 2002). Affinity sensors use the selective binding interaction between a target analyte and a biological component such as an antibody nucleic acid, or a receptor. Typically, electrochemical biosensors comprise different components (an analyte, receptors, signal generation, transducer, and data analysis system), and each component has its own distinctive features and working phenomenon within the biosensor. Each component of electrochemical biosensors use different materials for different purposes, such as (i) electrode materials and supporting substrate, (ii) materials for enhancing the electroanalytical performance, and (iii) materials for the immobilization of biological recognition elements and (iv) biological elements (Gauglitz, 2018; Karunakaran et al., 2015).

The progress in nanotechnology has guided the development of electrochemical biosensors utilizing various nanostructures as electrode materials, including carbon and metal-based nanomaterials. Generally, nanomaterials are used for electrode fabrication and as biomolecule tracers. Metal-based nanostructures are known to have excellent bio-sensing properties and they last longer because of their inorganic nature. However, most of the metal-based nanostructures are derived from precious metals like Au, Ag, etc., and therefore are difficult to synthesize on a large scale. Also, surface poisoning of these metal-based nanostructures drastically affects their catalytic as well as sensing capabilities. Metal-free materials, on the other hand, offer greater flexibility in terms of cost-effectiveness and ease of synthesis. In this context, carbonaceous nanomaterials and conducting polymers (CPs) have shown promising characteristics for electrochemical biosensor applications due to their unique structural and morphological properties. In fact, a wide variety of carbonaceous nanostructures are available, such as nanoparticles (NPs), nano-sheets, nano-onions, nanofibers, fullerenes, and nanotubes, which have been extensively used in analytical applications (Kuila et al., 2011; Yang et al., 2015). The biocompatibility of carbonaceous and polymer-based nanomaterials facilitates their application in electrochemical biosensors.

6.2 CARBON-BASED ELECTRODES FOR ELECTROCHEMICAL BIOSENSING

6.2.1 GRAPHENE (GN)-BASED ELECTROCHEMICAL BIOSENSORS

Graphene (GN) is a single-atom-thick planar sheet of sp^2 hybridized carbon atoms that are perfectly arranged in a two-dimensional (2D) honeycomb lattice. Currently, GN, unquestionably, is a promising candidate in the field of electrochemical biosensors, due to its high conductivity, large working potential window, chemical inertness, and suitability for various modes of sensing and detection. The large specific surface area of GN is capable of improving the surface loading of the desired biomolecules, and both high conductivity and small bandgap can be advantageous for facilitating electron transfer between biomolecules and the electrode surface. GN has great potential in the development of electrochemical biosensors, which depend on the direct electron transfer between the enzyme and the electrode surface (Song et al., 2016; Taniselass et al., 2019). In 2009, Shan et al. reported the first GN-based glucose biosensor using GN/poly ethyleneimine-functionalized ionic liquid nanocomposites modified electrode. Figure 6.1(a)) shows the TEM micrograph of PVP-protected GN, which reveals the formation of graphene nanosheets (GNs). The cyclic voltammograms of the GN-GOD-PFIL modified glassy carbon (GC) electrode were investigated at various scan rates (Figure 6.1(b)). The glucose biosensor exhibits a wide linear glucose response (2 to 14 mM, R = 0.994) with good reproducibility. Zhou et al. prepared chemically reduced graphene oxide (rGO) modified glassy carbon (CR-GO/GC) electrode for glucose biosensor applications (Zhou et al., 2009). Figure 6.1(c) depicts the SEM micrograph of graphite/GC, which shows the electrode formed by irregularly shaped and isolated flakes. Figure 6.1(d) represents the electrochemical response of the CR-GO/GC electrode to other biomolecules.

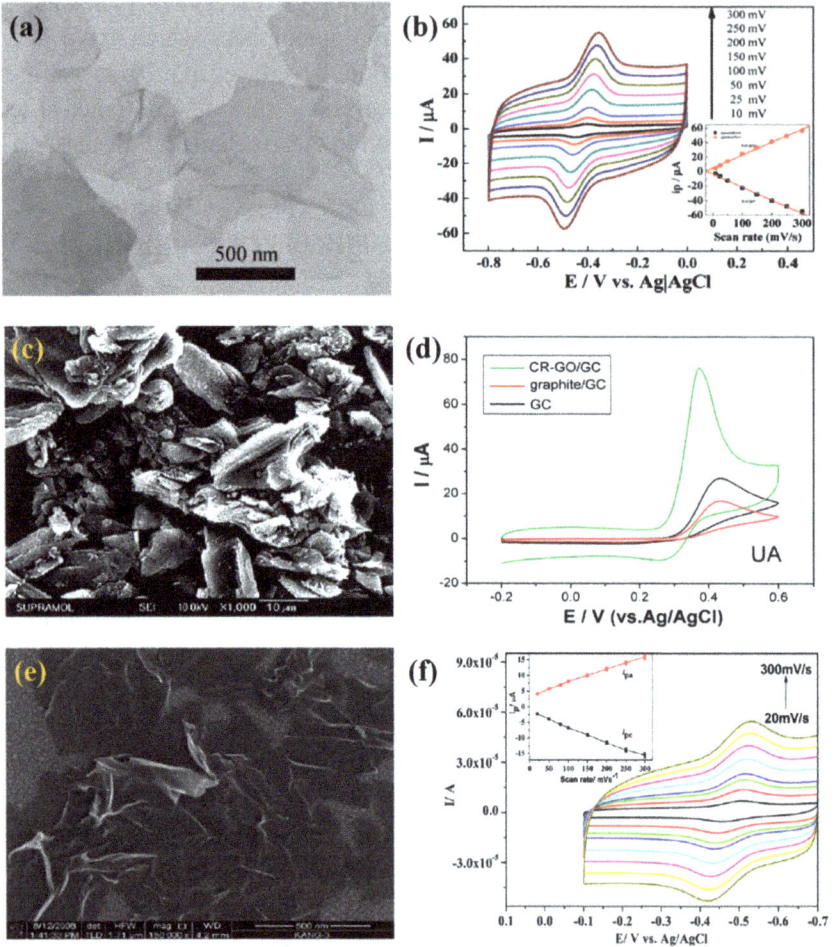

FIGURE 6.1   (a) TEM micrograph of PVP-protected graphene; (b) cyclic voltammetry profile of graphene-GOD-PFIL modified GC electrode at various scan rates; (c) SEM micrograph of graphite/GC electrode; (d) cyclic voltammetry profile of CR-GO/GC electrode to other biomolecules; (e) SEM micrograph of graphene chitosan composite; and (f) cyclic voltammetry profile of modified GCE with GOD-graphene-chitosan film in PBS with 0.1 M KCl electrolyte.

Source: Reproduced with permission from (a, b): Shan et al. (2009) @ American Chemical Society.; (c, d): Zhou, Zhai, and Dong (2009) © American Chemical Society.; (e, f): Kang et al. (2009) © Elsevier..

Similarly, Kang et al. employed biocompatible chitosan to disperse GN and prepared glucose biosensors (2009). The SEM micrograph of the GN chitosan composite deposited on the GCE surface is shown in Figure 6.1(e). The SEM micrograph indicates the typical crumpled and wrinkled GN sheet structure obtained on the rough surface of the film. Similarly, Figure 6.1(f) illustrates the cyclic voltammetry (CV) profile of a GCE, modified with GOD-GN-chitosan film, in PBS with 0.1 M KCl, at different scan rates. The GN-based enzymatic sensor exhibited excellent sensitivity and long-term stability for measuring glucose. Later on, Wu et al. fabricated a GOD/GN/Pt NPs/chitosan composite electrode material and used it for glucose sensing with a detection limit of 0.6 mM of glucose (Wu et al., 2009). These enhanced performances of GOD/GN/Pt NPs/ chitosan composite electrode can be attributed to the large surface area and good electrical conductivity of GN.

6.2.2   CARBON NANOTUBE (CNT)-BASED ELECTROCHEMICAL BIOSENSORS

Carbon nanotubes (CNTs), one of the allotropic modifications of carbon, were first discovered in 1991 by the Japanese scientist S. Iijima. CNTs have had a profound impact in the field of electrochemical biosensing applications, because of their unique physical, electronic, and chemical properties. Depending on the structure, CNTs are divided into two classes (i) single-walled carbon nanotubes (SWCNTs or SWNTs), and (ii) multi-walled carbon nanotubes (MWCNTs or MWNTs). SWNTs can be considered as one rolled-up GN sheet, while MWNTs are concentric tubes separated by about 0.34 nm of two or more rolled-up GN sheets (Jacobs et al., 2010; Vashist et al., 2011). In 2008, Sato et al. demonstrated the electrodeposited SWCNTs as an immobilization matrix for the construction of amperometric glucose biosensor applications (Sato and Okuma, 2008). The residual activity of the sensor was over 94% after 42 days, which indicates its usefulness for the determination of d-glucose. Rahman et al. utilized MWCNT to fabricate an amperometric glucose biosensor (2009). Figure 6.2(a) represents the structural schematic for the fabrication of Nafion/GO$_x$/MWCNT gold electrode for glucose sensing application. The CV profile of unmodified, MWCNT-modified, and Nafion/GO$_x$/MWCNT modified gold electrodes, in phosphate buffer solution (pH-7.4), have been shown in Figure 6.2(b). The interferences of the fabricated glucose biosensor were assessed with active biological biomolecules, and the long-term storage stability of the biosensor has been found to be excellent. Later on, Gao et al. developed a biosensor based on a nanocomposite made of a redox polymer into a multilayer system containing glucose oxidase (GO_x) and SWCNTs on a screen-printed carbon electrode (2011). Figure 6.2(c) illustrates the FESEM micrograph of glassy carbon (GC) electrode modified with nanocomposites, which reveals that the GC electrode was mostly covered with homogeneous, porous, and three-dimensional SWCNT films. Figure 6.2(d) represents the cyclic voltammogram profile of a screen-printed carbon electrode modified with GOx/SWCNT/PVI-Os layers (five layers) at different scan rates ranging from 5 to 200 mV/s. The fabricated biosensors showed a detection sensitivity of 16.4 $\mu A/(mM\ cm^2)$.

Baghayeri et al. reported the fabrication of functionalized multi-wall carbon nanotubes (fMWCNT) modified glassy carbon electrode (fMWCNT/GCE) for biosensing application (Baghayeri and Namadchian, 2013). The modified electrode was characterized as an electrochemical sensor and showed a large electrocatalytic activity for oxidation of levodopa (LD), acetaminophen (AC) and tyramine (TR). Li et al. developed an electrochemical biosensor for the detection of hydrogen peroxide, based on gold nanoparticles (AuNPs)/thionine (Thi)/AuNPs/MWCNTs-chitosan (Chits) composite film (2012). The SEM micrograph of AuNPs/MWCNTs-Chit/GCE is provided in Figure 6.2(e). Figure 6.2(f) illustrates the CV profile, and the effect of scan rates on peak current of the enzyme biosensor, investigated in 0.1 mol L^{-1} HAc-NaAc (pH 6.0).

6.2.3 CARBON DOT-BASED ELECTROCHEMICAL BIOSENSORS

Carbon dot is a 0-dimensional carbon-based nanostructure, which was discovered in 2004. Among various types of carbon dots, carbon quantum dot (QD) and GN QD have been widely used in electrochemical biosensors. The carbon QD is different from GN QD because of the nature of the precursor(s) used in the synthesis process. GN QDs consist of GN sheets having a size of less than 100 nm. GN QDs exhibit larger specific surface area, more surface-active sites, and more accessible edges than GN. GN QDs are mostly used in electrochemical biosensors due to the quantum confinement and edge effect, which make them a relevant transducer material to enhance or control the heterogeneous electron transfer for the

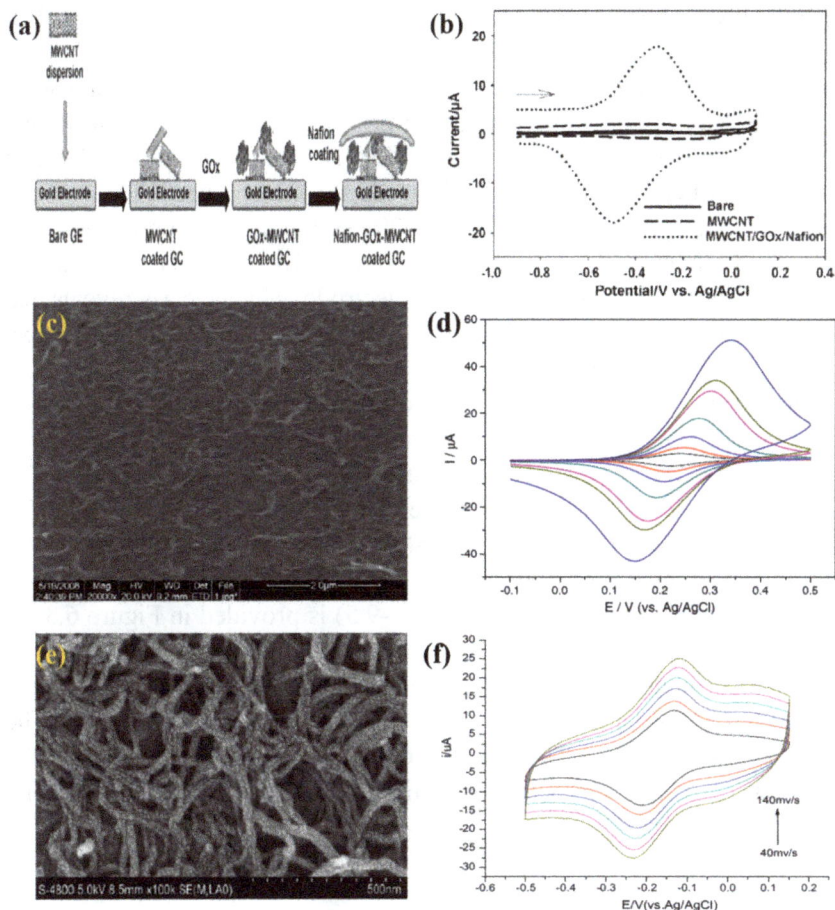

FIGURE 6.2 (a) Schematic illustration of the method by which an enzyme is co-immobilized into the MWCNT and Nafion films; (b) cyclic voltammograms profiles of MWCNT modified, and MWCNT/GOx/Nafion modified electrodes at a scan rate of 100 mV/s; (c) SEM micrograph of glassy carbon electrode, modified with SWCNT; (d) cyclic voltammograms of screen-printed carbon electrode, modified with GOx/SWCNT/PVI-Os layers, at various scan rate; (e) SEM micrograph of AuNPs/MWCNTs-Chit/GCE; and (f) cyclic voltammetry profile of the enzyme biosensor recorded at various scan rates in 0.1 mol L^{-1} HAc-NaAc (pH 6.0).

Source: Reproduced with permission from (a, b): Rahman, Umar, and Sawada (2009) © Elsevier.; (c, d): Gao et al. (2011) © Elsevier.; (e, f): Li et al. (2012) © Elsevier..

design of bio-electrochemical sensors (Dave and Gomes, 2019; Wang and Dai, 2015). In 2011, Zhao et al. designed an electrochemical biosensor by using GN QDs modified pyrolytic graphite electrode, coupled with specific sequence single-stranded DNA molecules, as probes. Figure 6.3(a) illustrates the schematic diagram for the fabrication process for GN QDs modified pyrolitic graphite electrode. Similarly, Figure 6.3(b) represents the differential pulse voltammograms profile for the GN QDs modified pyrolitic graphite electrode in 10 mM Tris-HCl buffer solution. Zhang et al. fabricated GN QDs on a gold electrode surface and used the GN QDs/Au electrode for sensing application (2013). Figure 6.3(c) represents the structural schematic for the fabrication of GN QDs/Au electrode. The CV profile (Figure 6.3(d)) of GN QDs/Au electrode, which clearly reveals that the current detected on the GN QDs/Au electrode was much higher than that on the bare Au electrode.

In order to explore the enzyme absorption ability of GN QDs, Razmi et al. developed GN QDs as a new substrate for the immobilization and direct electrochemistry of GO_x (2013). Figure 6.3(e), f represents the FE-SEM micrographs of GN QDs on carbon-ceramic electrode, which reveal that the formation of wrinkled GN QD sheets on the surface of the carbon-ceramic electrode. The CV profile of GO_x-GN QDs on the carbon-ceramic electrode in different pH solutions (3.4–9.5) is provided in Figure 6.3(g). Later on, Ganesh et al. designed a biosensor to detect H_2O_2 using electrochemical methods by utilizing a novel material based on horseradish peroxidase (HRP) immobilized green color emitting GN QDs (2014). The fabricated electrochemical biosensor exhibits a sensitivity value of 0.905 and 7.057 μA/mM and detection limits of ~530 nM and 2.16 μM along with response time of ~2–3 s.

6.2.4   CARBON NANOFIBER AND C_{60}-BASED ELECTROCHEMICAL BIOSENSORS

Carbon nanofibers (CNFs) have similar nanostructure, conductivity, and mechanical strength as observed in the case of CNTs. The key distinguishing characteristic of CNFs from CNTs is the stacking of GN sheets of different shapes in the case of the former, offering additional edge sites on the outer wall of CNFs, which can enhance the electron transfer of electroactive analytes. These unique properties (both chemical and physical) make CNFs extraordinary candidates for electrode materials and also as excellent substrates for the immobilization process (Huang et al., 2010). In 2006, Vamvakaki et al. demonstrated the utilization of highly

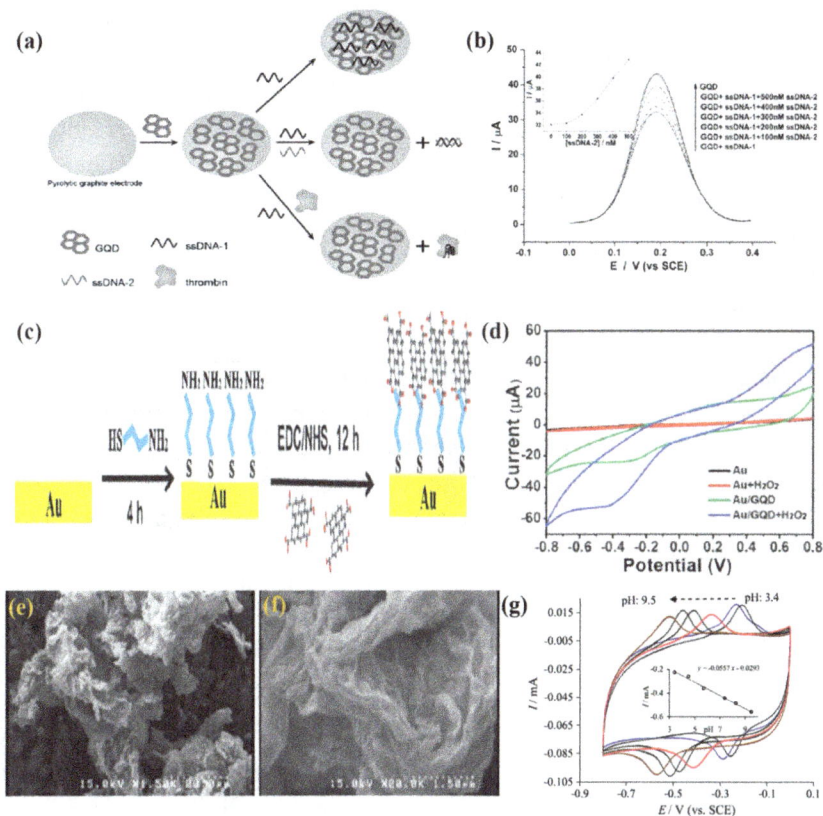

FIGURE 6.3 (a) Schematic diagram for the preparation of a graphene quantum dots modified pyrolitic graphite electrode; (b) differential pulse voltammograms profile of graphene quantum dots modified pyrolitic graphite electrode; (c) schematic diagram for the fabrication of graphene quantum dots/Au electrode; (d) cyclic voltammogram profiles of the Au electrode, and graphene quantum dots/Au electrode at a scan rate of 5 mV s^{-1}, (e and f) FE-SEM micrograph of graphene quantum dots on carbon-ceramic electrode; (g) cyclic voltammetry profile of glucose oxidase-graphene quantum dots on carbon-ceramic electrode at a scan rate of 300 mV s^{-1}.

Source: Reproduced with permission from (a, b): Zhao, Chen, Zhu, and Li (2011) © Elsevier.; (c, d): Zhang et al. (2013); (e–g): Razmi and Mohammad-Rezaei (2013) © Elsevier..

activated CNFs for the design of catalytic electrochemical biosensors. Figure 6.4(a) illustrates the SEM micrograph of CNFs, which reveals that the average diameter of CNFs is about 110 nm, while their length is in the order of few nanometers. In order to understand the electrochemical signal transduction ability of various types of CNFs, extensive CV studies have been carried out, as illustrated in Figure 6.4(b). Later on, Vamvakaki et al. utilized CNFs and bio-mimetically synthesized silica, for the development of a novel enzymatic electrochemical biosensor system (2008). The SEM micrograph of silica/CNFs is provided in Figure 6.4(c), which indicates that the immobilization of the enzyme on the surface of the fibers and further bio-silicification introduces silica particles along the fiber axis. Similarly, Figure 6.4(d) represents the stability of both free and silica stabilized enzyme, as calculated by the residual activity as a function of incubation time, and the biosensor shows extraordinary stability due to the composites of CNFs and silica.

Jia et al. reported the preparation of a novel biosensor platform based on palladium and helical CNF based hybrid nanostructures and GO_x with nafion (NF) on a glassy carbon electrode (GCE), for the sensing of H_2O_2 and glucose (2013). The TEM micrograph of the palladium decorated CNFs is shown in Figure 6.4(e), which represents that nano-sized palladium particles are highly dispersed and well anchored on the CNFs. The CV profile (Figure 6.4(f)) of Nafion/GOx/Pd-HCNFs/GCE, Nafion/GCE with and without one mM glucose in 0.1 M PBS has also been demonstrated. The fabricated bio-sensor illustrates very good long-term stability and high reproducibility, facilitated by the excellent properties of CNFs. Furthermore, Li et al. developed a novel phenolic biosensor on the basis of a composite of polydopamine (PDA)-laccase (Lac)-nickel nanoparticle loaded carbon nanofibers (NiCNFs), and it exhibited good repeatability, reproducibility, and stability, attributed to the excellent biocompatible microenvironment of the composite matrix (2014).

Fullerene (C_{60}), another zero-dimensional carbon allotrope, can exhibit rich electrochemical behaviors due to its unique dimensional and electronic structures. In early 2000, Gavalas et al. first reported a C_{60}-mediated amperometric biosensor. The biosensor was developed using C_{60}, assembly on a porous carbon electrode, which acted as a mediator for electron transfer. Later on, in 2014, Gao et al. reported the direct electrochemistry of a novel GO_x and hydroxyl fullerenes (GOD-HFs) nano-complex, which was self-assembled and immobilized on a GC electrode. Figure 6.5(a) represents the schematic diagram for the possible structure of GOD-HFs. Similarly, Figure 6.5(b) illustrates the CV profile of the chitosan/GOD HFs/GC electrode in 50 mM PBS (pH-7.0) at various scan rates, which reveals that the peak current increased linearly with increasing scan rates. Han et al. prepared a hydrophilic C_{60}-based nanomaterial and utilized it

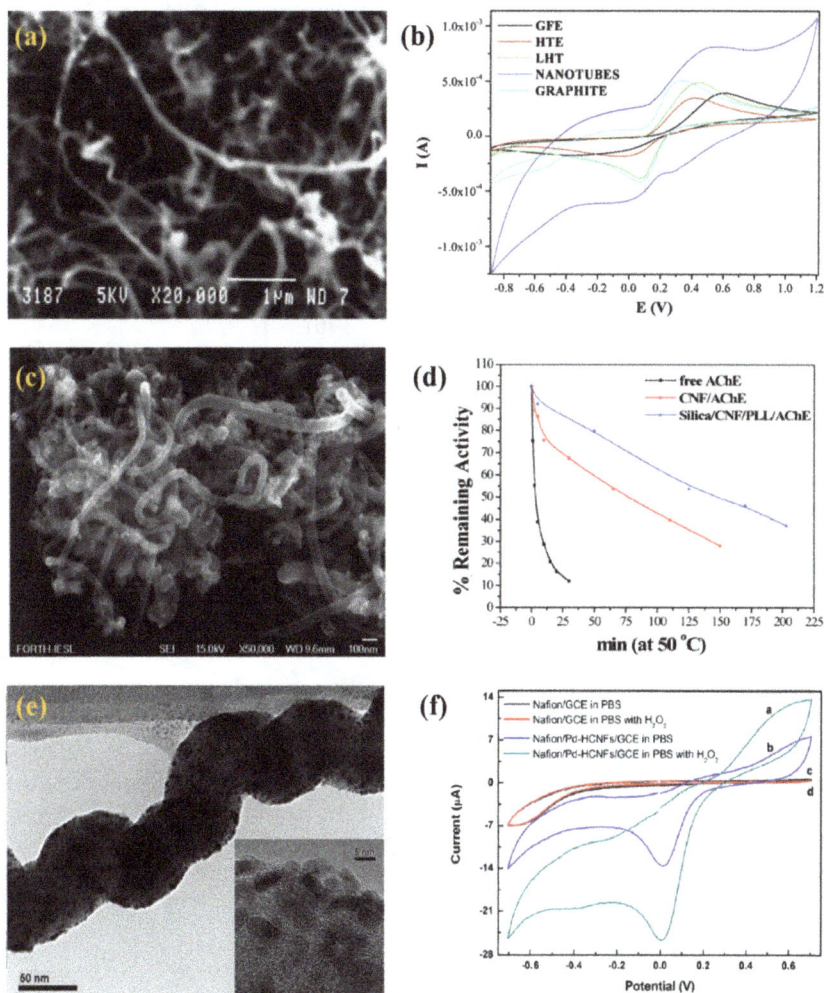

FIGURE 6.4 (a) SEM micrograph of carbon nanofibers; (b) cyclic voltammogram profile of various type carbon materials at a scan rate of 100 mV s^{-1}; (c) SEM micrograph of silica/carbon nanofibers composite; (d) the stability graph of free and immobilized acetylcholine esterase after incubation at 50°C acetylcholine esterase; (e) TEM micrograph of Pd decorated carbon nanofibers; (f) cyclic voltammograms of the Nafion/Pd-HCNFs/GCE (a, b) and Nafion/GCE (c, d) with and without 0.5 mM H$_2$O$_2$ in 0.1 M PBS (pH-7.0).

Source: Reproduced with permission from (a, b): Vamvakaki, Tsagaraki, and Chaniotakis (2006) © American Chemical Society; (c, d): Vamvakaki, Hatzimarinaki, and Chaniotakis (2008) © American Chemical Society; (e, f): Jia et al. (2013) © American Chemical Society.

as a new type of redox nano-probe to construct a sandwich-type immune sensor for erythropoietin detection (2015). The schematic diagram for an electrochemical immunoassay based on C_{60} is provided in Figure 6.5(c). Figure 6.5(d) represents the CV profile of developed immune sensor at various scan rates. The prepared immune sensor yielded good sensitivity, stability, and reproducibility, showing potential applications in doping control as well as bio-analysis.

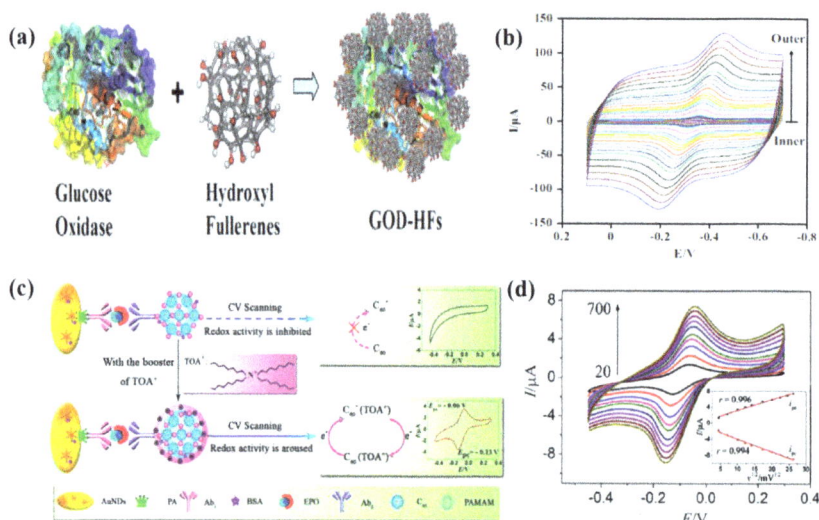

FIGURE 6.5   (a) Schematic diagram for the possible structure of GOD-HFs; (b) cyclic voltammetry profile of chitosan/GOD HFs/GC electrode in 50 mM PBS; (c) schematic diagram of an electrochemical immunoassay based on C_{60}; (d) cyclic voltammetry profile of the immune sensor at different scan rates.

Source: Reproduced with permission from (a, b): Gao et al. (2014) © Elsevier; (c, d): Han et al. (2015) © American Chemical Society.

6.2.5   CONDUCTING POLYMER (CP)-BASED ELECTROCHEMICAL BIOSENSORS

Among the various types of metal-free electrode materials, CPs-based electrochemical biosensors have acquired a considerable interest, as they provide excellent bio-sensing platforms, which are easy and cost-effective to fabricate, and can deliver a direct electrical readout for the presence of biological analytes with high sensitivity and selectivity (El-Said et al.,

2020; Moon et al., 2018). Yang et al. reported the fabrication and applications of PEDOT nanofibers for electrochemical detection of glucose based on the entrapment of the GO_x enzyme into the PEDOT nanofiber matrix (Yang et al., 2014). A schematic illustration of the fabrication process of the GO_x incorporated-PEDOT films (PEDOT F-GO_x) on the Pt substrate, by electrodeposition process, is provided in Figure 6.6(a). The CV profiles of PEDOT NF-GO_x, recorded at a potential increment of 700 mV (at various timestamps), have been shown in Figure 6.6(b). The prepared PEDOT nanofiber-based biosensor demonstrates a significant improvement in the overall performance, which includes sensitivity, limit of detection (LOD), and longevity. Munteanu et al. demonstrated a dual electrochemical sensor with optical microscopy as an opto-electrochemical sensor for detecting both hydrogen peroxide and glucose by drop-casting enzyme and redox polymer mixtures onto planar, optically transparent electrodes (2019). Figure 6.6(c) shows the digital image of ITO electrode arrays and the fabricated electrochemical cell facilitating the simultaneous optical and electrochemical investigation. The CV profiles of the modified FTO electrode, obtained at a scan rate of 0.010 V s^{-1}, in the absence and presence of hydrogen peroxide are shown in Figure 6.6(d). The as prepared biosensor, for hydrogen peroxide detection (with bright field reflected light microscopy), was able to determine hydrogen peroxide at concentrations as low as 12.5 μM. Aksou et al. fabricated electrochemical dopamine (DA) biosensor, using polyimide (PI) and polyimide-boron nitride (PI-BN) composites as a selective membrane, for DA detection (2017). The fabricated electrochemical biosensor exhibited wide linear ranges, excellent sensitivity, selectivity, reversibility, and low detection limits (4.10–8 M). Tancharoen et al. fabricated a new type of electrochemical biosensor for the detection of Zika virus using surface imprinted polymers (SIPs)/GN oxide composites (2018). Figure 6.6(e) depicts a schematic diagram for imprinted polymers (SIPs)/GN oxide composite electrodes, obtainable through various step-wise synthesis processes. The fabricated biosensor demonstrated a good LOD value, which is quite effective for real world applications including Zika virus detection.

6.3 PERSPECTIVES AND FUTURE DEVELOPMENT

This chapter emphasizes the development of electrochemical biosensors, based primarily on the metal-free electrode materials. We discuss here,

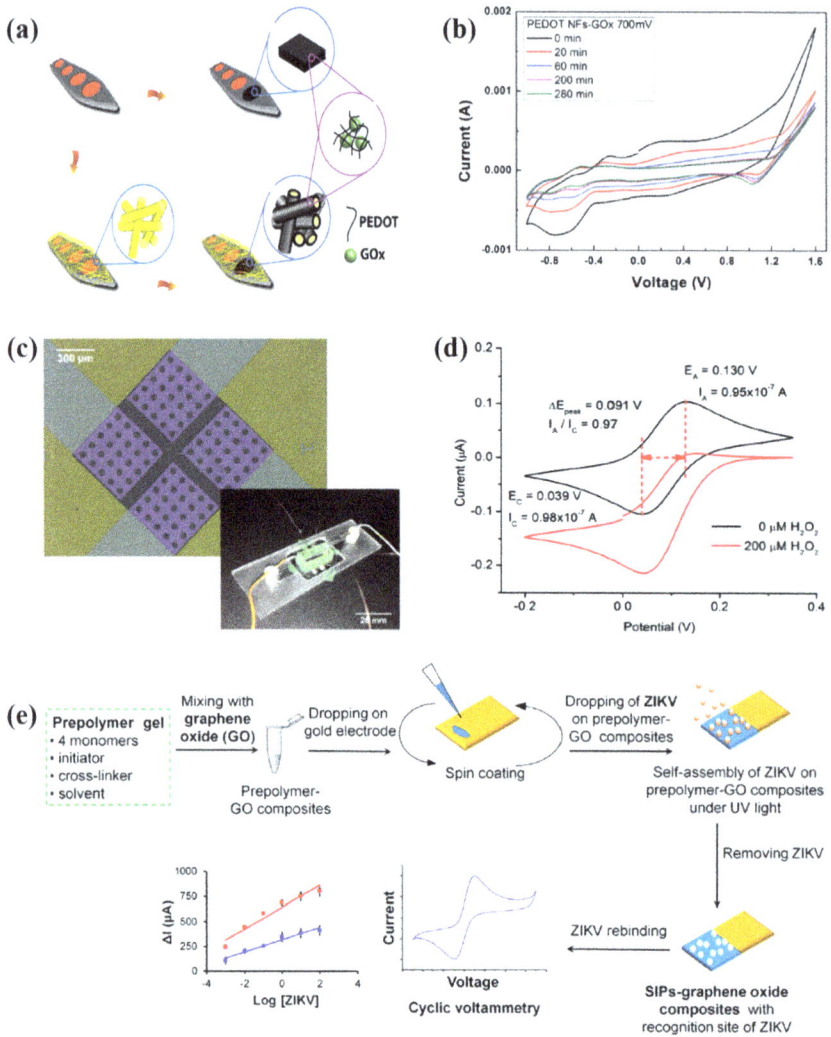

FIGURE 6.6 (a) Schematic diagram for the fabrication process of GO$_x$-incorporated PEDOT on the microelectrode array; (b) cyclic voltammetry profile of PEDOT NF-GO$_x$ electrode recorded in the scan rate of 700 mV s^{-1}; (c) digital image of as-fabricated ITO electrode arrays for biosensor applications; (d) cyclic voltammogram profiles of the modified FTO electrode obtained at a scan rate of 0.010 Vs^{-1}; (e) schematic diagram of surface imprinted polymers (SIPs)-graphene oxide composites preparation on a gold surface for fabrication Zika virus detection biosensor.

Source: Reproduced with permission from (a, b): Yang, Kampstra, and Abidian (2014) © John Wiley; (c, d): Munteanu et al. (2019) © Springer Nature; (e): Tancharoen et al. (2018) © American Chemical Society.

the various types of metal-free electrode materials, including the design, fabrication methods, and related theories on electrochemical biosensors. Carbonaceous nanomaterials and CPs offer a good approach for electrodes in electrochemical biosensors and result in improved detection of analytes. Although these metal-free electrode materials have enormous potential to simplify the manufacturing processes and reduce the overall cost associated with their metal counterparts, the current performance metrics are not at par with the commercially available bio-sensing methods, and thus lack the required thrust to be considered for clinical monitoring. Extensive research and development activities are, therefore, essential to bring further improvements to these metal-free bio-sensing techniques in order to have a significant impact on biosensor performances including selectivity, detection limit, response time and precision, etc. This can be achieved through devising novel electrode material assembly, mainly concerning the immobilization techniques, nanotechnology, miniaturization, and design of multi-sensor arrays.

KEYWORDS

- **carbon nanotube**
- **electrochemical bio-sensing**
- **glucose oxidase**
- **graphene**
- **multi-walled carbon nanotubes**
- **single-walled carbon nanotubes**

REFERENCES

Aksoy, B., Paşahan, A., Güngör, Ö., Köytepe, S., & Seçkin, T., (2017). A novel electrochemical biosensor based on polyimide-boron nitride composite membranes. *Int. J. Polym. Mater. Polym. Biomater., 66*, 203–212.

Baghayeri, M., & Namadchian, M., (2013). Fabrication of a nanostructured luteolin biosensor for simultaneous determination of levodopa in the presence of acetaminophen and tyramine: Application to the analysis of some real samples. *Electrochim. Acta, 108*, 22–31.

Dave, K., & Gomes, V. G., (2019). Carbon quantum dot-based composites for energy storage and electrocatalysis: Mechanism, applications and future prospects. *Nano Energy, 66,* 104093.

El-Said, W. A., Abdelshakour, M., Choi, J. H., & Choi, J. W., (2020). Application of conducting polymer nanostructures to electrochemical biosensors. *Molecules, 25,* 307.

Gao, Q., Guo, Y., Liu, J., Yuan, X., Qi, H., & Zhang, C., (2011). A biosensor prepared by co-entrapment of a glucose oxidase and a carbon nanotube within an electrochemically deposited redox polymer multilayer. *Bioelectrochemistry, 81,* 109–113.

Gao, Y. F., Yang, T., Yang, X. L., Zhang, Y. S., Xiao, B. L., Hong, J., Sheibani, N., et al., (2014). Direct electrochemistry of glucose oxidase and glucose biosensing on a hydroxyl fullerenes modified glassy carbon electrode. *Biosens. Bioelectron., 60,* 30–34.

Gauglitz, G., (2018). Analytical evaluation of sensor measurements. *Anal. Bioanal. Chem., 410,* 5–13.

Gavalas, V. G., & Chaniotakis, N. A., (2000). Fullerene-mediated amperometric biosensors. *Anal. Chim. Acta, 409,* 131–135.

Grieshaber, D., MacKenzie, R., Vörös, J., & Reimhult, E., (2008). Electrochemical biosensors-sensor principles and architectures. *Sensors, 8,* 1400–1458.

Han, J., Zhuo, Y., Chai, Y. Q., Xiang, Y., & Yuan, R., (2015). New type of redox nanoprobe: C60-based nanomaterial and its application in electrochemical immunoassay for doping detection. *Anal. Chem., 87,* 1669–1675.

Huang, J., Liu, Y., & You, T., (2010). Carbon nanofiber based electrochemical biosensors: A review. *Anal. Methods, 2,* 202–211.

Jacobs, C. B., Peairs, M. J., & Venton, B. J., (2010). Carbon nanotube based electrochemical sensors for biomolecules. *Anal. Chim. Acta, 662,* 105–127.

Jia, X., Hu, G., Nitze, F., Barzegar, H. R., Sharifi, T., Tai, C. W., & Wågberg, T., (2013). Synthesis of palladium/helical carbon nanofiber hybrid nanostructures and their application for hydrogen peroxide and glucose detection. *ACS Appl. Mater. Interfaces, 5,* 12017–12022.

Kang, X., Wang, J., Wu, H., Aksay, I. A., Liu, J., & Lin, Y., (2009). Glucose oxidase-graphene-chitosan modified electrode for direct electrochemistry and glucose sensing. *Biosens. Bioelectron., 25,* 901–905.

Karunakaran, C., Rajkumar, R., & Bhargava, K., (2015). Introduction to biosensors. In: *Biosensors and Bioelectronics* (pp. 1–68). Elsevier.

Kuila, T., Bose, S., Khanra, P., Mishra, A. K., Kim, N. H., & Lee, J. H., (2011). Recent advances in graphene-based biosensors. *Biosens. Bioelectron., 26,* 4637–4648.

Li, D., Luo, L., Pang, Z., Ding, L., Wang, Q., Ke, H., Huang, F., & Wei, Q., (2014). Novel phenolic biosensor based on a magnetic polydopamine-laccase-nickel nanoparticle loaded carbon nanofiber composite. *ACS Appl. Mater. Interfaces, 6,* 5144–5151.

Li, S., Zhu, X., Zhang, W., Xie, G., & Feng, W., (2012). Hydrogen peroxide biosensor based on gold nanoparticles/thionine/gold nanoparticles/multi-walled carbon nanotubes-chitosans composite film-modified electrode. *Appl. Surf. Sci., 258,* 2802–2807.

Moon, J. M., Thapliyal, N., Hussain, K. K., Goyal, R. N., & Shim, Y. B., (2018). Conducting polymer-based electrochemical biosensors for neurotransmitters: A review. *Biosens. Bioelectron., 102,* 540–552.

Munteanu, R. E., Ye, R., Polonschii, C., Ruff, A., Gheorghiu, M., Gheorghiu, E., Boukherroub, R., et al., (2019). High spatial resolution electrochemical biosensing using reflected light microscopy. *Sci. Rep., 9,* 1–10.

Muthurasu, A., & Ganesh, V., (2014). Horseradish peroxidase enzyme immobilized graphene quantum dots as electrochemical biosensors. *Appl. Biochem. Biotechnol., 174*, 945–959.

Pingarrón, J. M., Yanez-Sedeno, P., & González-Cortés, A., (2008). Gold nanoparticle-based electrochemical biosensors. *Electrochim. Acta, 53*, 5848–5866.

Pohanka, M., & Skládal, P., (2008). Electrochemical biosensors-principles and applications. *J. Appl. Biomed., 6.*

Rahman, M. M., Umar, A., & Sawada, K., (2009). Development of amperometric glucose biosensor based on glucose oxidase co-immobilized with multi-walled carbon nanotubes at low potential. *Sensors Actuators B Chem., 137*, 327–333.

Razmi, H., & Mohammad-Rezaei, R., (2013). Graphene quantum dots as a new substrate for immobilization and direct electrochemistry of glucose oxidase: Application to sensitive glucose determination. *Biosens. Bioelectron., 41*, 498–504.

Ronkainen, N. J., Halsall, H. B., & Heineman, W. R., (2010). Electrochemical biosensors. *Chem. Soc. Rev., 39*, 1747–1763.

Sato, N., & Okuma, H., (2008). Development of single-wall carbon nanotubes modified screen-printed electrode using a ferrocene-modified cationic surfactant for amperometric glucose biosensor applications. *Sensors Actuators B Chem., 129*, 188–194.

Shan, C., Yang, H., Song, J., Han, D., Ivaska, A., & Niu, L., (2009). Direct electrochemistry of glucose oxidase and biosensing for glucose based on graphene. *Anal. Chem., 81*, 2378–2382.

Song, Y., Luo, Y., Zhu, C., Li, H., Du, D., & Lin, Y., (2016). Recent advances in electrochemical biosensors based on graphene two-dimensional nanomaterials. *Biosens. Bioelectron., 76*, 195–212.

Tancharoen, C., Sukjee, W., Thepparit, C., Jaimipuk, T., Auewarakul, P., Thitithanyanont, A., & Sangma, C., (2018). Electrochemical biosensor based on surface imprinting for zika virus detection in serum. *ACS Sensors, 4*, 69–75.

Taniselass, S., Arshad, M. K. M., & Gopinath, S. C. B., (2019). Graphene-based electrochemical biosensors for monitoring noncommunicable disease biomarkers. *Biosens. Bioelectron., 130*, 276–292.

Vamvakaki, V., Hatzimarinaki, M., & Chaniotakis, N., (2008). Biomimetically synthesized silica-carbon nanofiber architectures for the development of highly stable electrochemical biosensor systems. *Anal. Chem., 80*, 5970–5975.

Vamvakaki, V., Tsagaraki, K., & Chaniotakis, N., (2006). Carbon nanofiber-based glucose biosensor. *Anal. Chem., 78*, 5538–5542.

Vashist, S. K., Zheng, D., Al-Rubeaan, K., Luong, J. H. T., & Sheu, F. S., (2011). Advances in carbon nanotube based electrochemical sensors for bioanalytical applications. *Biotechnol. Adv., 29*, 169–188.

Wang, Z., & Dai, Z., (2015). Carbon nanomaterial-based electrochemical biosensors: An overview. *Nanoscale, 7*, 6420–6431.

Wu, H., Wang, J., Kang, X., Wang, C., Wang, D., Liu, J., Aksay, I. A., & Lin, Y., (2009). Glucose biosensor based on immobilization of glucose oxidase in platinum nanoparticles/graphene/chitosan nanocomposite film. *Talanta, 80*, 403–406.

Yamanaka, K., Vestergaard, M. C., & Tamiya, E., (2016). Printable electrochemical biosensors: A focus on screen-printed electrodes and their application. *Sensors, 16*, 1761.

Yang, G., Kampstra, K. L., & Abidian, M. R., (2014). High performance conducting polymer nanofiber biosensors for detection of biomolecules. *Adv. Mater., 26*, 4954–4960.

Yang, N., Chen, X., Ren, T., Zhang, P., & Yang, D., (2015). Carbon nanotube-based biosensors. *Sensors Actuators B Chem., 207*, 690–715.

Yoon, H. C., Yang, H., & Kim, Y. T., (2002). Biocatalytic precipitation induced by an affinity reaction on dendrimer-activated surfaces for the electrochemical signaling from immunosensors. *Analyst, 127*, 1082–1087.

Zhang, Y., Wu, C., Zhou, X., Wu, X., Yang, Y., Wu, H., Guo, S., & Zhang, J., (2013). Graphene quantum dots/gold electrode and its application in living cell H_2O_2 detection. *Nanoscale, 5*, 1816–1819.

Zhao, J., Chen, G., Zhu, L., & Li, G., (2011). Graphene quantum dots-based platform for the fabrication of electrochemical biosensors. *Electrochem. Commun., 13*, 31–33.

Zhou, M., Zhai, Y., & Dong, S., (2009). Electrochemical sensing and biosensing platform based on chemically reduced graphene oxide. *Anal. Chem., 81*, 5603–5613.

CHAPTER 7

Noble Metal Nanoparticles-Based Composites for Gas Sensing: Progress and Perspective

SUDARSAN RAJ[1] and ANEEYA K. SAMANTARA[2]

[1]Institute of Materials and Systems for Sustainability, Nagoya University, Nagoya, Japan

[2]School of Chemical Sciences, National Institute of Science Education and Research, Bhubaneswar, Odisha–752050, India, E-mail: aneeya1986@gmail.com

ABSTRACTS

This chapter is useful for a wide range of readers who are interested in nanomaterial science and their current research trends in noble metal nanoparticles (NPs)-based composites from the perspectives of toxic gas sensor applications. In this chapter, we focus on recent trends in the synthesis of different types of noble metal NPs based composites and its gas sensor devices fabrication and mechanism. This chapter would be given a deep knowledge about different synthesis method of noble metal NPs based composites and the sensor devices internal architecture. There are wide ranges of noble metal NPs based composites including core@ shell, yolk@shell, noble metal support and noble metal doped nanostructures. Moreover, this chapter includes recent progress of selected nanomaterials over a broad range of toxic gas (CO, NO_x, H_2, VOC) sensor with higher response, sensitivity, and selectivity. Last but not least, this chapter concludes with the uses of nanotechnology to attain more efficient and cost-effective sensor devices. Issues relating to next generation sensor device architecture are discussed. With the extensive study of newly discovered noble metal NPs based composites used for sensor devices, this chapter will be interesting not only for researchers working in the field of noble metal-based sensor technology but also for wide range of academicians studying physics, chemistry, biology, material science and engineering, and nanotechnology.

7.1   OVERVIEW AND BACKGROUND

Environmental pollution due to gaseous pollutants has caused major concerns such as acid rain, human health hazard, greenhouse effect, and the ozone layer depletion (Zhang et al., 2019; Lee et al., 2001). There are enormous market potentials of gas sensors in environmental monitoring and personal safety. These days' gas sensors are becoming a crucial part of modern life with applications in air quality control in motor vehicles and buildings as well as the more traditional areas of toxic and explosive gas detection. The noble metal-based nanostructure with different morphology and gas sensing application are shown in Figure 7.1.

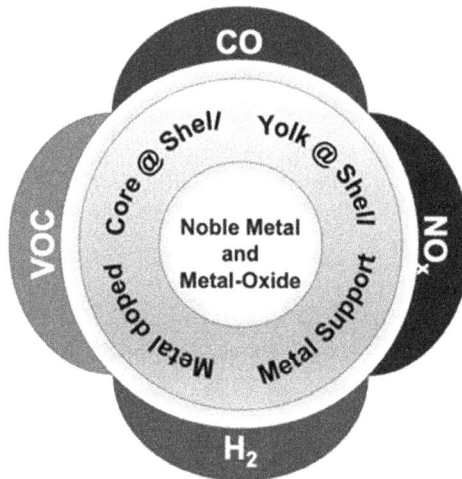

FIGURE 7.1   Schematic of noble metal and metal oxide-based nanostructure and its gas sensor applications.

There are different types of detectors having the same function are available in the market with the common accessories like monitor and alarming system. Out of which, chemiresistive metal oxide semiconductor

(MOS) sensors are widely used due to their small size, low cost, easy maintenance, and high sensitivity (Korotcenkov, 2007; Liu et al., 2019). The sensing mechanism based on the conductivity change in the sensor due to the surface chemical reaction between the surface of the sensor and the exposed target gases (Anand et al., 2017). Literature suggested that various parameters like morphology, size, and surface defects affect the interaction between the semiconductor metal oxide surface and target gas, which leads to affect their gas sensing properties (Xu et al., 1991; Rai et al., 2013; Spencer et al., 2012). There are ample of research showed many attempts to alter one or more of the above-mentioned parameters of semiconductor metal oxide by different methods like structure control, decoration with metal NPs, different noble metal doped metal oxide, and defects control synthesis to enhance the sensing properties of semiconductor metal oxide (Ahn et al., 2008; Li et al., 2011; Suo et al., 2015; Singh et al., 2016; Kim et al., 2019).

7.2 SYNTHESIS OF MORPHOLOGY CONTROLLED NOBLE METAL NPS COMPOSITES

In recent years, a variety of technologies has been employed to fabricate noble metal-based composites. Since the structure and morphology of the oxide materials and position of noble metals affect the functional properties, many attempts have been made to the production and design of noble metal NPs composites with different architectures. There are different methods like doping of metal oxide, decoration with metal NPs (metal support), structure control, and defects control synthesis for better gas sensing performances. There are many reports on noble metal-based NPs but here we mentioned some recent studied work of their synthesis with different morphology.

7.2.1 NOBLE METAL SUPPORTED COMPOSITES

Kim et al. recently reported the synthesis of SnO_2 nanowires (NWs) using a selective vapor-liquid-solid growth method and then decorated with Pd NPs by ultraviolet (UV) reduction method at room temperature (2019). Typically, the desired amount of $PdCl_2$ solution was prepared in a mixture of 8.5 g of isopropanol and 8.5 g propanol. The SnO_2 NWs dipped samples in the mentioned solution were irradiated by a UV light with a $\lambda = 360$ nm using a halogen lamp. The intensity of the UV light was 0.11 mW/cm^2 and the reduction was performed for 120 s followed by calcinations at 500°C for 1 h.

Figure 7.2(a) represents the FE-SEM image of bare SnO_2 NWs with a relatively smooth surface. Figure 7.2(b) shows the FE-SEM micrograph of Pd-decorated SnO_2 NWs. Fine Pd NPs was found on the surface of the SnO_2 NWs. The low magnification top-view images are shown in insets of Figures 7.2(a) and (b), which demonstrate the formation of dense NWs on the substrate. XRD pattern of the Pd-decorated SnO_2 NWs is represented in Figure 7.2(c). This reveals the weak metallic Pd peak along with a SnO_2 rutile peak.

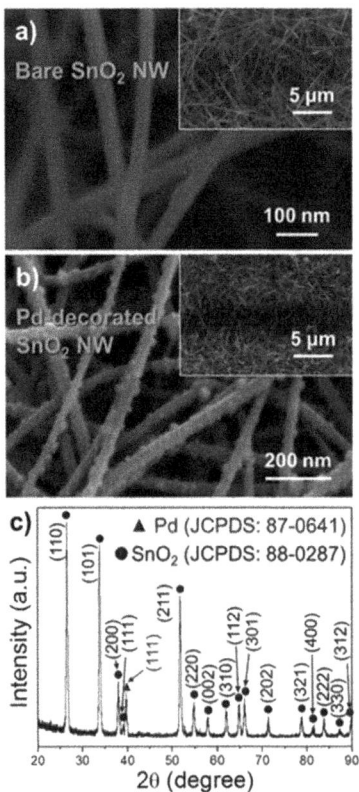

FIGURE 7.2   FE-SEM micrographs of (a) bare SnO_2 NWs; and (b) Pd-decorated SnO_2 NWs. Upper-right insets are top-view FE-SEM images. (c) XRD pattern of Pd decorated SnO_2 NWs.

Source: Reproduced with permission from: Kim, Mirzaei, Kim, and Kim (2019). © Elsevier.

7.2.2 NOBLE METAL DOPED COMPOSITES

Doping creates defects and gives preferential sites for the adsorption of gas molecules and dopant treated as a catalyst that promotes the surface reactions and adsorption leads to better sensor performance. Anand et al. synthesized Ag-doped In_2O_3 NPs with cubic bixbyite crystal phase by the co-precipitation method for acetone, methanol, ethanol, and LPG gas sensors at different operating temperatures (2017). Similarly, Singh et al. studied the sensing behavior with Ag NPs doped layer (2007). HCHO gas sensor studies were carried out by taking Ag-doped nanofiber Wang et al. (2009) and nano-flower Wang et al. (2014) metal oxide. Unlike Ag other metal dopants Au (Xu et al., 2011); Pt (Rout et al., 2006); Pd (Yang et al., 2010) are also used for different gas sensing applications.

7.2.3 NOBLE METAL CORE/YOLK SHELL COMPOSITES

The noble metalcore/yolk-shell NPs composites formation is a multistep process which required special care for nucleation and growth of the shell material on noble metal seeds. These processes are affected by a number of parameters, such as synthesis methods, reaction time, temperature, concentration, surfactant, lattice mismatch, interfacial energy, etc. The lack of chemical interaction and lattice mismatch between noble metals and metal oxides leads to a large interfacial energy between them. Synthesis of noble metalcore/yolk-shell NPs composites often fail due to the lattice mismatch between two materials. However, the use of ligand/surfactant can be tune the interface between two materials. The selection of a suitable ligand/surfactant is challenging; therefore, there are ample of reports about the synthesis of noble metalcore/yolk-shell NPs composites, although their corresponding pure oxides NPs are common. Therefore, here we are lighting more towards the synthesis of noble metalcore/yolk-shell NPs composites.

There are ample of research to prepare well-defined core@shell Ag@ZnO NPs (Aguirre et al., 2011; Liu et al., 2012; Yin et al., 2012). However, there is a lack of in-detailed information on the formation mechanism of core@shell NPs. Metal@ZnO core@shell NPs successfully synthesized by Sun et al., having a well-defined morphology and well presented a detailed growth mechanism (Figure 7.2) (Sun et al., 2013). It explained the important role of polyvinylpyrrolidone (PVP) and 4-mercaptobenzoic acid in the synthesis of Au@ZnO core@shell NPs. They found that

4-mercaptobenzoic acid can reduce the Au-ZnO interfacial energy (Zhu et al., 2012). However, in the absence of PVP, there was no well interaction between ZnO and the hydrophobic ligands on the Au surface. Which indicate that amphiphilicity of PVP was essential for ZnO encapsulation in the presence of hydrophobic ligands. Yang et al., implemented a similar strategy for synthesis of metal@ZnO core@shell NPs by using ascorbic acid (AA) to induce deposition of ZnO on different shaped and structured of cationic-surfactant-capped NP surfaces (2013). The metals used here were Pt, Pd, Au, Ag, and their bimetals, such as Pd@Pt, Au@Ag, Au@Pt, Pd@Au, etc. By implementing a similar strategy, CTAB or CTAC coated metal NPs in water medium can be prepared.

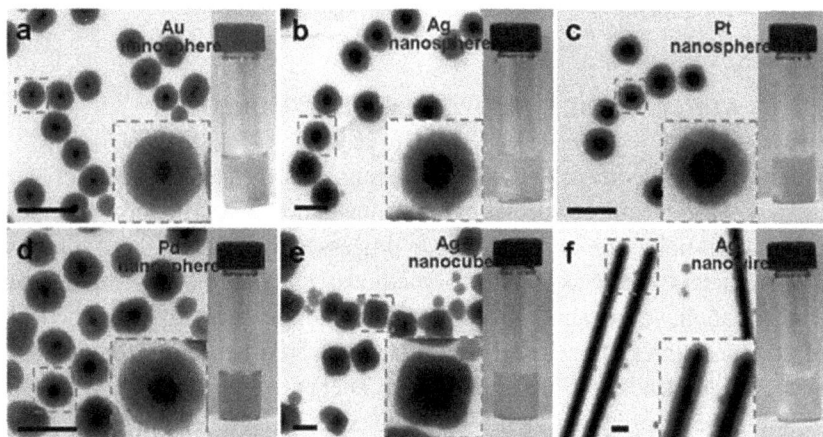

FIGURE 7.3 TEM images and photographs of metal@ZnO NPs that were synthesized from different noble metal cores: citrate-stabilized NPs, including: (a) Au nanospheres ($d_{Au} = 15$ nm); (b) Ag nanospheres ($d_{Ag} = 60$ nm); and (c) Pt nanospheres ($d_{Pt} = 40$ nm); and PVP-stabilized NPs, including: (d) Pd nanospheres ($d_{Pd} = 20$ nm); (e) Ag nanocubes ($d_{Ag} = 150$ nm); and (f) AgNWs ($d_{AgNW} = 120$ nm, lAgNW= 3–5 μm). Insets show magnified views of typical NPs. Scale bar: 200 nm.

Source: Reproduced with permission from: Sun et al. (2013). © American Chemical Society.

The yolk@shell nanostructures are a special class of core@shell structures having a well-defined core@void@shell configuration. The metal@ SiO_2 core@shell NPs template and metal@-carbon core@shell NPs template routes are an effective approach for the formation of yolk@shell nanostructure. The metal@-carbon core@shell NPs template routes were implemented for the synthesis of Au@NiO (Rai et al., 2014); Au@ZnO

(Li et al., 2014); Au@TiO$_2$ (Ngaw et al., 2014); yolk@shell nanostructure. Wang et al. (2013) synthesized Au@SnO$_2$ yolk@shell nanostructure by implementing the metal@SiO$_2$ core@shell NPs template route.

7.3 NOBLE METAL NPS COMPOSITES FOR GAS SENSOR APPLICATION

7.3.1 CO GAS SENSOR

The colorless, odorless, and tasteless CO gas detection and control in residential and industrial environments are necessary due to its potential threat to human health. Due to the incapability of human being to detect it directly, it is crucial to develop cost-effective smart CO sensing systems which can detect, and measure the gas. CO gas can be generated from natural as well as artificial sources. The vulnerability of CO gas usually occurred indoors, like kitchens, garages, etc. CO is produced during the combustion process which takes place in stoves, combustion engines, water heaters, lanterns, and generators, or during burning wood and charcoal (Goldstein, 2008). The fossil fuel burning leads to CO poisoning. Long-term CO exposure can also result from automotive exhaust, industrial sources, and constant exposure to smoke (Varon et al., 1999; Raub et al., 2000).

7.3.1.1 MOSS BASED CO SENSING

The MOS-based materials are widely used for CO detection. Researchers often investigated MOS sensors for CO gas detection with low fabrication cost, very high sensitivity, selectivity, stability, and reversibility, absorptivity (of oxygen), response (fast response/recovery time), and very low power consumption. The multistep sensing process involves the CO gas incorporation on the oxide layer surface which leads to a change in surface charge. In other words, the target gas is agitated by the interaction among the adsorbed oxygen molecules and the CO gas molecules. The variation of the e⁻ flow (electrical conductivity) on the oxide surface arises due to the oxygen adsorption. This results into a change in resistance of the oxide surface layer. The monitoring of variation in the resistance leads the material for sensing the CO gas. The whole reaction can be explained by the following expressions (Turja Nandy et al., 2018).

$$O_2 \leftrightarrow O_2^-$$
$$O_2^- + e^- \leftrightarrow 2O^-$$
$$O^- + e^- \leftrightarrow O^{2-}$$
$$2CO + O_2^- \rightarrow 2CO_2 + e^-$$
$$CO + O^- \rightarrow CO_2 + e^-$$
$$CO + O^{2-} \rightarrow CO_2 + 2e^-$$

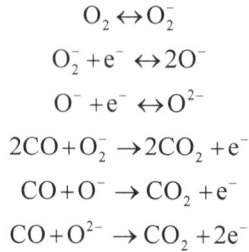

The O_2 adsorption increased on increasing the operating temperature (from O_2^- to O^- and O^{2-}). It has been observed that O_2^- active at < 150°C temperatures, O^- works at temperature between 150°C and 400°C and O_2^- works at temperature above 400°C. However, temperature should maintain optimal, because of its impact on the lifetime and reliability of the sensor. In addition to this, the adsorption also can be intensified by using the optimized amount of metal oxide doping and consequently increases the sensitivity. The n-type MOSs is more popular than p-type MOSs used for gas sensing applications (Kim et al., 2014). The summary of the noble metal-based materials for CO gas sensor is mentioned in Table 7.1.

7.3.1.2 *CORE@SHELL STRUCTURE FOR CO GAS SENSOR*

The existing and potential CO gas sensor applications are highlighted here by using the most effective core@shell structure NPs. Yu et al. (2011) first report the use of core@shell NPs in CO gas sensing. They investigated the CO (200–1000 ppm) gas sensing properties which showed higher response ($R_s = (R_a - R_g)/R_a$) for Au@SnO_2core@shell NPs compared to bare SnO_2 NPs. The electronic and chemical sensitization of core Au metal NPs causing the higher response of the Au@SnO_2core@shell NPs. The role of noble metals (Au, Ag, Pd) on sensing performance of Cu_2O in M@Cu_2Ocore@shell NPs was investigated by Lin et al. (2014) are shown in Figure 7.4. The response of pure Cu_2O, Au@Cu_2O, Ag@Cu_2O and Pd@Cu_2O nanocrystals, to 200 ppm of CO were found to be 1.66, 2.61, 1.80, and 2.06, respectively (Figure 7.4(e)). The difference in electron trapping capability of Au, Ag, and Pd NPs in metal@Cu_2O nanocrystals leads to difference in CO detection. The transfer of conduction band electrons of Cu_2O to noble metal with leaving abundant holes in Cu_2O to increase the hole mobility due to the high work function of Au (5.1 eV) and Pd (5.3 eV) as compared to Cu_2O (4.8 eV). The lower work function of Ag (4.3 eV)

TABLE 7.1 Summary of the Noble Metal-based Materials for CO Gas Sensor

Materials	Performance	Optimum Temperature (°C)	Advantage	References
Pd-ZnO nanofiber	Response time 25–29 s, recovery time 12–17 s	220	Low concentration detection and good selectivity	Wei et al. (2010)
Au/rGO loaded ZnO	Response (Ra/Rg) 35.8 Detection 5 ppm	400	Low concentration detection and good selectivity	Abideen et al. (2018)
Au-In$_2$O$_3$ nanomaterials	Response ~9, response, and recovery time ~30/30 s	25	Room temperature measurement and very good selectivity	Fu et al. (2017)
Pd-SnO$_2$ thin film	Sensitivity ~80%, response time ~50 m	450	Very high sensitivity	Menini et al. (2004)
Pd-SnO$_2$rGO	Detection 50–1600 ppm, response, and recovery time ~2 m, Response 1–9.5%	Room temperature	Room temperature measurement, quick response-recovery times	Shojaee et al. (2018)
Pt-SnO$_2$ porous nanosolid	Sensitivity (Ra/Rg) 64.5	Room temperature	Room temperature measurement and good selectivity	Wang et al. (2013)
Au-SnO$_2$ thin film	Sensitivity ~90%	Room temperature	Room temperature measurement, good selectivity and no humidity effect	Manjula et al. (2011)
Au@SnO$_2$ yolk-shell	5–100 ppm Response 0.3 s	210	Lower detection limit faster response	Wang et al. (2013)
Au-SnO$_2$/CO$_3$O$_4$	1000 ppm Response 186	100	High response	Choi et al. (2005)
Au/TiO$_2$	Response time <20 s, recovery time <20 s	230	–	Tan et al. (2006)

TABLE 7.1 *(Continued)*

Materials	Performance	Optimum Temperature (°C)	Advantage	References
Au/TiO$_2$	Detection 10–100 ppm, response time 10 s, recovery time 15 s Sensitivity (Ra/Rg) 3.4	300	Lower detection limit Faster response	Buso et al. (2008)
Pd/TiO$_2$	Detection 5–300 ppm, response time <20 s, sensitivity (Ra/Rg) 1.25	200	Lower detection limit faster response	Xu et al. (2013)
Pt/WO$_3$	Response (Ra/Rg) 10.1 Response-recovery time (16 s/1 s)	125	Low concentration Ultrashort response-recovery time and high selectivity	Junhao et al. (2018)

causing electron transfer from Ag to Cu_2O, in Ag@Cu_2O nanocrystals. The formation of Schottky barrier at the interface once the thermodynamic equilibrium was reached. The increased in response of metal@Cu_2O nanocrystals as compared to pure Cu_2O, due to change in resistance in the presence of Ag NPs.

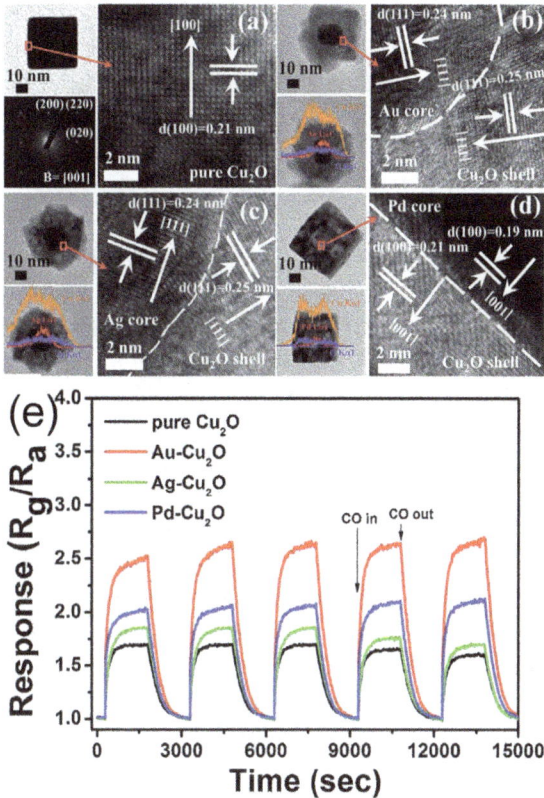

FIGURE 7.4 TEM, HRTEM images and EDS data of (a) pure Cu_2O; (b) Au-Cu_2O; (c) Ag-Cu_2O; and (d) Pd-Cu_2O nanocrystals; (e) responses of pure Cu_2O and metal-Cu_2O nanocrystals to 200 ppm of CO recorded at 200°C.

Source: Reproduced with permission from: Lin, Chiang, and Hsu (2014). © Elsevier.

7.3.1.3 YOLK@SHELL STRUCTURE FOR CO GAS SENSOR

The utilization of this special type of core@shell structured NPs as sensing materials in gas sensors may be limited by relatively low accessibility of metal NPs to gas molecules. The Au@SnO$_2$yolk@shell nano-spheres were synthesized by Wang et al. (2013) and applied for CO (up to 5 ppm) gas sensing, where AuNPs are effectively separated and highly accessible to gas molecules. Au@SnO$_2$ sensor displayed about fivefold enhancements in sensitivity compared to hollow SnO$_2$ with lower detection limit (5 ppm) and lower operating temperature (210°C), faster response (0.3 s) and better selectivity. The better sensing performances due to the electronic as well as catalytic effect of AuNPs along with unique features of yolk@shell nano-spheres, which has created a greater number of active sites.

7.3.2   NO$_2$ GAS SENSOR

Nitrogen dioxide (NO$_2$) is a toxic hazardous, dangerous gas which is produced during the combustion in motor vehicles, chemical plants, and thermal power plants industries, etc. The summary of the noble metal based MOS materials for NO$_2$ gas sensor is given in Table 7.2.

7.3.2.1   NOBLE METAL DOPING/SUPPORT NO$_2$ GAS SENSOR

The mechanism of NO$_2$ gas sensor is explained by Jaroenapibal et al. as shown in Figure 7.5. Herein, the NO$_2$ gas response is improved after the incorporation of noble metal, i.e., Ag due to the chemical sensitization and electronic excitement of the materials. The schematic representations of the sensing mechanism of WO$_3$ nanofibers are illustrated in Figure 7.5(a-b), which is related to the modulation of the conduction channel upon exposure to NO$_2$ gas. The introduction of NO$_2$ leads to the formation of surface acceptors on WO$_3$, as shown in Figure 7.5(a-b), due to which a decrease of the conduction channel volume has been observed with an increase in sensor's resistance. The optimum Ag-doped WO$_3$ nanofibers (Figure 7.5(b)), showed a relatively larger change in the conduction channel volume compared to that of the undoped WO$_3$ nanofibers (Figure 7.5(a)). Thus, Ag-doped WO$_3$ nanofibers sample with an optimum doping level gives a maximum gas response with enhanced electronic sensitization. Figure 7.5(c) showed the expansion of conduction channel after the injection of electrons from Ag into WO$_3$ due to the work function of Ag (4.26 eV) is smaller than that of WO$_3$ (5.05 eV) Halek et al. (2013). Ren et al. (2015) also enhanced the surface activities of WO$_3$ materials by

TABLE 7.2 Summary of the Noble Metal-based Materials for NO_2 Gas Sensor

Material	Performance	Optimum temperature (°C)	Advantages	References
PdO-SnO₂	Response ~20–30 Recovery time ~1.33 s	Room temperature	Higher response and faster response time	Teng et al. (2019)
Pt-N/WO₃	Response ($\Delta R/R_0$) = 4.8% at 5 ppm	50	Exceptional selectivity against interfering molecules,	Kim et al. (2018)
Pd-Si/WO₃	Response 5.2 Detection limit 0.25 ppm	Room temperature	Room temperature sensor	Qiang et al. (2018)
Pd-WO₃	Response 0.42 Detection limit 10 ppm	200	Lower detection limit	Penza et al. (1998)
Ag-WO₃	Response 44 detection limit of 100 ppb	75	—	Wang et al. (2016)
Ag-WO₃	Response (R_g/R_a) 90.3. detection of 5 ppm	225	High selectivity	Jaroenapibal et al. (2018)
Au-ZnO	Response 10.71 detection limit of 500 ppb	250	—	Navale et al. (2018)
Pd-In₂O₃	Response 4.05 Detection limit 5 ppm	110	Lower detection limit	Huang et al. (2015)
Au-In₂O₃	Response 472.4 detection limit of 10 ppb	65	High response, Low operating temperature	Li et al. (2018)
Au/rGO	Response 1.33 Recovery time 386 s	50	Low operating temperature	Zhang et al. (2016)
Au-SnO₂ NPs	Response (R_a/R_g) 25% = 100 ppm H_2 gas	250	—	Wang et al. (2017)

implementing Ag additives. Ag deposited WO_3 showed a higher (−1.41 eV) adsorption energy compared to that of a bare WO_3 surface (−0.48 eV) when polar molecules like NO binding to W. With the addition of Ag atoms, there will be a higher number of electrons transferred from the substrate to the adsorbed gas molecules. Thus, the enhanced gas response was found due to the higher numbers of electrons are extracted from the conduction band of WO_3. The interaction of NO_2 with the surface of MOS happens through the oxygen vacancy sites, and the charge transfer to the adsorbed NO_2 was strongly enhanced by the surface oxygen vacancies (Epifani et al., 2008). Thus, the gas response to NO_2 is obvious to enhance upon Ag doping. The existence of a thin layer of Ag_2O (Figure 7.5(b) left inset) present at the surface of Ag particles can assist the chemical sensitization effect. In this model, Ag_2O acts as a chemical sensitizer in the presence of NO_2. This causes a strong reduction reaction as shown in (Figure 7.5(b) right inset) took place according to the following equation:

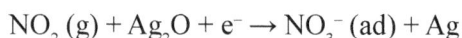

$$NO_2 \text{ (g)} + Ag_2O + e^- \rightarrow NO_3^- \text{ (ad)} + Ag$$

The so-called "spillover" mechanism occurs when gas molecules adsorbed at the metal cluster are excited and dissociate and then migrate to the metal oxide surface Kohl et al. (1990). A further decreased in the conduction channel volume leads to the improved gas response due to the larger number of electrons is extracted from WO_3. As mentioned by Bittencourt et al., this reaction causes a sharp increment in gas response of Ag-doped WO_3 materials (2004).

7.3.3   *H_2 GAS SENSOR*

Hydrogen (H_2) is a green and clean fuel and a tasteless, colorless, and odorless gas with explosive in nature. Moreover, the smallest molecular size and a high diffusion coefficient lead to easily leakage of it in a closed system. Therefore, it is highly essential the detection of H_2 gas during the transportation, leakage, and storage (Manikandan et al., 2019).

7.3.3.1   *NOBLE SUPPORTED/SURFACE FUNCTIONALIZATION*

Lupan et al. demonstrated the ultra-thin TiO_2 films have good selectivity to H_2 gas (2018). A response of ∼ 600% was achieved by the surface

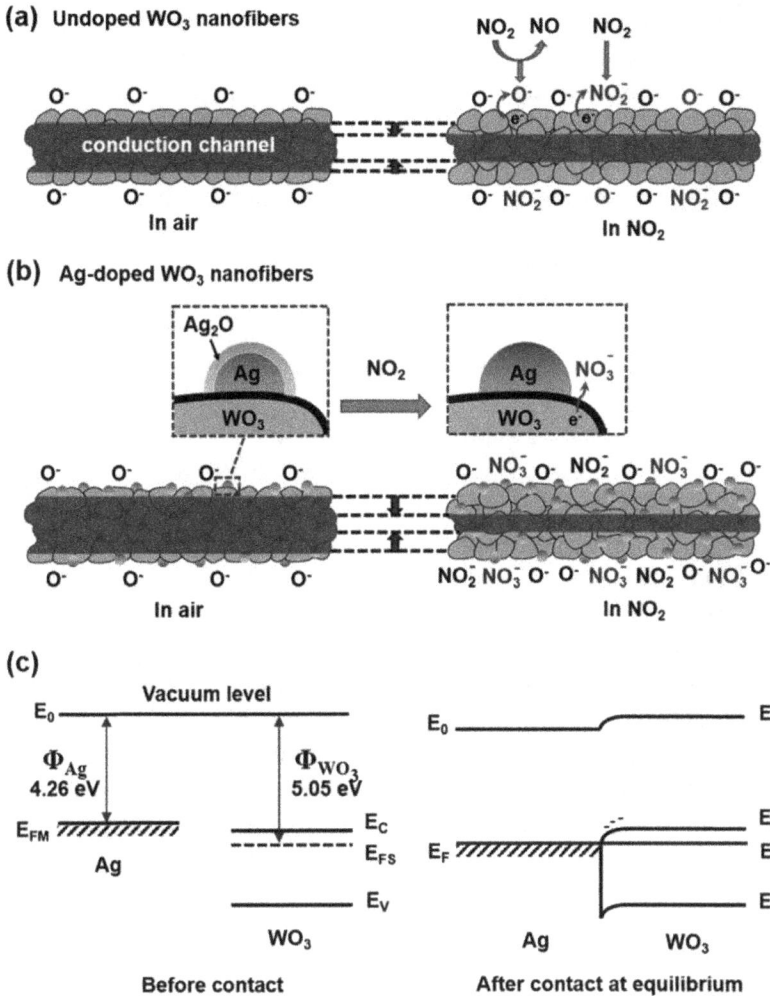

FIGURE 7.5 Schematic representations of (a) the NO_2 sensing mechanism of undoped WO_3 nanofibers; (b) the NO_2 sensing mechanism of Ag-doped WO_3 nanofibers; (c) the proposed energy band diagram of Ag-WO_3 before contact and after contact at equilibrium. *Source*: Reproduced with permission from: Jaroenapibal et al. (2018). © Elsevier.

functionalization with Au nano-dots samples having 15 nm thicknesses to 100 ppm of H_2 at 250°C operating temperature. Again Lupan et al. showed the influence of Pd nominal composition in Pd/ZnO nano-wire on the H_2 sensing (2018). The results demonstrate an ultra-high response and selectivity to H_2 gas at room temperature. They explain the H_2 gas sensors mechanism in details by using the most promising candidates of noble metals and their oxide nano-clusters. The high performances, especially the possibility to detect hydrogen gas at room temperature with the PdO-functionalized nanostructured ZnO films, can be explained by the interplay of different mechanisms dependent on the operating temperature. The general gas sensing mechanism of metal oxides is based on surface reactions (Yamazoe, 1991). Table 7.3 shows the summary of the noble metal-based materials for H_2 gas sensor.

7.3.4 AMMONIA (NH₃) GAS SENSOR

A recent study shows the application of Au-ZnO, Pt-WO_3, Pd-ITO nano-composites for NH_3 sensor (Atanasova et al., 2019; Wang et al., 2017; Kundu et al., 2019). The Pt-loaded WO_3 based sensor having higher sensitivity, quicker response-recovery rate (at 125°C) and better selectivity towards ammonia. It indicated that like Au@ZnO, Pt-loaded mesoporous WO_3 was also a potential ammonia gas sensor material. Seifaddini et al. studied the ammonia gas sensor using Au/graphene (GN) nanoribbon at room temperature (2019). These sensing materials showed a response of 34% for 25 ppm gas at room temperature with 224s/178s response and recovery time. Kundu et al. (2019) found that Pd incorporated ITO showed a significant enhancement in sensing response (~82%) at 300°C for 30 ppm ammonia gas. And also get a good sensing response (~43%) even at very low concentration (~ 3 ppm) of ammonia gas.

7.3.5 VOC GAS SENSOR

7.3.5.1 ETHANOL GAS SENSOR

Wu et al. have compared the sensing performances of Ag@SnO_2core@ shell NPs with bare SnO_2 and 1 wt.% Ag/SnO_2 nanocomposites for ethanol (200 ppm) gas sensor (2013). Xu et al. reported the Ag@2D-WO_3core@ shell have enhanced sensor performance as compared to both bared WO_3 and its composite due to generation and propagation of localized surface Plasmon (2014). The sensor response ($R_s = R_a/R_g$) for 500 ppm alcohol was increased from 44 for pure WO_3 to 52 for $Ag_{x-}WO_3$ mixture and

TABLE 7.3 Summary of the Noble Metal-based Materials for H_2 Gas Sensor

Material	Performance	Optimum temperature (°C)	References
Pd-WO$_3$ nanorods	Response 12% = (R$_g$/R$_a$) 200 ppm H$_2$ gas	300	Lee et al. (2018)
PdNP/carbon nanowires	Response 0.8% = ((R$_g$−R$_a$)/R$_a$) 700 ppm H$_2$ gas	Room temperature	Seo et al. (2017)
Pd-SnO$_2$/MoS$_2$	Response 18% = ((R$_g$−R$_a$)/R$_a$) 5000 ppm H$_2$ gas	Room temperature	Zhang et al. (2017)
Pd-PANI-rGO	Response 25% = ((R$_g$−R$_a$)/R$_a$) 10,000 ppm H$_2$ gas	Room temperature	Zou et al. (2016)
Pd thin film/carbon nanowires	Response 0.8% = ((R$_g$−R$_a$)/R$_a$) 100 ppm H$_2$ gas	100	Seo et al. (2015)
Pt/F-MWCNTs/SnO$_2$	Response 5.4% = ((R$_g$−R$_a$)/R$_a$) 50,000 ppm H$_2$ gas	Room temperature	Dhall et al. (2015)
Pd-Pt graphene	Response 4% = ((R$_g$−R$_a$)/R$_a$) 20,000 ppm H$_2$ gas	Room temperature	Kumar et al. (2011)
Pd-graphene composite	Response 7% = ((R$_g$−R$_a$)/R$_a$) 1000 ppm H$_2$ gas	Room temperature	Phan et al. (2014)
Ni/Pd composite	Response 11% = ((R$_g$−R$_a$)/R$_a$) 1000 ppm H$_2$ gas	Room temperature	Phan et al. (2014)
Au-SnO$_2$ NPs	Response 25% = (R$_a$/R$_g$) 100 ppm H$_2$ gas	250	Wang et al. (2017)
Pd-SnO$_2$ Thin films	Response 2.8% = (R$_a$/R$_g$) 25 ppm H$_2$ gas	300	Toan et al. (2016)
Pt-SnO$_2$ Thin films	Response 2.4% = (R$_a$/R$_g$) 25 ppm H$_2$ gas	300	
Au-SnO$_2$ Thin films	Response 2.4% = (R$_a$/R$_g$) 25 ppm H$_2$ gas	300	
Pd-SnO$_2$ NFs	Response 8.2% = (R$_a$/R$_g$) 100 ppm H$_2$ gas	280	Zhang et al. (2010)
Au-SnO$_2$	Response 12% = (R$_a$/R$_g$) 50 ppm H$_2$ gas	260	Borhaninia et al. (2017)
Pd-SnO$_2$ NWs	Response 16.95% = (R$_a$/R$_g$) 1 ppm H$_2$ gas	300	Kim et al. (2019)

154 for the $Ag_x@(2D\text{-}WO_3)$ core@shell structure. The optimum sensor working temperature lowered from 370°C to 340°C and also the recovery time shortened considerably from 15 s for pure WO_3, 7 s for the $Ag_x\text{-}WO_3$ mixture to and 4 s for the $Ag_x@(2D\text{-}WO_3)$ core@shell nanostructure. The better response in this core@shell structure due to the electron transfer from the WO_3 shell to Ag core leads to wider depletion zone formation due to the higher work function of Ag. The lower response of $Ag\text{-}WO_3$ mixture as compared to core@shell might be due to the poor Schottky junction formation achieved by relatively far distance between Ag and WO_3 NPs and/or the agglomeration of Ag and WO_3 NPs, as WO_3 powder and Ag NPs were prepared separately before being mixed together.

Anand et al. reported Ag-doped In_2O_3 for LPG (liquefied petroleum gas) and VOC (methanol, ethanol, and acetone) gas sensors (2017). Figure 7.6 showed the response of the In_2O_3 and (1%, 3%and 5%) Ag-doped In_2O_3 gas sensors to 50 ppm VOC and LPG, respectively with temperature varying from 200 to 450°C. The sensors response first increased with the increase in operating temperature and then decreased gradually on further increase of the operating temperature in case of pure and Ag-doped In_2O_3. Figure 7.6 clearly shows that, 3% Ag-doped In_2O_3 have a better response at each temperature in contrast to the pure In_2O_3. The noble metal present in doped In_2O_3 acts as a catalyst and enhanced the sensor response. The 3% Ag-doped In_2O_3 showed a response of 30.06 ± 0.42 towards ethanol at 300°C, 15.43 ± 0.51 towards acetone at 350°C and 16.53 ± 0.93 towards LPG at 400°C as compared to each other.

Liu et al. (2015) deposited the noble metal (Au, Pd, and Pt) NPs onto SnO_2 for demonstration of (methanol, ethanol, acetone, and THF (tetrahydrofuran)) gas sensor at high temperatures. The immobilization of noble metal NPs onto SnO_2 surfaces highly affects the sensitivity of such doped sensors versus bare/unmodified devices. For galvanic deposition of noble metal NPs, the as prepared metal oxide particles were first dispersed in 2 mL of $HAuCl_4/H_2PdCl_4/H_2PtCl_6$ (1 mM) precursor solution in required amount of 0.1 M AA under agitation for the preparation of Au-, Pd-or Pt-doped SnO_2 sensors, respectively. The reaction carried out for more than 4 h at room temperature for completion. The modified process leads to three specific hybrid sensors designed with 6 nm to 18 nm-sized noble metal particle size on the surface of {221} faceted octahedral SnO_2 nanostructures, as shown in Figure 7.7.

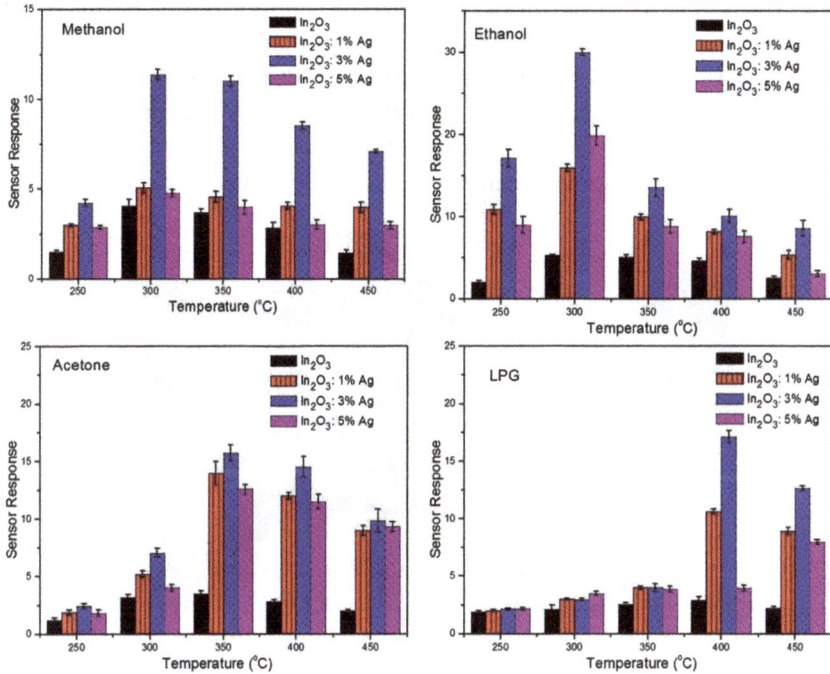

FIGURE 7.6 Histogram representing the sensor response versus operating temperature of In$_2$O$_3$ and Ag-doped In$_2$O$_3$ sensors towards (a) methanol; (b) ethanol; (c) acetone; and (d) LPG.

Source: Reproduced with permission from: Anand, Kaur, Singh, and Thangaraj (2017). © Elsevier.

7.3.5.2 ACETONE GAS SENSOR

Li et al. has made Au@ZnO yolk@shell nano-spheres for acetone sensor (2014). The response of the Au@ZnO nano-spheres was about two times higher than that of hollow ZnO nanostructures, for 100 ppm of acetone. Li et al. (2017) studied the gas sensor based on SnO$_2$/Au-doped In$_2$O$_3$ core-shell nanofibers exhibited a high response at 300°C and a good selectivity to acetone as compared to Au-doped In$_2$O$_3$ nanofiber. Guo et al. (2018) implemented ultra-small sizes (~ 3 nm) Pt NPs for highly sensitive acetone gas sensors. They found that the sensor based on Pt-ZnO-In$_2$O$_3$ nanofibers exhibit the better acetone response (R_a/R_g = 57.1 to 100 ppm at 300°C), ultra-fast response and recovery time (1/44s) and low detection limit (0.5 ppm). The excellent acetone gas response of Pt-ZnO-In$_2$O$_3$

nanofibers due to the chemical sensitization and electrical sensitization of Pt NPs, the p-n heterojunction between p-type PtO_2 and n-type In_2O_3 (ZnO) and the n-n heterojunctions between ZnO and In_2O_3. Saho et al. utilized $Au@WO_3$-SnO_2 nanofiber for acetone gas sensors (2019). It shows a response of 79.6 to 0.5 ppm of acetone gas at 150°C, which is a five times higher response than $Au@SnO_2$ based sensors.

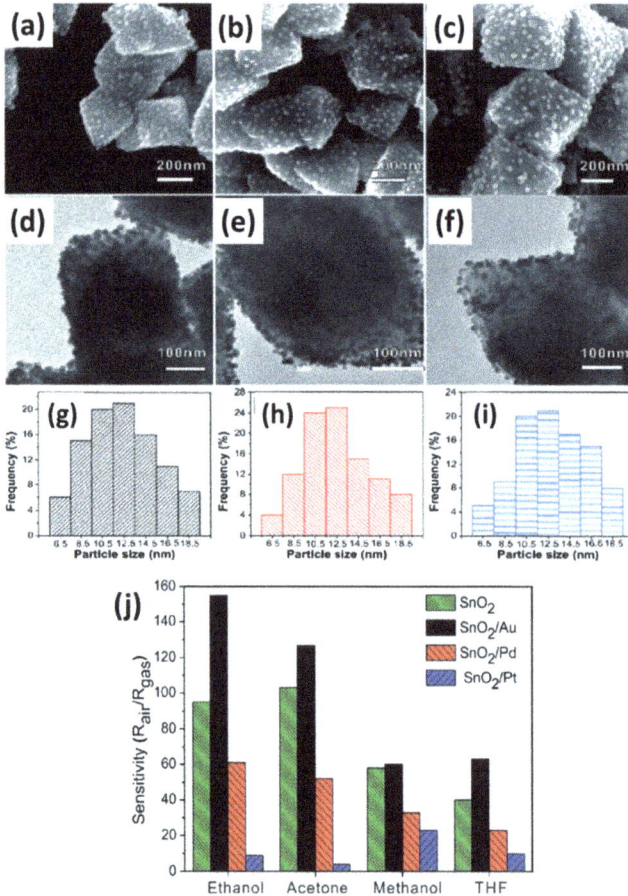

FIGURE 7.7 (a–c) SEM images and (d–f) TEM images of {221} SnO_2 structures decorated by Au, Pd, and Pt-NPs; (g–i) size distributions of Au, Pd, and Pt-NPs on the SnO_2 surface; comparison of the sensitivities of SnO_2, SnO_2/Au, SnO_2/Pd and SnO_2/Pt to various gases with 200 ppm concentration.

Source: Reproduced with permission from: Liu, Kuang, Xie, and Zheng (2015). © Royal Chemical Society.

7.3.5.3 METHANE (CH₄) GAS SENSOR

Methane (CH_4) is the major component of natural gas and coal mine tunnel gas which is highly inflammable and explosive in nature and it's a widely used raw chemical for industrial applications. The higher concentration (>5 vol.%) of CH_4 in air is dangerous in nature, which may lead to an explosion. In order to reduce the extent of risk, a suitable technique is required for detection of CH_4 at a low concentration to provide early alarm. On the other hand, CH_4 detection by traditional methods is more complicated, due to its colorless, odorless, and tasteless properties. Therefore, it is highly essential to develop a reliable, convenient, sensor device which detects the gas rapidly and effectively (Xue et al., 2019). Although different metal oxides are widely studied for methane sensor however the SnO_2 based sensor have attracted considerable attention due to its high mobility (160 cm² V⁻¹ s) good chemical stability and wide bandgap (3.6 eV) (Yang et al., 2018). Table 7.4 shows the noble metal-SnO_2 based sensing performances for CH_4 gas. Yang et al. illustrated the CH_4 gas sensor mechanism by implementing the noble metal Pd-on SnO_2 hollow sphere. The CH_4 sensor of Pd loaded SnO_2 hollow spheres (HS) are based on the chemi-resistivity change.

7.3.5.4 FORMALDEHYDE (HCHO) GAS SENSOR

Ma et al. utilized Pt doped nanosheet-assembled In_2O_3 hollow microspheres for formaldehyde (HCHO) gas sensor (2018). This sensing material showed a better performance toward HCHO gas with better selectivity, higher response, and short response-recovery time at a low operating temperature (120°C) compared to that of pure In_2O_3. The sensor response is increased three times after Pt loading for 10 ppm HCHO at 120°C. The response time is less than 2 s and recovery time is 51 s for 1 at% Pt-In_2O_3 composite. In addition to noble metal Pt, there are some reports on Au-In_2O_3 (Li et al., 2015; Zhang et al., 2017) and Ag-In_2O_3 (Wang et al., 2009, 2014; Lai et al., 2012; Dong et al., 2016) composites for HCHO sensing applications. Other than In_2O_3, noble metal-SnO_2 composites are also widely studied by many groups for HCHO sensing (Lin et al., 2015; Wang et al., 2014; Chen et al., 2016; Liu et al., 2019).

TABLE 7.4 The Brief Summary of Sensing Performance of the Noble Metal-SnO_2-based Materials of CH_4 Sensors

Material	Performance	Optimum temperature (°C)	References
Pt-SnO_2	Response 21% $(R_a-R_g)/R_g$ 500 ppm gas	350	Cabot et al. (2000)
Pd-SnO_2	Response 35% $(R_a-R_g)/R_g$ 1000 ppm gas	350	Cabot et al. (2002)
Pt-Ca/SnO_2	Response 2.3% (R_a/R_g) 5000 ppm gas	400	Min et al. (2005)
SnO_2-Pd	Response 20% $(R_a-R_g)/R_g$ 6600 ppm gas	400	Wagner et al. (2011)
Pd-SnO_2	Response 97.2% $(R_a-R_g)/R_g$ 200 ppm gas	220	Haridas et al. (2012)
Ag-SnO_2	Response 75% $(R_a-R_g)/R_g$ 2000 ppm gas	430	Horastani et al. (2015)
Pd/SnO_2-rGO	Response 9.5% $(R_a-R_g)/R_g$ 12000 ppm gas	Room temperature	Nasresfahani et al. (2017)
Pt-SnO_2	Response 4.48% (R_a/R_g) 1000 ppm gas	350	Lu et al. (2018)
Pd-SnO_2	Response 4.88% (R_a/R_g) 250 ppm gas	300	Yang et al. (2018)
Pt-SnO_2 with Au-CeZrO_2 filter	Response 35% (R_a/R_g) 500 ppm gas	400	Fateminia et al. (2019)

7.3.5.5   *H₂S GAS SENSOR*

Hydrogen sulfide (H_2S) is a flammable, poisonous, and corrosive gas with pungent rotten egg odor leads to disables olfactory senses at (> 50 ppm) higher concentrations and damage to lung tissue and blood circulation systems. The existence of trace amounts of highly toxic gases, like hydrogen sulfide (H_2S) at industrial environment is very dangerous and need early detection. Therefore, highly sensitive H_2S gas sensors are mandatory. For this many researches already done by taking different metal oxides. In a particular work Rai et al. used Au@NiO yolk@shell NPs for H_2S sensor (2014). They showed a fourfold increase in response as compared to pure NiO hollow nanospheres, along with a better selectivity than other interfering gases (NH_3, ethanol, CO, xylene, and H_2). The improvement in the performance of Au@NiO yolk@shell NPs was achieved due to the hollow spaces, which allowed the high accessibility of AuNPs to gas molecules. In addition to this, the electronic and chemical sensitization of AuNPs was also happened.

7.4   SUMMARY AND FUTURE PERSPECTIVE

In this chapter, we have categorically summarized the potential applications of noble metal decorated metal oxide NPs in gas sensing. In the past two decades, different synthesis approaches have been implemented for the preparation of core@shell, yolk@shell, noble metal support and noble metal doped NPs. There are ample of research contributions highlighted in this chapter, which includes various strategies for the synthesis of the above-mentioned NPs with controllable shapes, sizes, architectures, and compositions for different gas sensing applications. The noble metal-metal oxide NPs have shown better sensing properties as compared to pure metal. In the case of core@shell structure, the formation of metal oxide shell leads to thermal as well as chemical stability to noble metals. Due to the SPR of noble metals, further improvement of the gas sensing properties of core@shell NPs are achieved. In order to get the unique merit of core@shell, yolk@shell, noble metal support, and noble metal doped NPs, it is necessary to processes a general, facile method for synthesizing these high-quality NPs with controlled shape, size, structure, and fictionalization in an economical way. These noble metal-based metal oxide NPs are a promising platform for high performance gas sensors because of their unique physical and chemical properties, which can be tuned or designed separately.

KEYWORDS

- **core@shell**
- **gas sensor**
- **metal oxide semiconductor**
- **nanowires**
- **noble metal NPs**
- **yolk@shell**

REFERENCES

Abideen, U. Z., Kim, J. H., Mirzaei, A., Kim, H. W., & Kim, S. S., (2018). Sensing behavior to ppm-level gases and synergistic sensing mechanism in metal-functionalized rGO-loaded ZnO nanofibers. *Sensors and Actuators B, 255,* 1884–1896.

Aguirre, M. E., Rodríguez, H. B., Román, E. S., Feldhoff, A., & Grela, M. A., (2011). Ag@ ZnO core–shell NPss formed by the timely reduction of Ag$^+$ ions and zinc acetate hydrolysis in N,N-dimethylformamide: Mechanism of growth and photocatalytic properties. *J. Phys. Chem. C., 115,* 24967–24974.

Ahn, M. W., Park, K. S., Heo, J. H., Park, J. G., Kim, D. W., Choi, K. J., Lee, K. J., & Hong, S. H., (2008). Gas sensing properties of defect-controlled ZnO-nanowire gas sensor. *Appl. Phys. Lett., 93,* 263103.

Anand, K., Kaur, J., Singh, R. C., & Thangaraj, R., (2017). Preparation and characterization of Ag-doped In$_2$O$_3$ NPs gas sensor. *Chemical Physics Letters., 682,* 140–146.

Anand, K., Kaur, J., Singh, R. C., & Thangaraj, R., (2017). Temperature-dependent selectivity towards ethanol and acetone of Dy3+-doped In$_2$O$_3$ NPs. *Chem. Phys. Lett., 670,* 37–45.

Atanasova, G., Dikovska, A. O., Dilova, T., Georgieva, B., Avdeev, G. V., Stefanov, P., & Nedyalkov, N. N., (2019). Metal-oxide nanostructures produced by PLD in open air for gas sensor applications. *Applied Surface Science, 470,* 861–869.

Bittencourt, C., Llobet, E., Ivanov, P., Vilanova, X., Correig, X., Silva, M. A. P., Nunes, L. A. O., & Pieaux, J. J., (2004). Ag induced modifications on WO$_3$ films studied by AFM, Raman and x-ray photoelectron spectroscopy. *J. Phys. D: Appl. Phys., 37,* 3383–3391.

Borhaninia, A., Nikfarjam, A., & Salehifar, N., (2017). Gas sensing properties of SnO$_2$ NPs mixed with gold NPs. *Trans. Nonferrous Met. Soc. China, 27,* 1777–1784.

Buso, D., Post, M., Cantalini, C., & Mulvaney, P., (2008). Gold NPs-doped TiO_2 semiconductor thin films: Gas sensing properties. *Advanced Functional Materials, 18,* 3843–3849.

Cabot, A., Arbiol, J., Morante, J. R., Weimar, U., Bârsan, N., & Göpel, W., (2000). Analysis of the noble metal catalytic additives introduced by impregnation of as obtained SnO_2 sol-gel nanocrystals for gas sensors. *Sens. Actuators, B, 70,* 87–100.

Cabot, A., Vilà, A., & Morante, J. R., (2002). Analysis of the catalytic activity and electrical characteristics of different modified SnO_2 layers for gas sensors. *Sens. Actuators, B, 84,* 12–20.

Chen, Z., Lin, Z., Xu, M., Hong, Y., Li, N., Fu, P., & Chen, Z., (2016). Effect of gas sensing properties by Sn-Rh co-doped ZnO nanosheets. *Electron. Mater. Lett., 12,* 343–349.

Chiang, Y. J., Li, K. C., Yi-Chieh Lin, Y. C., & Pan, F. M., (2015). A mechanistic study of hydrogen gas sensing by PdO nanoflake thin films at temperatures below 250°C. *Phys. Chem. Chem. Phys., 17,* 3039–3049.

Choi, U. S., Sakai, G., Shimanoe, K., & Yamazoe, N., (2005). Sensing properties of Au-loaded SnO_2-Co_3O_4 composites to CO and H_2. *Sens. Actuator B Chem., 107,* 397–401.

Dhall, S., & Jaggi, N., (2015). Room temperature hydrogen gas sensing properties of Pt sputtered F-MWCNTs/SnO_2 network. *Sens. Actuators B, 210,* 742–747.

Dong, C., Liu, X., Han, B., Deng, S., Xiao, X., & Wang, Y., (2016). Non-aqueous synthesis of Ag-functionalized In_2O_3/ZnO nanocomposites for highly sensitive formaldehyde sensor. *Sens. Actuators B, 224,* 193–200.

Epifani, M., Prades, J. D., Comini, E., Pellicer, E., Avella, M., Siciliano, P., Faglia, G., et al., (2008). The role of surface oxygen vacancies in the NO_2 sensing properties of SnO_2 nanocrystals. *J. Phys. Chem. C, 112,* 19540–19546.

Fateminia, F. S., Mortazavi, Y., & Khodadadi, A. A., (2019). Au-promoted Ce-Zr catalytic filter for Pt/SnO_2 sensor to selectively detect methane and ethanol in the presence of interfering indoor gases. *Materials Science in Semiconductor Processing, 90,* 182–189.

Fu, H., Hou, C., Gu, F., Han, D., & Wang, Z., (2017). Facile preparation of rod-like Au/In_2O_3 nanocomposites exhibiting high response to CO at room temperature. *Sens. Actuators B Chem., 243,* 516–524.

Goldstein, M. (2008). Carbon monoxide poisoning. *Journal of Emergency Nursing, 34,* 538–542.

Guo, L., Chen, F., Xie, N., Kou, X., Wang, C., Sun, Y., Liu, F., et al., (2018). Ultra-sensitive sensing platform based on Pt-ZnO-In_2O_3 nanofibers for detection of acetone. *Sensors and Actuators: B. Chemical, 272,* 185–194.

Halek, G., Baikie, I. D., Teterycz, H., Halek, P., Suchorska-Woźniak, P., & Wiśniewski, K., (2013). Work function analysis of gas sensitive WO_3 layers with Pt doping. *Sens. Actuators B: Chem., 187,* 379–385.

Haridas, D., & Gupta, V., (2012). Enhanced response characteristics of SnO_2 thin film-based sensors loaded with Pd clusters for methane detection. *Sens. Actuators, B, 166,* 156–164.

Horastani, Z. K., Sayedi, S. M., Sheikhi, M. H., & Rahimi, E., (2015). Effect of silver additive on electrical conductivity and methane sensitivity of SnO_2. *Mater. Sci. Semicond. Process., 35,* 38–44.

Huang, M., Cui, Z., Yang, X., Zhu, S., Lia, Z., & Liang, Y., (2015). Pd-loaded In_2O_3 nanowire-like network synthesized using carbon nanotube templates for enhancing NO_2 sensing performance. *RSC Adv., 5*, 30038–30045.

Jaroenapibal, P., Boonma, P., Saksilaporn, N., Horprathum, M., Amornkitbamrung, V., & Triroj, N., (2018). Improved NO_2 sensing performance of electro spun WO_3 nanofibers with silver doping. *Sensors and Actuators B, 255*, 1831–1840.

Kim, D. H., Jung, J. W., Choi, S. J., Jang, J. S., Koo, W. T., & Kim, I. D., (2018). Pt NPs functionalized tungsten oxynitride hybrid chemiresistor: Low-temperature NO_2 sensing. *Sensors and Actuators: B. Chemical, 273*, 1269–1277.

Kim, H. J., & Lee, J. H., (2014). Highly sensitive and selective gas sensors using p-type oxide semiconductors: Overview. *Sens. Actuators B, 192*, 607–627.

Kim, J. H., Mirzaei, A., Kim, H. W., & Kim, S. S., (2019). Improving the hydrogen sensing properties of SnO_2 nanowire-based conductometric sensors by Pd-decoration. *Sensors and Actuators: B. Chemical, 285*, 358–367.

Kim, Y. S., Rai, P., & Yu, Y. T., (2013). Microwave assisted hydrothermal synthesis of Au@TiO_2 core–shell NPs for high temperature CO sensing applications. *Sens. Actuators B, 186*, 633–639.

Kohl, D., (1990). The role of noble metals in the chemistry of solid-state gas sensors. *Sens. Actuators B, 1*, 158–165.

Korotcenkov, G., (2007). Metal oxides for solid-state gas sensors: What determines our choice? *Mater. Sci. Eng. B., 139*, 1–23.

Kumar, R., Varandani, D., Mehta, B. R., Singh, V. N., Wen, Z., Feng, X., & Müllen, K., (2011). Fast response and recovery of hydrogen sensing in Pd-Pt NPs-graphene composite layers. *Nanotechnology, 22*, 275719.

Kundu, S., & Kumar, A., (2019). Low concentration ammonia sensing performance of Pd incorporated indium tin oxide. *Journal of Alloys and Compounds, 780*, 245–255.

Lai, X., Li, P., Yang, T., Tu, J., & Xue, P., (2012). Ordered array of Ag-In_2O_3 composite nanorods with enhanced gas-sensing properties. *Scripta Mater., 67*, 293–296,

Lee, D. D., & Lee, D. S., (2001). Environmental gas sensors. *IEEE Sensor Journal, 1*(3), 214–224.

Lee, Y. T., Lee, J. M., Kim, Y. J., Joe, J. H., & Lee, W., (2010). Hydrogen gas sensing properties of PdO thin films with nano-sized cracks. *Nanotechnol., 21*, 165503.

Li, F., Zhang, T., Gao, X., Wang, R., & Li, B., (2017). Coaxial electrospinning heterojunction SnO_2/Au-doped In_2O_3 core-shell nanofibers for acetone gas sensor. *Sensors and Actuators B, 252*, 822–830.

Li, S., Cheng, M., Liu, G., Zhao, L., Zhang, B., Gao, Y., Lu, H., et al., (2018). High-response and low-temperature nitrogen dioxide gas sensor based on gold-loaded mesoporous indium trioxide. *Journal of Colloid and Interface Science, 524*, 368–378.

Li, X., Liu, J., Guo, H., Zhou, X., Wang, C., Sun, P., Hua, X., & Lu, G., (2015). Au@In_2O_3 core-shell composites: A metal-semiconductor heterostructure for gas sensing applications. *RSC Adv., 5*, 545–551.

Li, X., Zhou, X., Guo, H., Wang, C., Liu, J., Sun, P., Liu, F., & Lu, G., (2014). Design of Au@ZnO yolk-shell nanospheres with enhanced gas sensing properties. *ACS Appl. Mater. Interfaces, 6*, 18661–18667.

Li, Y., Xu, J., Chao, J., Chen, D., Ouyang, S., Ye, J., & Shen, G., (2011). High-aspect-ratio single-crystalline porous In_2O_3 nanobelts with enhanced gas sensing properties. *J. Mater. Chem., 21,* 12852–12857.

Lim, Y., Lee, Y., Heo, J. I., & Shin, H., (2015). Highly sensitive hydrogen gas sensor based on a suspended palladium/carbon nanowire fabricated via batch microfabrication processes. *Sens. Actuators B, 210,* 218–224.

Lin, Y. K., Chiang, Y. J., & Hsu, Y. J., (2014). Metal-Cu_2O core-shell nanocrystals for gas sensing applications: Effect of metal composition. *Sens. Actuators, B, 204,* 190–196.

Lin, Y., Wei, W., Li, Y., Li, F., Zhou, J., Sun, D., Chen, Y., & Ruan, S., (2015). Preparation of Pd NPs-decorated hollow SnO_2 nanofibers and their enhanced formaldehyde sensing properties. *J. Alloy. Comp., 651,* 690–698.,

Liu, C., Kuang, Q., Xie, Z., & Zheng, L., (2015). The effect of noble metal (Au, Pd and Pt) NPs on the gas sensing performance of SnO_2-based sensors: A case study on the {221} high-index faceted SnO_2 octahedra. *Cryst. Eng. Comm., 17,* 6308–6313.

Liu, D., Pan, J., Tang, J., Liu, W., Bai, S., & Luo, R., (2019). Ag decorated SnO_2 NPs to enhance formaldehyde sensing properties. *Journal of Physics and Chemistry of Solids, 124,* 36–43.

Liu, H. R., Shao, G. X., Zhao, J. F., Zhang, Z. X., Zhang, Y., Liang, J., Liu, X. G., et al., (2012). Worm-like Ag/ZnO coreshell heterostructural composites: Fabrication, characterization, and photocatalysis. *J. Phys. Chem. C., 116,* 16182–16190.

Liu, X., Ling, Y., Huang, L., & Gao, W., (2013). A novel CO sensor based on the point contact between Pd decorated TiO_2 nanotubes array. *Journal of Nanoscience and Nanotechnology, 2,* 869–872.

Lu, W., Ding, D., Xue, Q., Du, Y., Xiong, Y., Zhang, J., Pan, X., & Xing, W., (2018). Great enhancement of CH_4 sensitivity of SnO_2 based nanofibers by heterogeneous sensitization and catalytic effect. *Sens. Actuators, B, 254,* 393–401.

Lupan, O., Chow, L., Pauporté, T., Ono, L. K., Roldan, B., & Chai, C. G., (2012). Highly sensitive and selective hydrogen single-nanowire nanosensor. *Sens. Actuators B, 173,* 772–780.

Lupan, O., Postica, V., Ababii, N., Reimer, T., Shree, S., Hoppe, M., Polonskyi, O., et al., (2018). Ultra-thin TiO_2 films by atomic layer deposition and surface functionalization with Au nanodots for sensing applications. *Materials Science in Semiconductor Processing, 87,* 44–53.

Lupan, O., Postica, V., Adelung, R., Labat, F., Ciofini, I., Schürmann, U., Kienle, L., Lee, C., Viana, B., & Pauporté, T., (2018). Functionalized Pd/ZnO nanowires for nano sensors. *Phys. Status Solidi RRL, 12,* 1700321.

Lupan, O., Postica, V., Hoppe, M., Wolff, N., Polonskyi, O., Pauporté, T., Viana, B., Majérus, O., Lorenz, K. L., & Adelung, R., (2018). PdO/PdO_2 functionalized ZnO: Pd films for lower operating temperature H_2 gas sensing. *Nanoscale, 10,* 14107–14127.

Lupan, O., Postica, V., Labat, F., Ciofini, I., Pauporté, T., & Adelung, R., (2018). Ultra-sensitive and selective hydrogen nanosensor with fast response at room temperature based on a single Pd/ZnO nanowire. *Sens. Actuators B, 254,* 1259–1270.

Ma, J., Ren, Y., Zhou, X., Liu, L., Zhu, Y., Cheng, X., Xu, P., et al., (2018). Pt NPs Sensitized Ordered Mesoporous WO_3 semiconductor: Gas sensing performance and mechanism study. *Adv. Funct. Mater., 28,* 1705268.

Ma, R. J., Zhao, X., Zou, X., & Li, G. D., (2018). Enhanced formaldehyde sensing performance at ppb level with Pt-doped nanosheet-assembled In_2O_3 hollow microspheres. *Journal of Alloys and Compounds, 732,* 863–870.

Manikandan, V., Kim, J. H., Mirzaei, A., Kim, S. S., Vigneselvan, S., Singh, M., & Chandrasekaran, J., (2019). Effect of temperature on gas sensing properties of lithium substituted nickel ferrite thin film. *Journal of Molecular Structure, 1177,* 485–490.

Manjula, P., Arunkumar, S., & Manorama, S. V., (2011). Au/SnO_2 an excellent material for room temperature carbon monoxide sensing. *Sens. Actuators B Chem., 152,* 168–175.

Ménini, P., Parret, F., Guerrero, M., Soulantica, K., Erades, L., Maisonnat, A., & Chaudret, B., (2004). CO response of a nanostructured SnO_2 gas sensor doped with palladium and platinum. *Sens. Actuators B Chem., 103,* 111–114.

Min, B. K., & Choi, S. D., (2005). Undoped and 0.1 wt.% Ca-doped Pt-catalyzed SnO_2 sensors for CH_4 detection. *Sens. Actuators, B, 108,* 119–124.

Nam, J., Lee, Y., Yang, Y., Jeong, S., Kim, W., Yoo, J. W., Moon, J. O., et al., (2018). Is it worth expending energy to convert biliverdin into bilirubin? *Applied Physics A, 124,* 232–240.

Nandy, T., Coutu, R. A., & Ababei, C., (2018). Carbon monoxide sensing technologies for next-generation cyber-physical systems. *Sensors, 18,* 3443.

Nasresfahani, S., Sheikhi, M. H., Tohidi, M., & Zarifkar, A., (2017). Methane gas sensing properties of Pd-doped SnO_2/reduced graphene oxide synthesized by a facile hydrothermal route. *Mater. Res. Bull., 89,* 161–169.

Navale, S. T., Liu, C., Yang, Z., Patil, V. B., Cao, P., Du, B., Mane, R. S., & Stadler, F. J., (2018). Low-temperature wet chemical synthesis strategy of In_2O_3 for selective detection of NO_2 down to ppb levels. *J. Alloy. Compd.,735,* 2102–2110.

Ngaw, C. K., Xu, Q., Tan, T. T. Y., Hu, P., Cao, S., & Loo, J. S. C., (2014). A strategy for *in-situ* synthesis of well-defined core-shell $Au@TiO_2$ hollow spheres for enhanced photocatalytic hydrogen evolution. *Chem. Eng. J., 257,* 112–121.

Noh, J. S., Kim, H., Kim, B., Lee, E., Cho, H. H., & Lee, W., (2011). High-performance vertical hydrogen sensors using Pd-coated rough Si nanowires. *J. Mater. Chem., 21,* 15935–15939.

Pauporté, T., Lupan, O., Zhang, J., Tugsuz, T., Ciofini, I., Labat, F., & Viana, B., (2015). Low-temperature preparation of Ag-doped ZnO nanowire arrays, DFT study, and application to light-emitting diode. *ACS Appl. Mater. Interfaces, 7,* 11871–11880.

Penza, M., Martucci, C., & Cassano, G., (1998). NOx gas sensing characteristics of WO_3 thin films activated by noble metals (Pd, Pt, Au) layers. *Sens. Actuators B, 50,* 52–59.

Phan, D. T., & Chung, G. S., (2014). Characteristics of resistivity-type hydrogen sensing based on palladium-graphene nanocomposites. *Int. J. Hydrogen Energy, 39,* 620–629.

Phan, D. T., & Chung, G. S., (2014). Reliability of hydrogen sensing based on bimetallic Ni-Pd/graphene composites. *Int. J. Hydrogen Energy, 39,* 20294–20304.

Qiang, X., Hu, M., Zhao, B., Qin, Y., Yang, R., Zhou, L., & Qin, Y., (2018). Effect of the functionalization of porous silicon/WO_3 nanorods with Pd NPs and their enhanced NO_2-sensing performance at room temperature. *Materials, 11,* 764.

Rai, P., Kwak, W. K., & Yu, Y. T., (2013). Solvothermal synthesis of ZnO nanostructures and their morphology-dependent gas-sensing properties. *ACS Appl. Mater. Interfaces, 5,* 3026–3032.

Rai, P., Yoon, J. W., Jeong, H. M., Hwang, S. J., Kwak, C. H., & Lee, J. H., (2014). Design of highly sensitive and selective Au@NiO yolk-shell nanoreactors for gas sensor applications. *Nanoscale, 6,* 8292–8299.

Raub, J. A., Mathieu-Nolf, M., Hampson, N. B., & Thom, S. R., (2000). Carbon monoxide poisoning: A public health perspective. *Toxicology, 145,* 1–14.

Ren, X., Zhang, S., Li, C., Li, S., Jia, Y., & Cho, J. H., (2015). Catalytic activities of noble metal atoms on WO3 (001): Nitric oxide adsorption. *Nanoscale Res. Lett., 10,* 1–6.

Rout, C. S., Govindaraj, A., & Rao, C. N. R., (2006). High-sensitivity hydrocarbon sensors based on tungsten oxide nanowires. *J. Mater. Chem., 16,* 3936–3941.

Seifaddini, P., Ghasempour, R., Ramezannezhad, M., & Nikfarjam, A., (2019). Room temperature ammonia gas sensor based on Au/graphene nanoribbon. *Materials Research Express, 6,* 045054.

Seo, J., Lim, Y., & Shin, H., (2017). Self-heating hydrogen gas sensor based on an array of single suspended carbon nanowires functionalized with palladium NPs. *Sens. Actuators B, 247,* 564–572.

Shao, S., Chen, X., Chen, Y., Lai, M., & Che, L., (2019). Ultrasensitive and highly selective detection of acetone based on Au@WO3-SnO2 corrugated nanofibers. *Applied Surface Science, 473,* 902–911.

Shojaee, M., Nasresfahani, M., & Sheikhi, H., (2018). Hydrothermally synthesized Pd-loaded SnO2/partially reduced graphene oxide nanocomposite for effective detection of carbon monoxide at room temperature. *Sensors and Actuators B, 254,* 457–467.

Singh, D., Kundu, V. S., & Maan, A. S., (2016). Structural, morphological, and gas sensing study of zinc doped tin oxide NPs synthesized via hydrothermal technique. *J. Mol. Struct., 1115,* 250–257.

Singh, V. N., Mehta, B. R., Joshi, R. K., Kruis, F. E., & Shivaprasad, S. M., (2007). Enhanced gas sensing properties of In_2O_3: Ag composite NPs layers; electronic interaction, size and surface-induced effects. *Sens. Actuators B, 125,* 482–488.

Spencer, M. J. S., Wong, K. W. J., & Yarovsky, I., (2012). Surface defects on ZnO nanowires: Implications for design of sensors. *J. Phys. Condens. Matter., 24,* 305001.

Sun, J., He, J., Wang, S., Zhang, Y., Liu, C., Sritharan, T., Mhaisalkar, S., et al., (2013). Investigating the multiple roles of polyvinylpyrrolidone for a general methodology of oxide encapsulation. *J. Am. Chem. Soc., 135,* 9099–9110.

Suo, C., Gao, C., Wu, X., Zuo, Y., Wang, X., & Jia, J., (2015). Ag-decorated ZnO nanorods prepared by photochemical deposition and their high selectivity to ethanol using conducting oxide electrodes. *RSC Adv., 5,* 92107–92113.

Tan, J., Wlodarski, W., Zadeh, K. K., & Livingston, P., (2006). Carbon monoxide gas sensor based on titanium dioxide nanocrystalline with a langasite substrate. *5th IEEE Conference on Sensors,* 228–231.

Teng, L., Liu, Y., Ikram, M., Liu, Z., Ullah, M., Ma, L., Zhang, X., et al., (2019). One-step synthesis of palladium oxide-functionalized tin dioxide nanotubes: Characterization and high nitrogen dioxide gas sensing performance at room temperature. *Journal of Colloid and Interface Science, 537,* 79–90.

Toan, N. V., Chien, N. V., Duy, N. V., Hong, H. S., Nguyen, H., Hoa, N. D., & Hieu, N. V., (2016). Fabrication of highly sensitive and selective H_2 gas sensor based on SnO_2 thin film sensitized with micro-sized Pd islands. *J. Hazard. Mater., 301,* 433–442.

Varon, J., Marik, P. E., Fromm, R. E. Jr., & Gueler, A., (1999). Carbon monoxide poisoning: A review for clinicians. *J. Emerg. Med., 17,* 87–93.

Wagner, T., Bauer, M., Sauerwald, T., Kohl, C. D., & Tiemann, M., (2011). X-ray absorption near-edge spectroscopy investigation of the oxidation state of Pd species in nanoporous SnO_2 gas sensors for methane detection. *Thin Solid Films, 520,* 909–912.

Wang, J. X., Zou, B., Ruan, S. P., Zhao, J., & Wu, F., (2009). Synthesis, characterization, and gas-sensing property for HCHO of Ag-doped In_2O_3 nanocrystalline powders. *Mater. Chem. Phys., 117,* 489–493.

Wang, J., Zou, B., Ruan, S., Zhao, J., Chen, Q., & Wu, F., (2009). HCHO sensing properties of Ag-doped In_2O_3 nanofibers synthesized by electrospinning. *Mater. Lett., 63,* 1750–1753.

Wang, K., Zhao, T., Lian, G., Yu, Q., Luan, C., Wang, Q., & Cui, D., (2013). Room temperature CO sensor fabricated from Pt-loaded SnO_2 porous nano solid. *Sens. Actuators B. Chem., 184,* 33–39.

Wang, L., Dou, H., Lou, Z., & Zhang, T., (2013). Encapsulated nanoreactors ($Au@SnO_2$): A new sensing material for chemical sensors. *Nanoscale, 5,* 2686–2691.

Wang, S., Xiao, B., Yang, T., Wang, P., Xiao, C., Li, Z., Zhao, R., & Zhang, M., (2014). Enhanced HCHO gas sensing properties by Ag-loaded sunflower-like In_2O_3 hierarchical nanostructures. *J. Mater. Chem. A., 2,* 6598–6604.

Wang, Y., Cui, X., Yang, Q., Liu, J., Gao, Y., Sun, P., & Lu, G., (2016). Preparation of Ag-loaded mesoporous WO_3 and its enhanced NO_2 sensing performance. *Sens. Actuat. B: Chem., 225,* 544–552.

Wang, Y., Zhao, Z., Sun, Y., Li, P., Ji, J., Chen, Y., Zhang, W., & Hu, J., (2017). Fabrication and gas sensing properties of Au-loaded SnO_2 composite NPs for highly sensitive hydrogen detection. *Sens. Actuators B, 240,* 664–673.

Wang, Z. L., & Song, J., (2006). Piezoelectric nanogenerators based on zinc oxide nanowire arrays, *Science, 312,* 242–246.

Wanga, Y., Liu, J., Cui, X., Gao, Y., Ma, J., Sun, Y., Sun, P., et al., (2017). NH_3 gas-sensing performance enhanced by Pt-loaded on mesoporous WO_3. *Sensors and Actuators B, 238,* 473–481.

Wei, S., Yu, Y., & Zhou, M., (2010). CO gas sensing of Pd-doped ZnO nanofibers synthesized by electrospinning method. *Mater. Lett., 64,* 2284–2286.

Wu, R. J., Lin, D. J., Yu, M. R., Chen, M. H., & Lai, H. F., (2013). $Ag@SnO_2$ core-shell material for use in fast-response ethanol sensor at room operating temperature. *Sens. Actuators, B, 178,* 185–191.

Xu, C., Tamaki, J., Miura, N., & Yamazoe, N., (1991). Grain size effects on gas sensitivity of porous SnO_2-based elements. *Sens. Actuators, B, 3,* 147–155.

Xu, L., Yin, M. L., & Liu, S. F., (2014). $Ag(x)@WO_3$ core-shell nanostructure for LSP enhanced chemical sensors. *Sci. Rep., 4,* 6745.

Xu, X., Fan, H., Liu, Y., Wang, L., & Zhang, T., (2011). Au-loaded In_2O_3 nanofibers-based ethanol micro gas sensor with low power consumption. *Sens. Actuators B., 160,* 713–719.

Xue, D., Zhang, S. S., & Zhang, Z., (2019). Hydrothermally prepared porous 3D SnO_2 microstructures for methane sensing at lower operating temperature. *Materials Letters, 237,* 336–339.

Yamazoe, N., (1991). New approaches for improving semiconductor gas sensors. *Sens. Actuators, B, 5,* 7–19.

Yanagimoto, T., Yu, Y. T., & Kaneko, K., (2012). Microstructure and CO gas sensing property of Au/SnO₂ core-shell structure NPs synthesized by precipitation method and microwave-assisted hydrothermal synthesis method. *Sens. Actuators, B, 166–167*, 31–35.

Yang, D. J., Kamienchick, I., Youn, D. Y., Rothschild, A., & Kim, I. D., (2010). Ultrasensitive and highly selective gas sensors based on electrospun SnO₂ nanofibers modified by Pd loading. *Adv. Funct. Mater., 20*, 4258–4264.

Yang, L., Wang, Z., Zhou, X., Wu, X., Han, N., & Chen, Y., (2018). Synthesis of Pd-loaded mesoporous SnO₂ hollow spheres for highly sensitive and stable methane gas sensors. *RSC Adv., 8*, 24268–24275.

Yang, Y., Han, S., Zhou, G., Zhang, L., Li, X., Zou, C., & Huang, S., (2013). Ascorbic-acid-assisted growth of high-quality M@ZnO: A growth mechanism and kinetics study. *Nanoscale, 5*, 11808–11819.

Yin, X., Que, W., Fei, D., Shen, F., & Guo, Q., (2012). Ag NPs/ZnO nanorods nanocomposites derived by a seed-mediated method and their photocatalytic properties. *J. Alloys Compd., 524*, 13–21.

Yu, Y. T., & Dutta, P., (2011). Examination of Au/SnO₂ core-shell architecture NPs for low temperature gas sensing applications. *Sens. Actuators B, 157*, 444–449.

Zhang, D., Sun, Y., Jiang, C., & Zhang, Y., (2017). Room temperature hydrogen gas sensor based on palladium decorated tin oxide/molybdenum disulfide ternary hybrid via hydrothermal route. *Sens. Actuators B, 242*, 15–24.

Zhang, D., Wu, J., & Cao, Y., (2019). Cobalt-doped indium oxide/molybdenum disulfide ternary nanocomposite toward carbon monoxide gas sensing. *Journal of Alloys and Compounds, 777*, 443–453.

Zhang, H., Li, Q., Huang, J., Du, Y., & Ruan, S. C., (2016). Reduced graphene oxide/au nanocomposite for NO₂ sensing at low operating temperature. *Sensors, 16*, 1152.

Zhang, H., Li, Z., Liu, L., Xu, X., Wang, Z., Wang, W., Zheng, W., et al., (2010). Enhancement of hydrogen monitoring properties based on Pd-SnO₂ composite nanofibers. *Sens. Actuators B, 147*, 111–115.

Zhang, S., Song, P., Li, J., Zhang, J., Yang, Z., & Wang, Q., (2017). Facile approach to prepare hierarchical Au-loaded In₂O₃ porous nanocubes and their enhanced sensing performance towards formaldehyde. *Sens. Actuators B, 241*, 1130–1138.

Zhu, L., Wang, H., Shen, X., Chen, L., Wang, Y., & Chen, H., (2012). Developing mutually encapsulating materials for versatile syntheses of multilayer metal-silica-polymer hybrid nanostructures. *Small, 8*, 1857–1862.

Zou, Y., Wang, Q., Xiang, C., Tang, C., Chu, H., Qiu, S., Yan, E., et al., (2016). Doping composite of polyaniline and reduced graphene oxide with palladium NPs for room-temperature hydrogen-gas sensing. *Int. J. Hydrogen Energy, 41*, 5396–5404.

CHAPTER 8

Nanoparticles: A Noble Metal for Ultrasensitive Electrochemical Biosensing Affinity

TAPAN KUMAR BEHERA[1], SNEHALATA PRADHAN[2],
CHINMAYEE ACHARYA[1], PRAMOD KUMAR SATAPATHY[1], and
PRIYABRAT MOHAPATRA[3]

[1]*North Orissa University, Baripada, Odisha–757003, India,
E-mail: tapankumarbeherachemistry@gmail.com (T. K. Behera)*

[2]*Government College Koraput, Landiguda, Odisha–764021, India*

[3]*C.V. Raman College of Engineering, Bhubaneswar, Odisha–752054, India*

ABSTRACT

Graphene (GN)/nanoparticles (NPs) composite holds an excellent transducer for electrochemical biosensor applications, since the electronic structures of both favors to target bio-sensing of even nano-molar quantity level of bio-analytes. The band engineering and outer shell electronic design of GN nanocomposite provides a unique tool for detection of bio-analytes than nano-crystalline semiconductors compared to that of other traditional techniques. The magnitude of redox property of GN nanocomposite caused for converting chemical energy into a measurable signal through electrochemical process. For a healthy society, the detection of essential biological molecule/bio-analytes in the field of pharmaceuticals, clinical, food beverage, human body, and environment in a sub-nanomolar range plays a challenging role to the current science. In this platform of bio-sensing, three main methods are used: (a) Photoelectrochemical; (B) electrochemical; and (c) optical sensor with each has its own advantage and disadvantage. Among these, the electrochemical bio-sensing by GN-nanoparticle hybrids composite have achievable sensitivities and selectivity compared to others. Because of its fascinating electronic, optical, and mechanical properties, GN nanocomposite acts a prominent transducer for electrochemical detection of bio-analytes like NADH, hydrogen peroxide (H_2O_2), glucose, uric acid (UA), ascorbic acid (AA) and nitrate in a sub- nano-molar range. This chapter covers the advantages of GN-supported NPs for electrochemical bio-sensing towards the detection of various bio-analytes.

8.1   INTRODUCTION

Monometallic (i.e., Au, Ag, Pt, Pd, Ru) and bimetallic (such as Pt-Pd, Pt-Au) noble metal nanoparticles (NPs) have emerged as a new class of compounds and received increasing attention in the field of biosensor owing to their unique electrical, magnetic, optical, and catalytic properties (Wu et al., 2011). Moreover, these noble metal nanomaterials have been made great contributions in catalysis, sensing, biomedical diagnosis and therapy, energy storage and conversion, and so on (Guo et al., 2011; Fang et al., 2010). Recent advances revealed that shape controlling the size, morphology, and composition of NPs provide the attractive opportunities to enhance their electrochemical catalytic activity functions like fuel cell and biosensing. Hybridization of these metal nanostructures with carbon nanomaterials increases the catalyst surface area, thereby facilitating the electrochemical reactions. Among various carbon-based materials such as carbon nanotubes (CNTs), graphene (GN), carbon nanohorns and carbon black; GN has been considered as a promising support for the catalytic activity (Sahu et al., 2016; Behera et al., 2018, 2019). The pioneer works of bio-analytes such as glucose, ascorbic acid (AA), uric acid (UA), nitrite, dopamine (DA), and hydrogen peroxide detection with nanoporous were often applied via incorporation with carbon nanotube, carbon nanofiber (CNF), polymer, and GN. GN, a two-dimensional single atomic planar sheet, possesses unique physicochemical properties, quantum hall effect, high electron carrier mobility, good optical transparency, high surface area (theoretically 2630 m^2/g for single-layer GN), high Young's modulus, excellent thermal and electric conductivity, and strong mechanical strength (Guo and Dong, 2011; Allen et al., 2010). The chemical reduction of graphene oxide (GO) to GN has been assumed as an efficient method for scalable preparation of GN and to apply in biosensors, electrochemical energy conversion, storage, and, etc. In addition, GO have abundant oxygen containing functional groups such as hydroxyl, epoxide, carbonyl, carboxyl, etc. Moreover, the integration of GN/noble metal hybrids has emerged as a new kind of nanocomposite to explore its multimodal applications.

GN-supported NPs play an excellent transducer to detect a particular target bio-analyte or family of analytes. Commonly in biosensors, the transducer is composed of reduction/oxidation of an electroactive bio-molecule by the sensing electrode into a measurable signal. Among electronic, electrochemical, and optical signals biosensors, the electro-chemical biosensor have evaluated as great sensitivity to the target(s), limit of detection (LOD), operational, and storage range, linear, and dynamic ranges, sensor's response time, reproducibility, and selectivity (Ronkainen et al., 2010; Kulia et al., 2011). GN-nanoparticle hybrids are particularly well-suited material for the development of electrochemical biosensors. Moreover, GN-NPs have enhanced achievable sensitivities by amplifying the obtained signal with increasing the available surface area for bio-analytes binding as well as improve their electrical conduc-tivity and electron mobility, thereby enhancing the achievable sensitivity and selectivity. Electrochemical biosensing possesses high sensitivities, spatial resolution for localized detection, easy miniaturization, and facile integration with standard semiconductor processing and real-time detection (Pingarron et al., 2008; Haun et al., 2010). In particular, the electrochemical sensors convert the biological recognition event to a measurable electronic signal. In addition, current flows along a trans-ducer path (the channel/working electrode) that connects two electrodes (the reference and the counter) through a protentional providing instru-ments (Potentiostat). Specifically, in electrochemical biosensors, the nanocomposite (transducer) is in direct contact with the sensing sample, which enhances the achievable sensitivity as single. Moreover, because of this high surface-to-volume ratio as well as signal amplification and enhanced electrical conductivity of nanocomposite caused a very lower LOD with more accurate of any bio-analytes (Liu and Guo, 2012; Lee et al., 2009). This chapter focuses on up-to-date electrochemical biosensing of bio-analytes by GN/noble metal hybrids and a simple approaches for the synthesis of GN-supported noble metal nanostructures such as *in-situ* and *ex-situ* solution based electrochemical method.

The rate of increasing population has caused demand for food and put up clinical and biological issues. The increased use of chemicals and fertilizers in croplands and our daily used materials is a matter of urgent concern for healthy family. The chemicals used beyond of permeable with very micromolar or nanomolar range in different fields like preservatives of materials for storage, washing, and much production of foodstuffs breaks our healthy society. So the sensitive and selective detection of such very lower range amount of bio-analytes/chemicals plays a vital role. And hence for a safe and healthy society, selective, and sensitive detection of hazardous bio-analytes is highly necessary. In this chapter, we elaborately discussed the synthesis of different shaped NPs in a green synthesis way and its composite with GN in both *in situ-ex situ* methods, its characterization and properties, and application to the accurate detection of bio-analytes like glucose, AA, UA, nitrate, NADH, and hydrogen peroxide through electrochemical method. In addition, we discussed on the biosensing capacity/range of semiconductor crystalline-like ZnS, CdS, etc. A real time detection of bio-analytes from natural sources like rainwater, hair color dye, blood sample analysis, milk packets, and a comparative study among these with different techniques will enlighten our research for a better future.

8.2   ELECTROCHEMICAL SENSING

Electrochemical sensors are the most accurate biosensing tool than other methods since it provides direct conversion of a biological recognition event to an electrical signal. A Typical electrochemical sensor consists of a working electrode, counter electrode, reference electrode, and with a biological recognition element and are separated by a layer of electrolytes. In this sensor the amount of analytes either reduced or oxidized at the working electrode (GN/NP) and produce electric signal in forms of cyclic voltammetry (CV), linear sweep, and amperometry (i-t) for the electrochemical detection of biomolecules (Sahu et al., 2016; Behera et al., 2018, 2019). NPs with GN plays an ideal material for electrochemical biosensors since the combination of both caused for excellent conductor availing a large number of electroactive sites. On comparing to other carbon-based materials, GN-based electrochemical sensors have superior performance to carbon nanotube (CNT) due to the presence of more planes and edge defects on the surface of GN. In addition to NPs metal oxide NPs and semiconductor NPs are widely used for electrochemical sensing applications (Pingarron et al., 2008; Luo et al., 2006). One advantageous property to electrochemical biosensors by using GN-nanoparticle hybrid is that GN sheets prevent aggregation of NPs on its surface and decorate to different shapes on it in certain cases. In the following subsections, discussion is presented on GN-nanoparticle hybrid composite structures towards the detection of biomolecules.

8.3 PERFORMANCE OF NANOPARTICLES (NPs) AND ITS COMPOSITE WITH GRAPHENE (GN) FOR DIFFERENT ELECTROCHEMICAL BIOSENSOR

The shape-controlled synthesis of different nanocomposite and their protentional study for detection by bioanalytes by electrochemical method are presented here. GN supported NPs shows higher catalytic activity than the only NPs in the electrochemical method. The detection of bioanalytes studied here are from different sources, which results the good operational stability, storage stability and very lower LOD by electrochemical method.

8.3.1 HYDROGEN PEROXIDE BIOSENSOR

The oxidizing property of hydrogen peroxide caused for a great application in the field of clinical, pharmaceuticals, food processing industry and also in our day-to-day life. It is used as a preservative for long term storage of food, in hair dyes, packing of milk, etc. Hydrogen peroxide could have adverse effect on the human health above the permissible level (Sahu et al., 2016; Behera et al., 2018, 2019). Therefore, effective, accurate, and precise value detection of hydrogen peroxide is more important. An electrochemical method nano-molar range of hydrogen peroxide can be detected by considering the both oxidation/reduction of hydrogen peroxide reaction current peaks as signal. The oxidative detection of hydrogen peroxide is preferred over the reductive detection to success in the interference taste. Electrochemical measurements used for sensitive detection of electro-active hydrogen peroxide species and provide a viable alternative to fluorescence, chemiluminescence based detection. Several reports described electrochemical biosensors for in vitro and in vivo detection of hydrogen peroxide. Hazhir et al. developed a one-step synthetic route of Fe_3O_4 magnetic NPs/RGO/GCE electrode for electrocatalytic behaviors of H_2O_2. The nanocomposite possesses electrocatalytic activities toward H_2O_2 reduction analytes because of the synergistic integration of the two nanomaterials (Teymourian et al., 2013). This synthesized material shows positive interference taste with other bioanalytes like AA, UA and DA. This sample acts as a best for all the analytes. Wang et al. have synthesized hybrid hematite α-Fe$_2$O$_3$/rGO NPs through a simple one-step hydrothermal method without the addition of reducing agents, and the important fact is that here Fe^{2+} present in the sample acts a self-reducing agent. From the characterized data of as prepared hematite hybrid material signified the well dispersed hematite NPs on GN sheet of size 21 nm and the electrochemical data of CV and amperometry data revealed the catalytic performance toward the reduction of H$_2$O$_2$ with a linear sweep range of 5.0–4495.0 µM (R = 0.9998), a low detection limit of 1.0 µM, and a high sensitivity of 126.9 µA cm^{-2}mM^{-1} to the detection of H$_2$O$_2$ (2014). Gold nanoparticles (AuNPs) are the cheapest and easily available NPs and the properties of AuNPs attract more researchers for electrocatalytic bio-sensing. Fang et al. build the self-assembly of GNs/Au NPs heterostructure by use of cationic polyelectrolyte poly(diallyl dimethyl ammonium chloride) (PDDA) functionalized cationic 2D graphene nanosheets (GNs) for electrochemical catalytic (2010). The use of PDDA did both altering the electrostatic charges of GN as well as hybridization of GN to Au NPs. The hybrid materials employed as the electrochemical enhanced material of wide linear ranges from 0.5 µM to 50 mM and low detection limits (LOD) of 0.22 µM. In contrast to the reported, this interesting LOD and linear range by using such 2D GN with AuNPs was the lowest value on comparing to GN with other NPs and also with the carbon nanotube (Liu et al., 2008; Li et al., 2009; Zhao et al., 2009). The composite of GN with carbon nanotube shows excellent electrocatalytic properties than the individual GN or CNT. Veerappan et al. synthesized novel nano-bio-composite, reduced GN oxide-multiwalled CNTs-platinum NPs for the application towards determination of hydrogen peroxide (2014). The synthesized material possesses a three-dimensional hierarchical arrangement, large surface area, high conductivity, long-term stability, outstanding electrocatalytic, and anti-interference abilities. This biosensor displayed the lowest detection limit of 6 pM with a linear range of 10 pM–0.19 nM with a sensitivity of 1.99 µA pM^{-1} cm^{-2}, which is the lowest LOD ever achieved for the detection of H$_2$O$_2$ by such synthesized materials.

Different NPs with different shape have different linear sweep range, LOD and current values. Since NPs are highly contaminated to the glass-wares so to avoid interference of different NPs in electrochemical sensitivity and selectivity, the best practice is to use all the chemicals in 99% purity, and glassware should be free from any other chemical traces and dust. For this, all the glassware should be perfectly rinsed with freshly prepared aqua regia, then thoroughly washed with Millipore water and dried prior to use *(Caution! aqua regia is a powerful oxidizing agent and it should be handled with extreme care)*. Considering the different shaped NPs, there is a report on branched Pt GN nanocomposite and its application for the detection of H_2O_2 with very lower LOD till 2018 and made the practical source detection of hydrogen peroxide from rainwater (Behera et al., 2016). Here the from the TEM and HRTEM study (Figure 8.1), branched Pt NPs well spread over the GN sheet and from XRD, XPS data has been concluded that the Pt NPs formed are highly crystalline and from FTIR data the reduction of GO to RGO has been confirmed. This work shown the oxidation peak at an ultra-low potential value of +0.37 V for RGO/Pt/GCE and showed a sensitivity of 811.26 µA/mm cm^2 including a very fast response and stable current. In another report, hydrogen peroxide reduction experiment employed by fabricated Pt/RGO/GCE electrode. The characterization data showed the Pt size of 1–4 nm and well dispersed on the surface of reduced GN oxide. The transducer showed excellent hydrogen peroxide detection efficiency of linear response range was from 2 µM to 710 µM with correlation coefficient of 0.9989. And the LOD of H_2O_2 was found to be 0.5 µM with signal to noise ratio (SNR) greater than three (Xu et al., 2011).

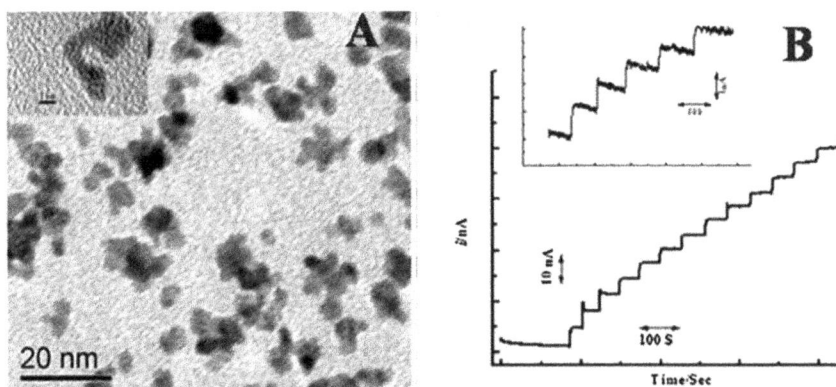

FIGURE 8.1 (A) HRTEM and TEM image of branched Pt nanoparticles. (B) Amperometric i-t technique employed for branched Pt nanoparticles of 5 nM in 0.1 M PBS solution at 7.2 pH value.
Source: Reproduced with permission from: Sahu et al. (2016). © Royal Chemical Society.

On comparing to Pt NPs, Palladium NPs used as more electrocatalytic biosensing, fuel cell activity due to none evolve of poisons CO_2 at Pd electrode as in Pt (Sahu et al., 2013). Sahu et al. synthesized the unique porous Pd structure and found to show excellent electrocatalytic activity towards the reduction of H_2O_2. The unique porous Pd nanostructures (PPd NS) decorated over the GN sheet uniformly show highly catalytically active. The reduction of hydrogen peroxide by RGO-Pd/GCE electrode, yielding a current density of 445.267 $\mu A/cm^2$ with electrode potential value at 0.126 V. This achieved unique potential may be due to the interesting morphology of the porous palladium NPs with very lower LOD of 1 nM. This LOD value considered as the lowest limit sensing capacity value till 2016 by Pd NPs.

Both Pt and Pd NPs shown good operational and storage stability. For example, after two weeks of storage, only a 3% decrease in the current value has been observed in case of the RGO-Pt/GCE and RGO/Pd/GCE electrode (Sahu et al., 2016; Behera et al., 2016). Except these two, all rest sample shown above possess only <10% percentage decrease in current after 2–3 weeks. From the interference study data, for bioanalytes like AA, UA, DA, and glucose (Glu) shown no interference with any other analytes and confirmed the selectivity of the nanomaterials for H_2O_2 biosensing. In addition Behera et al. did the rainwater experiment for detection of bioanalytes by their prepared NPs composite. As we know hydrogen peroxide is one of the most important oxidants present in the troposphere and playing a major role in controlling the chemical composition of the atmosphere at trace gas levels. First, rainwater samples were filtered and then put forward to electrochemical analysis of the bioanalytes. By correlating the current and total concentration of H_2O_2 in rainwater was found to be in the range of 50 nM to 100 nM. The concentration of hydrogen peroxide in rainwater varies from place to place, depending on the weather condition and periodical sampling throughout the day.

8.3.2   GLUCOSE BIOSENSOR

From day to day, the accurate detection of glucose in blood and food becoming a more challenging research area due to the increase in diabetics patients. Among several methods, electrochemical biosensors have attracted considerable attention due to their excellent selectivity, simplicity, and low cost (Bahmani et al., 2010; Yazdanpanah et al., 2015). As like in the case of hydrogen peroxide sensing, Palladium NPs are the most dominating material than others due to its excellent uniform size and even distribution were prepared on GN oxide (Pd NPs/GO). Wang et al. developed Pd NPs/GO nanocomposite by using a simple and environmentally friendly ultrasonic method, in which no additional reductant was used and applied for non-enzymatic biosensor for the determination of glucose (2012). The thickness of GO obtained AFM image is about 0.8 nm and Pd nanoparticle size of nearly 4 nm after 15-minute sonication of the sample and more interestingly the nanoparticle size increases on increasing the sonication time for synthesis of sample, i.e., approx. 1 nM size increases on each time increase in sonication of 10 min.

The nanocomposite exhibited high electrochemical activity for electro-catalytic oxidation of glucose as a non-enzymatic biosensor with a linear range of 0.2–10 mM, correlation coefficient of 0.9897 at detection potential of 0.4 V (Figure 8.2). This range is nearly insusceptible to common electro active interfering species of AA, UA, DA, etc. Chen et al. did the use of same Pd NPs-FCNTs-NF modified electrode Pd nanoparticle with CNT support for electrochemical detection of glucose bio-analytes (2010). Direct glucose oxidation on the modified electrode was investigated using CV and amperometry methods with a linear concentration range of glucose (0–46 mM) with a sensitivity of 11.4 $\mu A\ cm^{-2}\ ml\ mol^{-1}$. The oxidation of glucose at 0.40 V in the presence of 0.2 M NaCl and showed excellent resistance for interfering species as AA, UA. Again Chen et al. did the use of same Pd nanoparticle without GN support for electrochemical detection of glucose bio-analytes (2016). The synthesized material, Pd NPs-PDDA-TiO_2 NTs/GCE was electrochemically treated with H_2SO_4 and NaOH and the glucose oxidation current at –0.05 V in the presence of 0.1 M NaCl. The hold here was the most efficient to showed excellent resistance toward interference poisoning from interfering species such as AA, UA, and urea. In a similar fashion, Lu et al. have developed Pd NPs/Nafion/RGO/GCE by an *in-situ* method using hydrazine hydrate as reducing agent for non-enzymatic glucose sensor. This fabricated electrode shown a very high electrochemical activity for electrocatalytic oxidation of glucose in alkaline condition with a wide linear range covering from 10 μM to 5 mM (R = 0.998) with a low LOD limit of 1 μM. The experiment exhibits good reproducibility and long-term stability with high selectivity with noninterference with other competing bio-analytes (Lu et al., 2011). In another report, Cheng et al. used palladium NPs/reduce graphene oxide (Pd/RGO) nanocomposite and explored its bio-sensor application (2012).

By using the ecofriendly hydrazine as a reducing agent, they prepared the reduced GN oxide with simultaneously accomplished from the reduction of dispersed solution of $PdCl_2$. The fabricated nanocomposite exhibits high electrocatalytic activities towards the oxidation of H_2O_2 with a short response time (3 s), high sensitivity (14.1 μA/mM), and low detection limit (0.034 mM) and good stability under the optimized experimental conditions. In addition, due to the lower potential value, the catalytic ability of the presence of Pd NPs shows no inference tests.

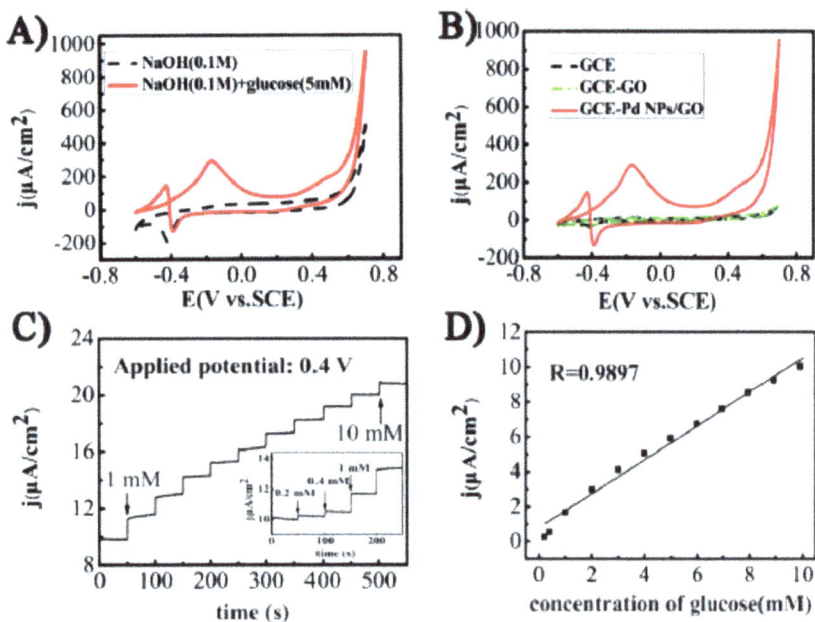

FIGURE 8.2 (A) CV of Pd NPs/GN (reaction time: 15 min; volume ratio of GO and Pd 20:1) modified electrode in 0.1 M NaOH solution with and without 5 mM glucose. (B) CVs of GC electrode, GO modified GCE and Pd NPs/GO/GCE in a 5 mm glucose solution with 0.1 NaOH. Scan rate: 10 mV s^{-1}. (C) Typical current density time dynamic response of as-synthesized Pd NPs/Go-Nafion modified GCE towards successive addition of 1 mM glucose in NaOH (0.1 m) at 0.4 V, the right inset is amplified curve. (D) The calibration curve for glucose detection.

Source: Reproduced with permission from: Wang et al. (2012). © Royal Chemical Society.

Subsequently, Wu et al. did the experiment by Pt NPs supported on GN NPs for non-enzymatic detection of glucose bio-analytes (2013). The synthesized platinum nano-flowers supported on graphene oxide

(Pt NFs-GO) using a nontoxic, rapid, Low-cost green solvent ethanol for the reductant. Here 2D carbon material-GO nanosheet played as the stabilizing material. The modified electrode exhibited strong and sensitive amperometry responses to glucose within 5 seconds. The optimal detection potential hold at 0.47 V vs. calomel electrode caused no interference effects for AA and UA analytes. The Pt NFs-GO modified electrode performed a two-current response at a broad concentration range from 2 mM to 20.3 mM with correlation coefficient 0.9968 and at 10.3 mM to 20.3 mM with a sensitivity of 0.64 mA mM^{-1} cm^{-2} with correlation coefficient 0.9969. The modified electrode was investigated both using voltammetric and amperometry methods with a very accurate LOD of 2 mM was lower than many non-enzymatic electrochemical glucose sensors. This value may be owing to its highly active surface area and the synergistic effect of the GO and Pt NFs. The proposed no enzymatic sensor provided good reproducibility for glucose determination in real samples such as glucose injection solution. Again the bimetallic work did by Hossain et al. in 2014 give a new blow to the detection of glucose biosensor. The platinum and palladium NPs/RGO electrode exhibited high electrocatalytic activities toward H_2O_2, with a linear range from 0.5 to 8 mM ($R^2 = 0.997$) and high sensitivity of 814×10^{-6} A/mM cm^2. Furthermore, on drop-casting glucose oxidase (GO_x) with active material on the RGO/PdPt NPs surface the as-prepared biosensor showed good amperometry response to glucose in the linear range from 2 mM to 12 mM, with a sensitivity of 24×10^{-6} A/mM cm^2, a low detection limit of 0.001 mM, and a short response time (5 s).

On a recent report, AuNPs decorated on GN applied for electrochemical ultrasensitive glucose biosensor. This synthesized process avoids complicated polymer-transfer processes of GN and affords AuNPs (Yuan et al., 2019). The improved electrochemical performance may be due to the low background current of single-layer GN-supported AuNPs. The sensor has a wider detection range of 0.1 nM to 5 mM with a lower detection limit of 0.1 nM, good storage and operational stability, anti-interference capability.

8.3.3 ASCORBIC ACID (AA) BIOSENSOR

Ascorbic acid (AA), known as vitamin C plays an important role in the human body as a biological protector to the human cells. It acts as a reducing agent, antioxidant for the protection of the human body against to side effects of the oxidation process. In addition, AA also involved in the cell development, bone-cartilage, and as an effective agent for the prevention and treatment of various diseases, including cancer, mental illness, AIDS, infertility, activities of living structures such as blood vessels synthesis and healing of burns and wounds (Tsai et al., 2012; Zhu et al., 2018). So the selective and sensitive detection of bioanalytes is more important, and the topic should be more discussed. On a recent report in 2020, Demirkan et al. have designed the electrodes modified with rGO/ Pd@PPy NPs for the individual AA and simultaneous detection of AA, DA, and UA. The prepared rGO/Pd@PPy NPs on the electrodes exhibited excellent electrocatalytic performance, good stability and a wide linear concentration range 1×10^{-3} to 1.5×10^{-2} M and LOD value 4.9×10^{-8} M (Demirkan et al., 2020).

Apart from this, the detection of AA in biological samples such as blood sample, urine, saliva for the safety of human being for a healthy society is a challenged matter. An increase or decrease in concentration from the permit able level of AA in human sample caused for different health issues. In a recent report, Pichaimuthu et al. developed non-enzymatic Silver nanoparticle-supported on GN oxide (Ag NPs-GO) nanocomposite for the detection of AA in Human Urine Sample by electrochemical method (2018).

From the characterization data, the spherical shape Ag NPs size was from 50–60 nM and the presence of C, O, and Ag on the surface of RGO clearly made the more electronic synergic increase in electrocatalytic value (Figure 8.3). The real sample analysis by Ag NP-GO electrode in human urine and vitamin c tablet was found that the recovery results observed ranged between 98.5% and 96.7%, respectively. Hence the result proved that the fabricate electrode Ag NPs-GO acts as a simple, inexpensive better transducer electrode for real sample analysis. The fabricated sensor showed the LOD value of 25 nM, with a sensitivity of 1.71 μA mM^{-1} cm^{-2} ($R^2 = 0.9967$) in the linear range of 1–210 μM.

In another work, Kumar et al. made an excellent experiment by fabricating platinum NPs decorated on graphene (GPt NPs) nanocomposite toward the electrochemical determination of AA. From the CV experiment determination of AA exhibited linearity range from 300 mM to 20.89 mM and exhibited low detection limits of 300 μM (Kumar et al., 2019). Apart from the GN supported, ongoing through the recent reports, carbon nanotube (CNT) supported NPs also were employed for the detection of AA by electrochemical method. But the linear range and LOD value shows not good result on comparing to GN-supported NPs. Though in 2014, GN

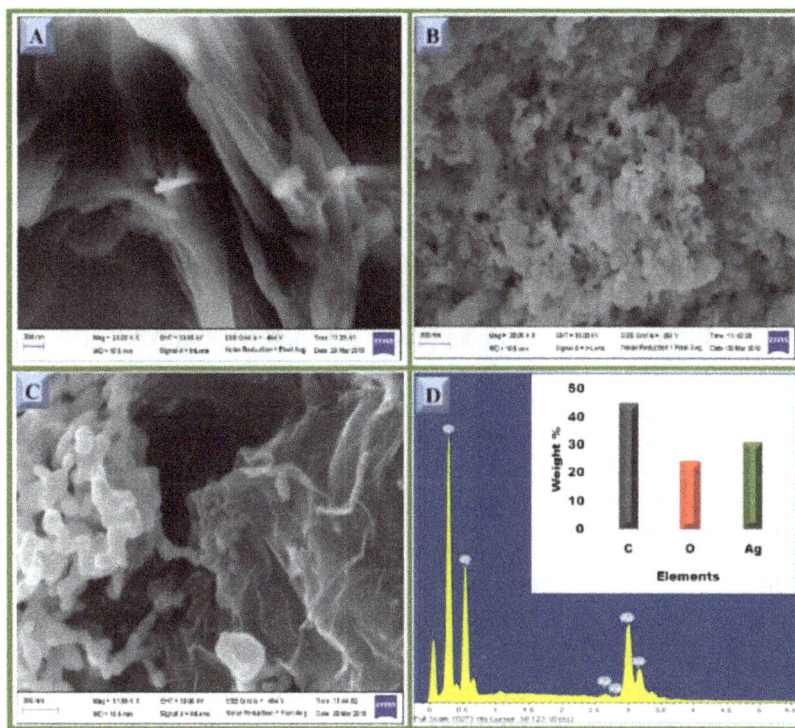

FIGURE 8.3 (A) FESEM image of GO; (B, C) Ag NPs-GO nanocomposite; (D) EDX spectra of nanocomposite.

Source: Reproduced with permission from: Pichaimuthu et al. (2018). © 2018 The Authors. Published by ESG (www.electrochemsci.org) (http://creativecommons.org/licenses/by/4.0/).

has made its own identity on electrocatalytic application still Filik et al. did a sensitivity detection of AA by using AuNPs (2015). The proposed sensor was made by multi-walled CNTs/AuNP composites (Nafion/AuNPs/MWCNTs) for the simultaneous determination of AA, DA, UA, and tryptophan by electrochemical sensor. The modified electrode showed excellent electrocatalytic activity toward AA oxidation and results showed from CV, the linear response range 300–10,000 lM, and the detection limits were 16 lM, (S/N= 3). The proposed and fabricated electrode promises for simple, rapid, selective, and cost-effective analysis of AA. As the glucose and hydrogen peroxide, AA detection by bi-metallic also carried out for its detection. The morphology of both NPs co-relates to enhancing the electronic enlarged the sensing area and increased the sensitivity of the electrode. The morphology featured of Ni-Pt electrode caused for high sensitivity and reliability in this study. The crystallization nature of the Ni-Pt alloy was able to sense AA by oxidation resulted from charge transfer from Pt rather than from Ni. The Pt/Ni alloy electrode exhibited sensitivity of 333 μA cm^{-2} mM^{-1} for AA sensing. This electrode was tested for reproducibility of the sensitivity by storage stability, operational stability, endurance, and no interference experiment (Weng et al., 2011). Jo et al. also synthesized another bi-metallic electrode for detection of AA (2014). They reported a new fabricated electrode hollow Au/Ru nano-shells for non-enzymatic amperometric detection of AA. The hollow structure of Au-Ru electrode exhibits catalytic activities and showed sensitivity of 426 μA mM^{-1} cm^{-2}, linear dynamic range of <5 μM to 2 mM AA at physiological pH. The LOD was 2.2 μM with response time 1.6 s. Furthermore, the Au-Ru/GC electrode displayed no interference taste including glucose, UA, DA. Overall, the hollow Au-Ru nano-shells possessed a potential candidate material for a non-enzymatic AA sensor.

In addition Pt NPs show excellent electrocatalytic activity toward AA bio-sensing. Sun et al. studied on GN/Pt-modified GC electrode nanocomposite and size of Pt nanoparticle with a mean diameter of 1.7 nm (2011). In comparison to the protentional of CV data, results the use of the GN/Pt nanocomposite is essential to the distinguishing of other bioanalytes like UA, glucose, and hydrogen peroxide. The observed detection limits for AA was 0.15 μM, in amperometry current-time measurements. An optimized adsorption of size-selected Pt colloidal NPs on the GN surface results in a good platform for the routine analysis of AA, DA, and UA (Sun et al., 2011). Wu et al. studied on electrochemical detection of AA sensor on a GC electrode modified with palladium NPs supported on GN oxide (Pd NPs-GO) (2012). From TEM, HRTEM data Pd NPs with a mean diameter of 2.6 nm were homogeneously deposited on GO. From the CV and amperometry, the potential hold at 0.006 V for Pd NPs-GO modified electrode exhibited a rapid response to AA within 5 s and a broad range from 20 μM to 2.28 mM with a correlation coefficient of R = 0.9991. Moreover, the proposed sensor was applied to the real sample analysis of AA in vitamin C tablet samples. In addition, the fabricated electrode proposed the no interference taste with other bioanalytes and the sensor was promising for the AA determination (Wu et al., 2012). Wang et al. also studied on Pd NPs for AA detection on GN support carbon materials (2013). The fabricated Pd NPs/GR/GCE electrode displayed excellent electrochemical catalytic activities towards AA with no inference taste with DA and UA. The peak potential at 252 mV for AA having limits of detection (S/N = 3) of 20 μM showed many merits insensitivity, facility, and economy.

8.3.4 DOPAMINE (DA) BIOSENSOR

DA (3, 4-dihydroxyphenylalanine) plays an important biological role in human metabolism, cardiovascular, signal transmissions to the brain, central nervous, renal, and hormonal systems (Kim et al., 2018). The normal concentration of DA is between 10 and 1000 nM L^{-1} (Fazio et al., 2018; Owesson et al., 2012). Deviation in concentration to this level can lead to many disorders in the human body such as schizophrenia, hypertension, and attention deficit hyperactivity disorder (ADHD) (Seeman, 1980; How et al., 2014). Therefore, the detection of DA in a biological sample has become a more research interest today. As like the AA, Glucose, and hydrogen peroxide, the detection of bioanalytes by most used NPs such as Pt, Pd, Au, bimetallic Pt-Au, etc., also employed for sensitivity and selectivity detection of DA bioanalytes. In a recent report, Park et al. synthesized RGO sheet/Au by spin coating rGS on a bare gold electrode (2017). The detection of DA by electrochemical sensor with modified electrode of RGO sheet (rGS)-AuNPs complexes to within a range of 0.1–100 μM and the LOD was 0.098 μM. More amazing fact was that, this sensor method showed quite an accurate linear range similar to the *in vivo* DA level. And hence this developed neurotransmitter fabricated sensing system could be useful to integrate *in vivo* implant to control the accurate location inside the brain for detection of neuronal disease.

In a recent report, though GN acts a best supporting carbon-based materials to enhance the electrocatalytic activity, still in a very recent report in 2019, an electrochemical sensor based on modification of the AuNPs was fabricated with Nafion (NF), β-cyclodextrin (CD) for the determination of DA in biological fluids. The catalytic activity of the sensor with NF, β-cyclodextrin (CD), enhances the electron transfer rate and was achieved determination of DA in real urine samples in a range 0.05–280 μM with a low detection limit of 0.6 nM (Atta et al., 2019). Here the synergy existed between AuNPs, β-CD and NF, facilitated surface pre-concentration of DA by ion selectivity and accumulation of DA in the hydrophilic regions (which played as a host-guest inclusion complex with

DA) enhanced the electron-transfer kinetics. Liu et al. also used AuNPs without the GN support studied the DA detection (2019). They synthesized Ag@C core-shell with AuNPs by one-pot hydrothermal method on Au NPs *in situ* reduction process. The electrochemical investigations indicated that Ag@C/Au nanocomposite possessed intriguing properties towards DA. The synergistic effect of Ag@C with enhanced substrate accessibility and conductivity attributed with surface of negative charges. Furthermore, the electrochemical sensor showed a wider liner range was 0.5 µM to 27.5 µM, with detection limit was 0.21 µM (S/N = 3) and a favorable selectivity in the presence of interferents such as AA and UA and glucose. In general, the work could provide a promising possibility to develop excellent electrochemical sensors for DA detection. But that LOD value could able to showed better result than gold with GN supported.

For detection of DA, silver nanoparticle supported with GN oxide also employed for the enhanced electrochemical detection of DA. For the first time, shin et al. fabricated silver nanoparticle (SNP) supported by GN oxide and the most interestingly, the surface of indium tin oxide (ITO) electrode was modified using SNPs and then followed by GN oxide through the electrochemical deposition method (2017). This technique showed the amperometry (i-t) DA concentrations ranging from 10 µM to 100 µM and LOD value of 0.2 µM. This newly developed biosensor could provide a method to monitor neurological diseases through electrochemical signal enhancement at low DA concentrations. In the current year, silver-platinum GN nanocomposite modified electrode suggest a new research idea for the electrochemical detection of DA. From the TEM image, the GN sheets were decorated with small spherical Ag and Pt NPs of approx. size of Pt, Ag is 6.50 nm and 4.0 nm, respectively. The small size of the NPs on GN support plays a significant role in the sensitivity detection of NPs. The platinum-silver graphene (Pt-Ag/Gr) nanocomposite modified electrode were performed by CV and differential pulse voltammetry (DPV) study. The synergistic effects between the platinum-silver NPs and GN showed the enhanced electrocatalytic activity towards DA oxidation of a linear concentration range between 0.1 and 60 mM with a LOD of 0.012 mM. The Pt-Ag/Gr/GCE showed satisfactory reproducibility, stability, and selectivity performance for DA. Another bimetallic in the previous year shows also excellent electrocatalytic highly activity for DA sensor based on Pt-Au supported with the most interestingly excellent and most dominating, laser-induced graphene (LIG)/poly dimethyl siloxane (PDMS)

(Hui et al., 2019). The fabricated Pt-AuNPs/LIG electrode sensor showed a sensitivity value of approximately 865.80 µA/mM cm² and LOD of 75 nM. The current peaks at 0.11 V caused for no interference taste for other bioanalytes like AA, glucose, UA, etc. Not only the noble metal nanostructures, but also the non-noble metal nanostructures like molybdenum (Mo) NPs on supported with multi walled carbon nanotube exhibited DA detection. Keerthi et al. reported novel Mo NPs on self-supported with multi walled CNTs nanomaterials for electrochemical DA detection and clearly explained the electrochemical detection of neurotransmitter in biological sample (Figure 8.4).

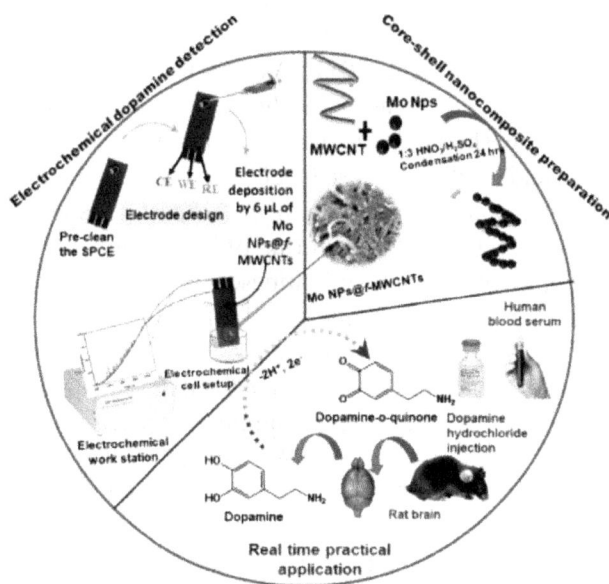

FIGURE 8.4 Schematic representations for the preparation of core-shell Mo NPs@ MWCNT hybrid nanocomposite and its electrochemical detection of neurotransmitter in biological sample.

Source: Reproduced with permission from: Keerthi et al. (2019). © Springer Nature.

The MoNPs@*f*-MWCNTs hybrid material possesses tremendous superiority in the DA detection. The fabricated electrode having NPs range with an average diameter of 40–45 nm was be the best developed for DA biosensor with amazing LOD value 1.26 nM, excellent linear response of 0.01 µM to 1609 µM with good sensitivity of 4.925 µA µM^{-1} cm^{-2}.

This LOD value was the lowest till ever, and the linear range of such small-sized NPs would consider as the best materials for electrochemical detection of DA. This sample employed for the real sample analysis of rat brain, human blood serum attracts more research interest for this (Keerthi et al., 2019).

8.3.5 NITRITE BIOSENSOR

Nitrite generally used as a preservative, dyeing agent, fertilizer, and food additive (gives the cured products and their characteristic red color and flavor) in our daily life. Nitrites can interact with amines to form carcinogenic nitrosamines, which oxidize hemoglobin to methemoglobin (Li et al., 2014; Calfuman et al., 2011). As we know methemoglobin causes the methemoglobinemia disease. And hence the technology of accurate detection of nitrite should be a matter of attention for public health, environmental, and food industries. Quantitative analysis of nitrite (NO^{2-}) has becoming more attracted attention in the past decades and reliable methods for the detection and monitoring of it. Among several techniques such as spectrophotometry, chemiluminescence, spectrofluorimetry, and electrochemical methods are employed for detecting nitrite (Pourreza et al., 2012; Lin et al., 2011; Azad et al., 2014; Yuan et al., 2014; Afkhami et al., 2014). However, each have their own advantage and disadvantage like using toxic reagents, requiring time-consuming sample preparation process, and suffering of interference-effect. Among them, the electrochemical method has considered as the more attractive method due to low cost, low detection limit and high accuracy (Rocha et al., 2002; Fu et al., 2014).

In current years, metal NPs and metal oxide NPs have been used to detect nitrite, such as Au, Pd, Ag, Fe_3O_4, Fe_2O_3 and so on (Jiang et al., 2014; Zhang et al., 2013; Qin et al., 2013; Absalan et al., 2015; Radhakrishnan et al., 2014). All have advantages of improvement of the mass transport, outstanding catalytic performance, unique size, high effective surface area, and biocompatibility (Liu et al., 2017; Thanh et al., 2016). Among all palladium NPs due to relatively low cost, high electrocatalytic activity and chemical inertness to oxygen and moisture have most widely used (Pham et al., 2014). Fu et al. fabricated a novel and sensitive electrochemical nitrite sensor Pd NPs and reduced GN oxide supported on a glassy carbon electrode (GCE) (2015). Moreover, the agglomeration of RGO prevented due to the incorporation of Pd in between RGO sheets effectively. The Pd/

RGO modified electrode exhibited significant the more oxidation of nitrite with increased current response due to synergistic catalytic effect of RGO and Pd NPs. The developed nitrite sensor showed excellent selectivity, reproducibility, and stability and had a linear response in the concentration range of 1–1000 μM with LOD value of 0.23 μM. The oxidation peak potentials of G/Pd/RGO were measured to be 0.829 V. This potential is the more negative potential range in comparison with G/Pd and only RGO. Moreover, the shift of anodic peak to a more negative potential and the higher current response concludes that the G/Pd/RG is an effective promoter for electrochemical process of nitrite. The constructed sensor is highly selective for nitrite determination, with excellent non-interference test experiment, repeatability, and more stability. In another report, Pd NPs fabricated by cobalt phthalocyanine (Pd/CoPc) followed by using a facile methanol-mediated method (Song et al., 2017). Pd/CoPc/GC used for a sensitive and selective electrochemical nitrate sensor. Cobalt phthalocyanines are two-dimensional (2D) organic macrocyclic molecular catalysts similar to porphyrin exhibits excellent electronic and optical property (Sorokin et al., 2013). The spherical Pd particles of 4–6 nm exhibited enhanced electrocatalytic behavior in comparing to commercial activated carbon-supported palladium. The fabricated sensor exhibits the excellent electrocatalytic performance for nitrite in linear range from 0.2 to 50 μM and from 500 to 5000 μM with a low detection limit of 0.10 μM nitrite and a sensitivity of 0.01 μA μM^{-1} (S/N = 3). Moreover, compared with the other reported values previously on nitrite-based sensor, the Pd/CoPc/GCE exhibits a better electrocatalytic activity excellent detection of nitrite and would be a promising material in fabricating sensors for nitrite of food.

8.3.6 URIC ACID (UA) BIOSENSOR

Uric acid (UA, $C_5H_4N_4O_3$) is another important and antioxidant biological analytes present in our body fluids as an end-product of metabolism process of the purine nucleotide and imbalance in percentage levels of UA (i.e., 0.1–0.4 mM in blood and 1.5–4.4 mM in urine) can cause the several diseases such as gout, kidney diseases, hypertension, and cardiovascular diseases (Arora et al., 2011; Sun et al., 2011; Ping et al., 2012). These facts caused thus making it important to monitor UA regularly. In the current year 2020, electrochemically sensors based on without use of NPs on GN supported surface but nitrogen-doped reduced GN oxide used for detection of UA blow a more research interest on it. GN-based materials have caused for high surface area, high chemical stability, and unique electronic and mechanical properties and hence show immense prospects in the field's sensors. Introduction of heteroatoms such as N, B, P, S into surface matrix of GN could able to tunable high conducting properties since bonding configurations in carbon with nitrogen play an important role in physical and chemical properties of N-doped GN. Zhang et al. fabricated nitrogen-doped GN for UA sensor (2020). The characterization data revealed the presence of nitrogen in GN sheet also shows the reduction of GN oxide to GN. This sample showed good sensing performances for detection of UA in the linear ranges of 1 mM–30 mM with LOD value 0.2 mM. This work provides a highly effective approach for the preparation of GN-based materials for electrochemical sensing applications. Nowadays, synthesis of nanocomposite by greenway mechanism has been becoming main motto in the research field. The 12 principles of green chemistry will make our society a more and hygienic one day. For example, $NaBH_4$ acts a best reducing agent for reduction of NPs (from its cationic form to neutral form) and also GN oxide but it has more adverse effect to the society. On replacing this hazardous reducing agent, rutin, a tree extract, and Phyllanthus acids, a fruit extract adopted for the same purpose.

Recently, Nayak et al. did a green synthesis of silver NPs with reduced GN oxide (Ag-rGO) nanocomposite for electrocatalytic activity towards oxidation of UA by using the aqueous fruit extract of *Phyllanthus acidus* in basic medium as a reducing agent and also as a good stabilizing agent. The Ag-rGO modified electrode produced almost four times higher anodic current compared to a bare GCE with a narrow linear range from a concentration 10–130 μM (R^2 = ¼ 0.9896) with potential value 0.27 V (Ag@AgCl electrode) and detection limit of 1 μM (S/N = 3). This simple, highly specific and economical to obtain improved results, modification to the surface of electrodes is very essential. For this, materials prepared using green methods are being explored to a great extent since the process is cost-effective and environment friendly. This prepared electrode in greenway shows best selectivity, stability, and reproducibility towards sensing UA. Pang et al. developed a simple strategy to construct of gold nano-clusters (Au NCs) and quantum dots (QDs) (2019). Here they used bovine serum albumin-capped Au NCs for the stabilizers to prepare CdS QDs. The synthesized bovine serum albumin-capped Au NCs and CdS QDs nanohybrid (BSA-Au NCs/QDs) displayed with the linear range from 0.67

to 60 μmol L^{-1} and the detection limit of 0.21 μmol L^{-1}. In a recent report, Immanuel et al. reported an electrochemical biosensor based on Au-SiO$_2$ nanocomposite for the detection of UA (2019). The nanocomposite was prepared by a simple wet chemical process and CV was used to assess the electrocatalytic response of Au-SiO$_2$/GCE towards UA detection. The detection of DA and UA was performed linear ranges from 200 μM–500 μM and detection limit of 2.58 μM. The detection of UA was carried out which showed a peak of 215 mV. The sensor showed excellent sensitivity for DA and UA with good stability and reproducibility and further for UA in serum sample analysis with satisfactory recovery values (Jaina et al., 2019). Though GN was used for detection of UA still Aryal et al. used CNF with reduced graphite oxide (rGO) for detection of UA simultaneously with AA, DA also (2020). The electrode material was prepared with CNF modified with rGO, for electrochemical detection of AA, DA, and UA. The modified electrode displayed oxidation peaks of UA at 0.32 V with DPV with sensitivities of 0.14 μA/μM. The modified CNF-RGO electrode was investigated showed excellent performances and attributed to large electrochemical active surface area and increased reactivity obtained from synergic effect of CNF and RGO. The synthesis of modified CNFRGO electrode was very simple and easy and expected that modified electrode could be applied for biosensor application tremendously.

In addition to Pd, Pt, Ag, and Au NPs for electrocatalytic activity Cu$_2$ZnSnS$_4$ (CZTS) NPs films have been proposed as a novel material for enzyme-based electrochemical biosensors (Jaina et al., 2019). This nanoparticle provides a non-toxic, low-cost alternative for the other NPs due to its tunability of the bandgap of CZTS by varying the cation ratio and size of NPs enables to possess desirable electrical properties electro-chemical analyzes. The modified uricase/CZTS/ITO/glass electrode with spherical CZTS NPs of size 15–16 nm and bandgap 2.65 eV exhibits good linearity over a wide range of 0–700 μM with a LOD of 0.066 μM. Thus, this report confirms the promising application for an electrochemical biosensor.

8.4 CONCLUSION

Electrochemical bio-sensing has been one of the most interested topics in the biological entities for a healthy environment. Different carbon-based materials with their unique properties, ranging from CNTs, nanorods (NRs), and nano-wires, have been analyzed and compared with the most attracting GN for electrochemical biosensor applications. This chapter highlights the importance of electrochemical biosensor than other techniques and developed a most demanding method. GN, with its unusual properties, makes an ideal platform for fabricating a series of GN-based functional nanomaterials for biosensors. We have highlighted GN with various NPs, and their different shaped hybrids structures can bring synergistic advantages to a wide variety of electrochemical biosensor applications with minimize costs and lead to its commercialization. Hopefully, this book chapter will inspire various disciplines that will benefit from the development of GN-nanoparticle hybrids for biosensor applications.

ACKNOWLEDGMENTS

One of the author's PM acknowledges financial support from Science and Engineering Research Board (SERB), Department of Science and Technology (DST), Government of India, New Delhi, vide File No. EMR/2016/003370 under EMR Scheme.

KEYWORDS

- ascorbic acid
- biosensor
- carbon nanotube
- glucose
- graphene
- hydrogen peroxide
- nanoparticles
- nitrate
- uric acid

REFERENCES

Absalan, G., Akhond, M., Bananejad, A., & Ershadifar, H., (2015). Green synthesis of Pd/Fe$_3$O$_4$ composite based on poly DOPA functionalized reduced graphene oxide for electrochemical detection of nitrite in cured food. *J. Iran Chem. Soc., 12*, 1293–1301.

Afkhami, A., Soltani-Felehgari, F., Madrakian, T., & Ghaedi, H., (2014). A modified carbon paste electrode based on Fe$_3$O$_4$@multi-walled carbon nanotubes@polyacrylonitrile nanofibers for determination of imatinib anticancer drug. *Biosensors and Bioelectronics, 51*, 379–385.

Allen, M. J., Tung, V. C., & Kaner, B. R., (2010). Honeycomb carbon: A review of graphene. *Chem. Rev., 110*, 132–145.

Arora, K., Tomar, M., & Gupta, V., (2011). Highly sensitive and selective uric acid biosensor based on RF sputtered NiO thin film. *Biosensors and Bioelectronics, 30*, 333–336.

Aryal, K. P., & Jeong, H. K., (2020). Carbon nanofiber modified with reduced graphite oxide for detection of ascorbic acid, dopamine, and uric acid. *Chemical Physics Letters, 739*, 136969.

Atta, N. F., & Galal, A., (2019). Novel design of a layered electrochemical dopamine sensor in real samples based on gold nanoparticles/β-cyclodextrin/Nafion modified gold electrode. *ACS Omega, 4*, 17947–17955.

Azad, U. P., Turllapati, S., Rastogi, P. K., & Ganesan, V., (2014). Tris (1, 10-phenanthroline) iron(II)-bentonite film as efficient electrochemical sensing platform for nitrite determination. *Electrochimica Acta, 127*, 193–199.

Bahmani, B., Moztarzadeh, F., Rabiee, M., & Tahriri, M., (2010). Rotating ring-disk enzyme electrode for surface catalysis studies. *Synthetic Metals, 160*, 2653–2657.

Behera, T. K., Sahu, S. C., Satpati, B., Bag, B. P., Sanjay, K., & Jena, B. K., (2016). Branched platinum nanostructures on reduced graphene: An excellent transducer for nonenzymatic sensing of hydrogen peroxide and biosensing of xanthine,. *Electrochimica Acta, 206*, 238–245.

Behera, T. K., Satpathy, P. K., & Mohapatra, P., (2018). *Nanoparticles: Excellent Transducer for Electrochemical Biosensor* (Vol. 1, pp. 215–249). Arcler Publishing. ISBN 978-1-77361-539-4.

Behera, T. K., Satpathy, P. K., & Mohapatra, P., (2019). *Methanol and Formic Acid Oxidation: Selective Fuel Cell Processes*. Apple Academic Press (AAP), Inc., Canada, a Taylor & Francis Group, ISBN hard: 978-1-77188-885-1.

Calfumán, M., Aguirre, J., Cañete-Rosales, P., Bollo, L. R., & Isaacs, M., (2011). Electrochemical reduction of nitrite and nitric oxide catalyzed by an iron-alizarin complex one adsorbed on a graphite electrode. *Electrochimica Acta, 56*, 8484–8491.

Chen, X., Gang, L., Zhang, G., Houb, K., Pan, H., & Du, M., (2016). Applications of hierarchically structured porous materials from energy storage and conversion, catalysis, photocatalysis, adsorption, separation, and sensing to biomedicine. *Materials Science and Engineering C, 62*, 323–328.

Cheng, N., Wang, H., Li, X., Yang, X., & Zhu, L., (2012). Single-, few-, and multilayer graphene not exhibiting significant advantages over graphite microparticles in electro-analysis. *American Journal of Analytical Chemistry, 3*, 312–319.

Demirkan, B., Bozkurt, S., & Cellat, K., (2020). Palladium supported on polypyrrole/ reduced graphene oxide nanoparticles for simultaneous biosensing application of ascorbic acid, dopamine, and uric acid. *Sci. Rep., 10*, 2946.

Fang, Y., Guo, S., Zhu, C., Dong, S., & Wang, E., (2010). Synthesis of graphene-supported noble metal hybrid nanostructures and their applications as advanced electrocatalysts for fuel cells. *Langmuir, 26*, 17816–17820.

Filik, H., Aslıhan, A., & Asiye, A., (2016). Photosensitized growth of silver nanoparticles under visible light irradiation: A mechanistic investigation. *Arabian Journal of Chemistry, 9*, 471–780.

Fu, L., Lai, G., Mahon, P., Wang, J., Zhu, D., Jia, B., Malherbe, F., & Yu, A., (2014). Electrodeposition of Au nanoparticles on poly(diallyl dimethylammonium chloride) functionalized reduced graphene oxide sheets for voltammetric determination of nicotine in tobacco products and anti-smoking pharmaceuticals. *RSC Advances, 4*, 39645–39650.

Fu, L., Shuhong, Y., Thompson, L., & Yu, A., (2015). Development of a novel nitrite electrochemical sensor by stepwise in situ formation of palladium and reduced graphene oxide nanocomposites. *RSC Adv., 5,* 40111–40116.

Giorgio, F. E., Spadaro, S., & Lavanya, N., (2018). Molybdenum oxide nanoparticles for the sensitive and selective detection of dopamine. *J. Electroanal. Chem., 814*, 91–96.

Guo, S., & Dong, S., (2011). Graphene nanosheet: Synthesis, molecular engineering, thin-film, hybrids, and energy and analytical applications. *Chem. Soc. Rev., 40*, 2644–2672.

Guo, S., & Wang, E. (2011). Functional micro/nanostructures: Simple synthesis and application in sensors, fuel cells, and gene delivery. *Acc. Chem. Res., 44*, 491–500.

Guo, S., & Wang, E., (2011). Noble metal nanomaterials: Controllable synthesis and application in fuel cells and analytical sensors. *Nano Today, 6*, 240–264.

Haun, J. B., Yoon, T. J., Lee, H., & Weissleder, R., (2010). Magnetic nanoparticle biosensors. *Nanomed. Nanobiotechnol., 2*, 291.

Hazhir, T., Abdollah, S., & Somayeh, K., (2013). Fe_3O_4 magnetic nanoparticles/reduced graphene oxide nanosheets as a novel electrochemical and bio-electrochemical sensing platform. *Biosensors and Bioelectronics, 49*, 1–8.

Hossain, M. F., & Jae, Y., (2014). Amperometric glucose biosensor based on Pt-Pd nanoparticles supported by reduced graphene oxide and integrated with glucose oxidase. *Electroanalysis, 26*, 940–951.

How, G. T. S., Pandikumar, A., Ming, H. N., & Ngee, L. H., (2014). Highly exposed {001} facets of titanium dioxide modified with reduced graphene oxide for dopamine sensing. *Sci. Rep., 4*, 5044.

Hui, X., Xuan, X., Kim, J., & Park, J. Y., (2019). Solid-state ion recognition strategy using 2D hexagonal mesophase silica monolithic platform: A smart two-in-one approach for rapid and selective sensing of Cd^{2+} and Hg^{2+} ions. *Electrochimica Acta, 328*, 135066.

Immanuel, S., Aparna, T. K., & Sivasubramanian, R., (2019). Graphene-based electrochemical sensors for biomolecules. *Micro and Nano Technologies*, 113–138.

Jaina, S., Verma, S., Singh, S. P., & Sharma, S. N., (2019). An electrochemical biosensor based on novel butylamine capped CZTS nanoparticles immobilized by uricase for uric acid detection. *Biosensors and Bioelectronics, 127*(15), 135–141.

Jiang, J. J., Fan, W. J., & Du, X. Z., (2014). Electrochemical synthesis of gold nanoparticles decorated flower-like graphene for high sensitivity detection of nitrite. *Biosens. Bioelectron., 51*, 343–348.

Jo, A., Kang, M., Cha, A., Jang, H. S., Shim, J. H., Lee, N. S., Kim, M. H., et al., (2014). An efficient electrochemical sensor driven by hierarchical hetero-nanostructures consisting of RuO_2 nanorods on WO_3 nanofibers for detecting biologically relevant molecules. *Analytica Chimica Acta, 819*, 94–101.

Keerthi, M., Boopathy, G., Chen, S. M., Chen, T. W., & Lou, B. S., (2019). A core-shell molybdenum nanoparticles entrapped f-MWCNTs hybrid nanostructured material based non-enzymatic biosensor for electrochemical detection of dopamine neurotransmitter in biological samples. *Sci. Rep., 9*, 13075.

Kim, D., Kang, E., Seungho, B., Sung, S., Yong, H., Donghyun, L., & Junhong, M., (2018). Electrochemical detection of dopamine using periodic cylindrical gold nanoelectrode arrays. *Sci. Rep., 8*, 14049.

Kuila, T., Bose, S., Khanra, P., Mishra, A. K., Kim, N. H., & Lee, J. H., (2011). Recent advances in graphene-based biosensor technology with applications in life sciences. *Biosensor. and Bioelectronics, 26*, 4637.

Kumar, M. A., Lakshminarayanan, V., & Ramamurthy, S. S., (2019). Platinum nanoparticles-decorated graphene-modified glassy carbon electrode toward the electrochemical determination of ascorbic acid, dopamine, and paracetamol. *Comptes Rendus Chimie, 22*(1), 58–72.

Lee, C. S., Kim, S. K., & Kim, M., (2009). Ion-sensitive field-effect transistor for biological sensing. *Sensors, 9*, 7111.

Li, M. Y., Zhao, G. Q., Yue, Z. L., & Huang, S. S., (2009). A third-generation hydrogen peroxide biosensor based on horseradish peroxidase cross-linked to multi-wall carbon nanotubes. *Microchim. Acta, 167*, 167.

Li, Y., Wang, H., Liu, X., Guo, L., Ji, X., Wang, L., Tian, D., & Yang, X., (2014). Nonenzymatic nitrite sensor based on a titanium dioxide nanoparticles/ionic liquid composite electrode. *Journal of Electroanalytical Chemistry, 719*, 35–40.

Lin, W., Xue, H., Chen, J., & Lin, M., (2011). Simple and sensitive fluorescent and electro-chemical trinitrotoluene sensors based on aqueous carbon dots. *Analytical Chemistry, 83*, 8245–8251.

Liu, S., & Guo, X. F., (2012). Carbon nanomaterials field-effect-transistor-based biosensors. *NPG Asia Mater., 4*, 1.

Liu, X., Fu, Y., Sheng, Q., & Zheng, J., (2019). Recent advances in chemiluminescence for reactive oxygen species sensing and imaging analysis. *Microchemical Journal, 146*, 509–516.

Liu, Y., Lei, J., & Ju, H., (2008). Amperometric sensor for hydrogen peroxide-based on electric wire composed of horseradish peroxidase and toluidine blue-multiwalled carbon nanotubes nanocomposite. *Talanta, 74*, 965.

Liu, Z., Xue, Q., & Guo, Y., (2017). Sensitive electrochemical detection of rutin and isoquercitrin based on SH-β-cyclodextrin functionalized graphene-palladium nanoparticles. *Biosensors and Bioelectronics, 89*(1), 444–452.

Lu, L. M., Li, H, B., Qu, F., Zhang, B. X., Shen, L., & Yu, Q., (2011). In situ synthesis of palladium nanoparticle-graphene nanohybrids and their application in nonenzymatic glucose biosensors. *Biosensors and Bioelectronics, 26*, 3500–3504.

Luo, X. L., Morrin, A., Killard, A. J., & Smyth, M. R., (2006). Application of nanoparticles in electrochemical sensors and biosensors. *Electroanalysis, 18*, 319.

Ming-Yan, W., Shen, T., Wang, M., Zhang, D., Tong, Z., & Jun, C., (2014). Fabrication of an Au@SnO_2 core–shell structure for gaseous formaldehyde sensing at room temperature. *Sensors and Actuators B, 190,* 645–650.

Nayak, S. P., Ramamurthy, S. S., & Kumar, J. K., (2020). Green synthesis of silver nanoparticles decorated reduced graphene oxide nanocomposite as an electrocatalytic platform for the simultaneous detection of dopamine and uric acid. *Materials Chemistry and Physics, 252,* 123302.

Owesson, W., Roitman, M. F., & Somber, L. A., (2012). Sources contributing to the average extracellular concentration of dopamine in the nucleus accumbens. *J. Neuro Chem., 121,* 252–262.

Pang, S., (2019). A ratiometric fluorescent probe for detection of uric acid based on the gold nanoclusters-quantum dots nanohybrid. *Spectrochimica Acta Part A: Molecular and Biomolecular Spectroscopy, 222,* 117233.

Park, D. J., Choi, J. H., Lee, W. J., Um, S. H., & Oh, B. K., (2017). Effect of interface roughness on electrical properties of Ag cathode and the role of the LiF layer to organic light-emitting devices. *Nanosci. Nanotechnol., 17,* 11.

Pham, X. H., Li, C. A., Han, K. N., Huynh-Nguyen, B. C., Le, T. H., Ko, E., Kim, J. H., & Seong, G. H. (2014). Electrochemical detection of nitrite using urchin-like palladium nanostructures on carbon nanotube thin-film electrodes. *Sensor Actuat. B Chem., 193,* 815–822.

Pichaimuthu, K., Keerthi, M., Chen, S. M., Chen, T. W., & Su, C., (2018). Silver nanoparticles decorated on graphene oxide sheets for electrochemical detection of ascorbic acid (AA) in human urine sample. *Int. J. Electrochem. Sci., 13,* 7859–7869.

Ping, J., Wu, J., Wang, Y., & Ying, Y., (2012). Simultaneous determination of ascorbic acid, dopamine and uric acid using high-performance screen-printed graphene electrode. *Bioelectronics, 34,* 70–76.

Pingarron, J. M., Yanez-Sedeno, P., & Gonzalez-Cortes, A., (2008). Gold nanoparticle-based electrochemical biosensors. *Electrochim. Acta, 53,* 5848.

Pourreza, N., Fathi, M. R., & Hatami, A., (2012). Colorimetric determination of hydrazine and nitrite using catalytic effect of palladium nanoparticles on the reduction reaction of methylene blue. *Microchemical Journal, 104,* 22–25.

Qin, C., Wang, W., Chen, C., Bu, L. J., Wang, T., Su, X. L., Xie, Q. J., & Yao, S. Z., (2013). Carbon dots prepared for fluorescence and chemiluminescence sensing. *Sensor Actuat. B-Chem., 181,* 375–381.

Radhakrishnan, S., Krishnamoorthy, K., Sekar, C., Wilson, J., & Kim, S. J., (2014). A highly sensitive electrochemical sensor for nitrite detection based on Fe_2O_3 nanoparticles decorated reduced graphene oxide nanosheets. *Appl. Catal. B-Environ., 148,* 22–28.

Rocha, J. R., Angnes, L., Bertotti, M., Araki, K., & Toma, H. E., (2002). Simultaneous determination of acetaminophen and tyrosine using a glassy carbon electrode modified with a tetraruthenated cobalt(II) porphyrin intercalated into a smectite clay. *Analytica Chimica Acta, 452,* 23–28.

Ronkainen, N. J., Halsall, H. B., & Heineman, W. R., (2010). Electrochemical biosensors. *Chem. Soc. Rev., 39,* 1747.

Sahu, S. C., Behera, T. K., Dash, A., Jena, B., Ghosh, & Jena, B. K., (2016). Highly porous Pd nanostructures and reduced graphene hybrids: Excellent electrocatalytic activity towards hydrogen peroxide. *New J. Chem., 40,* 1096–1099.

Sahu, S. C., Samantara, A. K., Dash, A., Juluri, R. R., Sahu, R. K., Mishra, B. K., & Jena, B. K., (2013). Graphene-induced Pd nano dendrites: A high performance hybrid nano electrocatalyst. *Nano Research, 6*, 635–643.

Seeman, P., (1980). Brain dopamine receptors. *Pharmacological Reviews, 32*, 229–313.

Shin, J., Kim, K. J., Yoon, J., Jo, J., El-Said, W. A., & Choi, J. W., (2017). Fabrication of gold/graphene nanostructures modified ITO electrode as highly sensitive electrochemical detection of aflatoxin B1. *Sensors, 17*, 2771.

Song, X., Gao, L., Yamin, L., Mao, L., & Yang, J. H., (2017). A sensitive and selective electrochemical nitrite sensor based on a glassy carbon electrode modified with cobalt phthalocyanine-supported Pd nanoparticles. *Anal. Methods, 9*, 3166–3171.

Sorokin, A. B., (2013). Phthalocyanine metal complexes in catalysis. *Chem. Rev., 113*, 8152–8191.

Sun, C. L., Lee, H. H., Yang, J. M., & Wu, C. C., (2011). The simultaneous electrochemical detection of ascorbic acid, dopamine, and uric acid using graphene/size-selected Pt nanocomposites. *Biosensors and Bioelectronics, 26*, 3450–3455.

Sun, C. L., Leea, H. H., Yanga, J. M., & Wu, C. C., (2011). Sandwich-structured nanoparticles-grafted functionalized graphene-based 3D nanocomposites for high-performance biosensors to detect ascorbic acid biomolecules. *Biosensors and Bioelectronics, 26*, 3450–3455.

Thanh, D., Balamurugan, J., Lee, S. H., Kim, N. H., & Lee, J. H., (2016). A novel hierarchical 3D N-Co-CNT@NG nanocomposite electrode for non-enzymatic glucose and hydrogen peroxide sensing applications. *Biosens. Bioelectron., 85*, 669–678.

Tsai, T. H., Thiagarajan, S., Chen, S. M., & Cheng, C. Y., (2012). Ionic liquid assisted synthesis of nano Pd-Au particles and application for the detection of epinephrine, dopamine and uric acid. *Thin Solid Films, 520*, 3054–3059.

Veerappan, M., Bose, D., Shen-Ming, C., & Ramiah, S., (2014). Direct electrochemistry of myoglobin at reduced graphene oxide-multiwalled carbon nanotubes-platinum nanoparticles nanocomposite and biosensing towards hydrogen peroxide and nitrite. *Biosensors and Bioelectronics, 53*, 420–427.

Wang, Q., Cui, X., Chen, J., Zheng, X., Liu, C., Xue, T., Wang, H., et al., (2012). Well-dispersed palladium nanoparticles on graphene oxide as a non-enzymatic glucose sensor. *RSC Advances, 2*, 6245–6249.

Wang, X., Wu, M., Tang, W., Zhu, Y., Wang, L., Wang, Q., He, P., & Fang, Y., (2013). Facile synthesis of porous bimetallic alloyed Pd/Ag nanoflowers supported on reduced graphene oxide for simultaneous detection of ascorbic acid, dopamine, and uric acid. *Journal of Electroanalytical Chemistry, 695*, 10–16.

Weng, Y. C., Lee, Y. G., Hsiao, Y. L., & Lin, C. Y., (2011). *Electrochimica Acta, 56*, 9937–9945.

Wu, B., Kuang, Y., Zhang, X., & Chen, J., (2011). Noble metal nanoparticles/carbon nanotubes nanohybrids: Synthesis and applications. *Nano Today, 6*, 75–90.

Wu, G., Song, X., Wu, Y., Chen, X., Luo, F., & Chen, X., (2013). Non-enzymatic electrochemical glucose sensor based on platinum nanoflowers supported on graphene oxide. *Talanta, 105*, 379–385.

Wu, G., Wu, Y., Liu, X., Chen, M., & Chen, X., (2012). Methods of non-enzymatic determination of hydrogen peroxide and related reactive oxygen species. *Analytica Chimica. Acta, 745*, 33–37.

Xiao, C., Zhi, L., De, C., Tian, J., Cai, Z., Wang, X., Chen, X., et al., (2010). Biocompatible graphene oxide-based glucose. *Biosensors and Bioelectronics, 25*, 1803–1808.

Xu, F., Sun, Y., Zhang, Y., Yan, S., Wen, Z., & Li, Z., (2011). Electrochemical sensing of hydrogen peroxide using metal nanoparticles: A review. *Electrochemistry Communications, 13*, 1131–1134.

Yawen, Y., Yishi, W., Hua, W., & Shifeng, H., (2019). Gold nanoparticles decorated on single-layer graphene applied for electrochemical ultrasensitive glucose biosensor. *Journal of Electroanalytical Chemistry, 855*, 113495.

Yazdanpanah, S., Rabiee, M., Tahriri, M., Abdolrahim, M., & Tayebi, L., (2015). A novel electrochemical biosensor based $OnFe_3O_4$ nanoparticles-polyvinyl alcohol composite for sensitive detection of glucose. *TrAC Trends in Analytical Chemistry, 72*, 53–67.

Youxing, F., Shaojun, G., Chengzhou, Z., Yueming, Z., & Erkang, W., (2010). Self-assembly of cationic polyelectrolyte-functionalized graphene nanosheets and gold nanoparticles: A two-dimensional heterostructure for hydrogen peroxide sensing. *Langmuir, 26*, 11277–11282.

Yuan, B., Xu, C., Liu, L., Shi, Y., Li, S., Zhang, R., & Zhang, D., (2014). Sensitive detection of hydrogen peroxide and nitrite based on silver/carbon nanocomposite synthesized by carbon dots as reductant via one-step method. *Sensors and Actuators B: Chemical, 198*, 55–61.

Zhang, H., & Liu, S., (2020). Electrochemical sensors based on nitrogen-doped reduced graphene oxide for the simultaneous detection of ascorbic acid, dopamine and uric acid. *Journal of Alloys and Compounds, 842*, 155873.

Zhang, Y., Zhao, Y. H., Yuan, S. S., Wang, H. G., & He, C. D., (2013). Highly sensitive and selective amperometric nitrite sensor based on electrochemically activated graphite modified screen-printed carbon electrode. *Sensor Actuat. B-Chem., 185*, 602–607.

Zhao, W., Wang, H., Qin, X., Wang, X., Zhao, Z., Miao, Z., Chen, L., et al., (2009). A novel nonenzymatic hydrogen peroxide sensor based on multi-wall carbon nanotube/ silver nanoparticle nanohybrids modified gold electrode. *Talanta, 80*, 1029.

Zhu, J., Li, P. Y., Guo, Z., & Zou, R., (2018). Synthesis of micro/nano-scaled metal-organic frameworks and their direct electrochemical applications. *Coordination Chemistry Reviews, 359*, 80–101.

Index

For Product Safety Concerns and Information please contact our EU
representative GPSR@taylorandfrancis.com
Taylor & Francis Verlag GmbH, Kaufingerstraße 24, 80331 München, Germany

www.ingramcontent.com/pod-product-compliance
Lightning Source LLC
Chambersburg PA
CBHW060335220326
41598CB00023B/2717